PRAISE FOR
WOVEN ROOTS

"Impressive in scope, fascinating in detail, this compendium of stories and heretofore lost knowledge is a genuine contribution to our herbal libraries."

> —ROBIN ROSE BENNETT, herbalist and author of *The Gift of Healing Herbs, Healing Magic, A Green Witch's Pocket Book of Wisdom,* and *The Young Green Witch's Guide to Plant Magic*

"The peaceful and mutually beneficial interaction between Jews and non-Jews was for centuries the norm throughout central Europe. Deatra Cohen and Adam Siegel's *Woven Roots* is a fascinating tale of that interaction and a must-read for anyone interested in traditional herbal remedies."

> —PAUL ROBERT MAGOCSI, John Yaremko Chair of Ukrainian Studies at the University of Toronto and author of *Historical Atlas of Central Europe, A History of Ukraine,* and *With Their Backs to the Mountains*

"This book is a remedy, one I will keep on the altar of my kitchen table and return to again and again. . . . [It] made me weep with the joy of coming home, of remembering healing traditions dedicated to collective thriving, in deep reverence and love with the flowering, green world."

> —DORI MIDNIGHT, community care practitioner, herbalist, and ritual leader

"Marvelous . . . a rich picture of little-known healing practices and folk beliefs."

> —MAX DASHU, founder and director of the Suppressed Histories Archives and author of *Witches and Pagans*

"*Woven Roots* is so much more than a book about the world of plants. This botanical atlas of Eastern Europe is also an encyclopedia of folk medicine and a testament to the many connections between the cultures that inhabited the region in the nineteenth and early twentieth centuries. . . . It is a fascinating journey."

> —MAREK TUSZEWICKI, deputy director of the Institute of Jewish Studies at Jagiellonian University in Kraków and author of *A Frog Under the Tongue*

"*Woven Roots* is aptly named for its digging deeper into the fertile soils of our ancient human connection—to the earth and to each other. . . . [It illuminates] some ways n which our diverse practices have always served and continue to serve our personal health and well-being and contribute to the much-needed healing of our world."

—JESSE WOLF HARDIN, founder of Animá and editor and publisher of *Plant Healer Quarterly*

"*Woven Roots* reminds us that collective health depends on a flow of knowledge across boundaries. It invites us to cultivate solidarity and recover lost healing wisdom by following the plants."

—YARDEN KATZ, assistant professor of American culture at the University of Michigan and author of *Artificial Whiteness*

"An essential reference for magical practitioners and those interested in the folk history of Eastern Europe and the important role of Jewish people in this history. . . . You will find, as I do, that this is a reference that you will return to again and again."

—MADAME PAMITA, Ukrainian-American witch, teacher, and author of *Baba Yaga's Book of Witchcraft* and *The Witch's Guide to Animal Familiars*

"By shining a light into the dank and foggy corners of Eastern European Jewish folklore, Deatra Cohen and Adam Siegel have illuminated a verdant herbal underworld that reveals the ways in which all manner of flora was used and shared by Jewish and other ethnic herbalists throughout this region. . . . *Woven Roots* opens the door to an unexpected interface of Jewish folklife, healing practices, and the generous natural world that surrounded the Jews of this place and time."

—EDDY PORTNOY, academic advisor and director of exhibitions at YIVO Institute for Jewish Research and author of *Bad Rabbi*

"*Woven Roots* is setting a high bar and an example for other scholars to follow and will influence generations of herbalists, writers, and researchers to come."

—NAOMI SPECTOR, ethnoherbalist and author of *The Jewish Book of Flowers*

"In *Woven Roots*, Cohen and Siegel delve into Ashkenazi Jewish herbalism with signature depth and sincerity. Their rigorous scholarship illuminates the ethic of communal care that flourished in the Pale of Settlement, crossing religious and ethnic divides. . . . A vital contribution to the understanding of our diasporic and syncretic herbal tradition!"

—BRUNEM WARSHAW, clinical herbalist and co-creator of the Ashkenazi Herbalism workshop series

"A must-read for any of us attuning to and listening deeply for the knowing whispers that weave us back to the hands of our ancestors who tended the villages. In a time of profound collective need for ecosystems of healing, regenerating Jewish plant medicine could not be more crucial."

—DEVORAH BROUS, herbalist, ritualist, and creator of FromSoil2Soul

"This is a healing balm of a book for divided times! Through detailed and generous monographs, Cohen and Siegel lead us through a world of cross-cultural plant healing in pre-World War Eastern Europe. This is an essential read as we weave together cultures of healing today."

—BEN LEVINE NAHAR, chief herbalist and co-founder at Rasa and jewishherbalism.com

"For anyone seeking a window into the earth-reverent embodied practices of the peoples of the Pale of Settlement, and any wanting to learn about and rekindle relationships with ancestral plants and healing ways of these lands, *Woven Roots* is not to be missed, an absolute treasure."

—TAYA SHERE, host of the *Jewish Ancestral Healing* podcast, professor of multireligious ritual, and co-author of *The Hebrew Priestess*

PRAISE FOR
ASHKENAZI HERBALISM

ᕲᑐᙦᕲ

"*Ashkenazi Herbalism* is an important addition to the canon of herbal literature, bequeathing to us a tradition of herbal practice that, but for [Cohen's and Siegel's] efforts, would have remained lost to the world."

—JUDITH BERGER, writer, herbalist, and author of *Herbal Rituals*

"A brilliant work that captures an important but long-ignored facet of traditional herbal healing practices."

—ROSEMARY GLADSTAR, herbalist and author of *Rosemary Gladstar's Medicinal Herbs* and *Rosemary Gladstar's Herbal Recipes for Vibrant Health*

"A delightfully written and highly original work that sheds new light on a woefully understudied aspect of Eastern European Jewish folk culture."

—NATHANIEL DEUTSCH, Baumgarten Professor of Jewish Studies at the University of California, Santa Cruz, and author of *The Jewish Dark Continent* and *The Lost World of Russia's Jews*

"Whether you are an avid herbalist, history buff, or plant lover, you'll find something in this book to satisfy your soul. What a gift to us all."

—PHYLLIS D. LIGHT, herbalist and author of *Southern Folk Medicine*

"Whether you're in it for the gender analysis, the Bubbecore aesthetic, or because your inner Goth can't wait to use a spider web as a bandage, [*Ashkenazi Herbalism*] is a project that offers important answers, and questions, for a time that needs all the healing it can get."

—ROKHL KAFRISSEN, *Tablet* magazine

"Part botanical guide and part folk history, [*Ashkenazi Herbalism*] details the most common natural cures employed in the Pale of Settlement and explores the interplay between religious leaders, shamans, barber surgeons and midwives who provided medical care to Jewish communities."

—IRENE KATZ CONNELLY, *The Forward*

WOVEN ROOTS

ALSO BY
DEATRA COHEN AND ADAM SIEGEL

Ashkenazi Herbalism: Rediscovering the
Herbal Traditions of Eastern European Jews

Woven Roots

Recovering
the Healing Plant Traditions
of Jews and Their Neighbors
in Eastern Europe

DEATRA COHEN
AND ADAM SIEGEL

ILLUSTRATED BY DEATRA COHEN

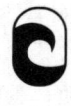

North Atlantic Books
Huichin, unceded Ohlone land
Berkeley, California

North Atlantic Books
Huichin, unceded Ohlone land
2526 Martin Luther King Jr Way
Berkeley, CA 94704 USA
www.northatlanticbooks.com

Cover design by Amanda Weiss
Book design by Happenstance Type-O-Rama

Printed in Canada

Woven Roots: Recovering the Healing Plant Traditions of Jews and Their Neighbors in Eastern Europe is sponsored and published by North Atlantic Books, an educational nonprofit based in the unceded Ohlone land Huichin (Berkeley, CA) that collaborates with partners to develop cross-cultural perspectives; nurture holistic views of art, science, the humanities, and healing; and seed personal and global transformation by publishing work on the relationship of body, spirit, and nature.

North Atlantic Books's publications are distributed to the US trade and internationally by Penguin Random House Publisher Services. For further information, visit our website at www.northatlanticbooks.com.

MEDICAL DISCLAIMER: The following information is intended for general information purposes only. Individuals should always see their health care provider before administering any suggestions made in this book. Any application of the material set forth in the following pages is at the reader's discretion and is their sole responsibility.

Library of Congress Cataloging-in-Publication data.
Names: Cohen, Deatra, 1964- author illustrator | Siegel, Adam, 1966- author
Title: Woven roots : recovering the healing plant traditions of Jews and
    their neighbors in Eastern Europe / Deatra Cohen and Adam Siegel ;
    illustrated by Deatra Cohen.
Description: Berkeley, California : North Atlantic Books, 2025. | Includes
    bibliographical references and index. | Names of plants given in
    Yiddish, Polish, Ukrainian, Belarusian, Lithuanian, Russian, German, and
    Hebrew. | Summary: "A guide to the medicinal plants and folk healers of
    Eastern Europe's Pale of Settlement from 1600 through the present that
    maps the interwoven histories of Ashkenazi Jews and their neighbors"--
    Provided by publisher.
Identifiers: LCCN 2024056227 (print) | LCCN 2024056228 (ebook) | ISBN
    9781623179625 trade paperback | ISBN 9781623179632 ebook
Subjects: LCSH: Medicinal plants--Europe, Eastern | Medicine, Popular |
    Jews--Medicine--Europe, Eastern--History | Ethnobotany--Europe,
    Eastern--History | Ashkenazim--History.
Classification: LCC QK99.E852 C64 2025 (print) | LCC QK99.E852 (ebook) |
    DDC 581.6/3409437--dc23/eng/20250303
LC record available at https://lccn.loc.gov/2024056227
LC ebook record available at https://lccn.loc.gov/2024056228

The authorized representative in the EU for product safety and compliance is Eucomply OÜ, Pärnu mnt 139b-14, 11317 Tallinn, Estonia, hello@eucompliancepartner.com, +33757690241

1 2 3 4 5 6 7 8 9 FRIESENS 30 29 28 27 26 25

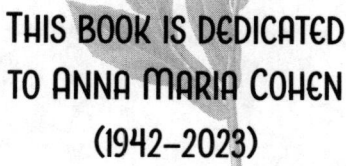

THIS BOOK IS DEDICATED
TO ANNA MARIA COHEN
(1942–2023)

CONTENTS

AUTHORS' NOTE

THIS BOOK IS THE PRODUCT of a great deal of research in source materials that are primarily ethnographic in nature, being accounts of plant and magical healing practices among various peoples, ethnic groups, and religious communities of Eastern Europe. (In the nineteenth century, this would have included territory in the Russian, Austro-Hungarian, German, and Ottoman Empires.)

Our recovery of these lost practices should be read as a descriptive history rather than a prescriptive guide. Nothing presented in this book should be taken as advisory. Anyone interested in working with any plant should take great care and consult with a trained, certified, or licensed herbal practitioner.

The Healers

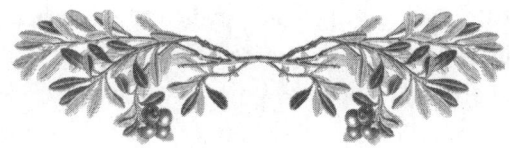

There is no field of science in which cooperation between Jews and non-Jews took place to a greater extent than in medicine. In spite of all social, political and religious restrictions—as far as Christian Europe is concerned—in cases of illness non-Jews sought remedies from Jews and Jews asked non-Jews for help. This applies to all classes of the population and to all centuries. Medicine alone did not respect any boundary.

H. J. ZIMMELS, *Magicians, Theologians, and Doctors: Studies in Folk-Medicine and Folk-Lore As Reflected in the Rabbinical Responsa*

As in other shtetlekh, folk medicine in all its many manifestations thrived for centuries in Eishyshok, and would continue to coexist with conventional medicine right up until the end. Some practitioners of the art cured with "words alone"—magic spells—while others supplemented them with concoctions of herbs and other elements. Each ailment had its corresponding magic spells. Reflecting Jewish mystical traditions as well as Christian and Muslim sources, they were recited in various languages, including Hebrew, Yiddish, Russian, and several local dialects, especially Tataric, since the Muslim Tatars were considered the best of all the folk practitioners.

YAFFA ELIACH, *There Once Was a World: A Nine-Hundred-Year Chronicle of the Shtetl of Eishyshok*

EARLY ON, WHILE WE WERE UNDERTAKING RESEARCH for our first book, these extraordinary statements seized our attention, and the beautiful senti-ments they express have haunted us ever since. *Ashkenazi Herbalism* focused on recovering the hidden or nearly lost traditions of our Eastern European ancestral folkways. But as we worked through the historical and comparative evidence, we knew, intuitively (and increasingly empirically), that people's reliance on the healing powers of plants and their rituals that accompanied both the act and the art of healing were, in many communities, inter-ethnic and/or inter-confessional affairs. In the yizkor memory books, we read of towns with Jewish and Christian healers (midwives, feldshers, bobes, or opshprekherns) sought for treatment by everyone in these often highly integrated communi-ties, regardless of the ethnicity or religion of either healer or patient. We were so inspired by this discovery that we resolved to explore the phenomenon at greater length.

With this book, we wish to emphasize just how crucial communal care across Eastern Europe has been, both for Jew and non-Jew, and how peoples' common faith in shared traditions had the power to restore and maintain a balance and a commonweal among the many ethnic groups and faiths of the region, to ensure their collective health.

That Jew and non-Jew (Pole, Ukrainian, Belarusian, Rusyn, Russian, Lith-uanian, Latvian, Tatar, Romanian, Roma) shared plant knowledge and plant healing modalities and cared for one another should come as a surprise to no one. But it often does. Even while we were drafting this book, it was obvious to us that almost everyone—ourselves included—has continued to maintain an image of Eastern Europe before the Shoah as one of constant pogroms, threats, hatreds, and ceaseless ethnic conflict.

Which is not to say that prejudice, violence, and discrimination were not prevalent—they were. But this was generally not the case in every or even most places, neither all nor most of the time. Again and again, we have encoun-tered anecdotes like this one, concerning Pesya Feyge, the opshprekherin of Mikulintsy (now Mykulyntsi), Ukraine: "Everyone liked, respected, and admired her. Nobody would ever forget to wish her well on Sabbaths and hol-idays. Not only Jews would come to her, but also non-Jews from neighboring villages in wagons and carriages. She would help everyone and never turned anyone away. She would give advice, a hot compress, or other assistance." Or from the shtetl of Zawiercie, Poland, whose yizkor honors the memory of the community midwife, a Christian woman whom they called "di zhandarin" (being the widow of the local gendarme); she lived among the Jews and delivered their children, comforting fearful parents in fluent Yiddish. Stories such as these are legion, and testify to the intimacy of this world.

Why might this be? We believe it was due to these communities' proximity to the natural world and the plant realm. The plant realm is a sovereign one that spans the planet. This realm has thrived on Earth for hundreds of millions of years. In a way, plants are our true ancestors and benefactors, and we humans, along with other animals, have depended upon their generosity and abundance to supply us with almost everything we need both to survive and to thrive: air, food, shelter, fuel, clothing, medicine, and so much more.

This relationship is not exclusive to modern *Homo sapiens sapiens*. In 2018 paleoanthropologists reported that Neanderthals had been so sufficiently knowledgeable about the healing properties of plants that they looked to specific herbs to address their health issues, such as fever management, wound care, and other ailments. Among the likely preferred remedies for the cave-dwelling Neanderthals in the Caucasus Mountains of modern Georgia were *Achillea millefolium* (yarrow) and *Artemisia absinthium* (wormwood), both extremely important plants for herbalists all over the world.

Neanderthals and *Homo sapiens sapiens* (us) coexisted and even procreated, so it isn't very difficult to imagine that they must have shared knowledge, including how to care for one another with healing plants. Findings such as this suggest that our human dependence upon the healing power of plants is timeless and universal. It's thrilling to contemplate that a good portion of our collective herbal wisdom may descend directly from these prehistoric ancestors and cousins in our shadowy past.

For the vast span of our hominin history, this plant knowledge has been passed down orally. By the time modern humans invented the technology of writing and began to memorialize and document plants, such knowledge had been gathered, sorted, stored, and transmitted from person to person for tens of thousands of years—as is still the case for many, if not most, of the world's plant healing cultures today.

But writing did revolutionize the transmission of plant knowledge, as it did all other types of knowledge. As far back as the Ebers Papyrus, an Egyptian materia medica dated to approximately 1500 BCE, the world's civilizations have committed to writing extensive botanical and medical information. Other early historical records of medicinal plant knowledge have come down to us from ancient Mesopotamia, Greece, South Asia, Mesoamerica, and China.

The invention of writing provided humans with an inexhaustible array of benefits, but in this instance, the written record has allowed us to draw inferences about the interconnectedness of herbal practices across far-flung cultures. We can pinpoint the exact moment, give or take a couple of years, when New World plants such as *Theobroma cacao* (chocolate) and *Nicotiana tabacum* (tobacco) arrived in Europe (given our terminus ante quem, the "point before which," of 1492, this would have been no earlier than the very beginning of the sixteenth century), and voluminous records left by the Spanish and Portuguese conquistadores inventory the many plants and minerals (especially gold and silver) they carried with them back to Europe.

The written record is scantier when it comes to transmission of knowledge throughout the "old world" (Eurasia and Africa). When did the first Europeans drink tea? When did the first Chinese taste coffee? How ancient is the spice trade between East and West? (See our *Myristica fragrans* (nutmeg) monograph in *Ashkenazi Herbalism*.)

Much of the history we uncover here derives from plant migrations, whether via trade routes, either silk (from East Asia across central Asia and Siberia into Eastern Europe) or spice (from South Asia via the Black and Red Seas and the Caucasus). Along these storied trade routes came goods and knowledge. Among the traders, translators, and mediators in medicinal plants and plant knowledge were Jews who, across their diaspora, often acted as intermediaries, bridging East and West. There is so much to this trade that we know little about, but it's apparent that, in many parts of Europe, the economic life of Jewish communities was wrapped up in it.

Some of the history we consider here is barely "history" at all—it's the unwritten and undocumented movement of plants into Eastern Europe from elsewhere: How did rosemary come to the Pale of Settlement? When and how did sweet flag (*Acorus calamus*) arrive? Were sanicle's healing powers commonly known in the region, despite its natural scarcity east of the Vistula River?

So, too, much of this history of plant healing among Eastern European Jews has remained undiscovered due to language barriers, political realities, cultural misunderstandings, historical tragedies, and the patriarchal cultures of Jewish communities in the Pale and beyond. Here we must underscore the fact that, although the Ashkenazim have predominated in Eastern Europe, theirs is not the only Jewish community in the region. Eastern Europe has been home to significant Sephardic populations, particularly in southeastern Europe (Bulgaria, Serbia, Bosnia and Herzegovina, Greece), Karaim Jews of Poland and Lithuania, Mountain Jews of the Caucasus, Bukharan Jews of central Asia, and Georgian Jews. Referring back to the importance of writing in the transmission of plant knowledge, we can say that the role of Jewish science and medicine, particularly in the Islamic(ate)/Muslim world (e.g., Moorish Spain, the Ottoman Empire), ensured that Hebrew-literate Jews of Eastern Europe possessed, retained, and transmitted plant knowledge from Greek, Latin, Arabic, Persian, Chinese, and even Indian (Sanskrit, Pali, and so on) healing traditions.

But this is, of course, an instance of "official" knowledge, belonging to educated classes or those able to travel freely across Eastern Europe and beyond. The career of Tobias ha-Kohen (1652–1729), who carries many appellations with many spellings, but whom we shall refer to as ha-Kohen, is instructive. His grandfather emigrated to Kraków from Safed, Palestine, and his parents fled what is now western Ukraine to western Europe to escape the Xmel'nyc'kyj pogroms of the mid-seventeenth century. Ha-Kohen himself was born in Metz, France, spent part of his childhood in Poland, began his medical studies in Frankfurt an der Oder in Germany, completed them in Padova, Italy, and entered into medical service in Ottoman Europe (Edirne and possibly Crimea), before settling in Istanbul. He traveled to Venice to oversee the publication of his book *Ma'aseh Tuviyah* (The Work of Tobias) and ultimately retired to Jerusalem, where he died. Such a peripatetic curriculum vitae is not atypical for a Jewish physician of his era.

Even recapitulating the stations of ha-Kohen's life, we are reminded that some obscured traditions, such as the lives of male healers, actually do get documented, particularly if their careers bring them into the orbit of state power.

Conversely, historians have rarely acknowledged or examined the herbal healing practices of Jewish women of Eastern Europe, who weren't employed by
sultans, emirs, emperors, princes, or dukes. The practices of these folk healers
were almost never committed to writing. Their wisdom was passed down via
direct experience, by word of mouth from one generation to the next. In other
words, much like prehistoric humans (whether *sapiens sapiens* or *neandertha-
lensis*) did thousands of years ago. Women folk healers from throughout the
world regard the act of healing as treating the individual who is suffering and
bringing them from a state of dis-ease back into ease, to comfort and restore
balance within them, and, by extension, within and for their communities.

In this manner, the folk medicinal practices of Eastern European Jewish
women differed from those of their male counterparts in a number of significant ways. As we've said, their traditions were mostly undocumented, were
handed down in vernacular languages rather than the loshn koydesh ("holy
tongue" in Yiddish) of Hebrew, and generally focused on women's and children's health. They often foregrounded healing treatments different from those
found in Hebrew or Yiddish remedy books (Yiddish segules, "charms," and
refues, "remedies"). And their social role in the region was far larger than that
of women healers in other parts of Europe: because the infrastructure of official medicine (clinics, hospitals, pharmacies, doctors, nurses, etc.) across much
of Eastern Europe (especially Russia) was very limited in scale for centuries,
communal reliance on the village midwife or opshprekherin persisted right up
until the Second World War (and afterward, especially in many regions of the
Soviet Union).

Women healers were held in higher regard than their male counterparts
for monitoring pregnancies, delivering children, and treating postpartum and
childhood illnesses and complaints, owing to their greater skill in these areas
of care, as well as in the more magical aspects of healing, such as divination,
removing an evil eye, curing fear and other psychosomatic illnesses, and treating common complaints such as erysipelas. They healed with plants, minerals,
and other natural substances and were versed in hundreds of (ancient) remedies.

Although men constituted a large number of the folk healers of Eastern
Europe (from the ba'alei shem, the "masters of the name" or practical kab-
balists, to barber-surgeons, feldshers, bonesetters, eye-lickers, doctors, and

opshprekhers, most of whom we profiled in *Ashkenazi Herbalism*), we hold that intercommunal folk healing was far more common among female healers than male practitioners.

Traditional healers and herbalists the world over have tended to be women. Wolf-Dieter Storl, the herbalist, cultural anthropologist, and ethnobotanist, has even asserted that the materiae medicae we associate with Dioscorides and other male physicians of classical antiquity who documented the herbal knowledge of their time were actually "borrowed" from what was originally wise women's knowledge, the wisdom never set down in writing but passed down across the generations by word of mouth. To give this assertion credence, we look back to Ukraine in the 1920s and 1930s, where the majority of informants interviewed by the interwar Soviet ethnobotanical surveys were women, and the plants they described for field researchers were mainly relied upon for gynecological health. Even contemporary studies on herbal medicine in Eastern Europe—including the herbal medicine of the region's surviving Jewish communities—reveal that women, rather than men, have tended to practice folk and plant medicine, not only for women's (reproductive) health, but for everyone in their communities.

It may come as a surprise to learn that a majority of Ashkenazi Jewish communities in prewar Eastern Europe professed a deep love and reverence for the natural world in general and for the landscape they occupied, cared for, tilled, and harvested for at least a thousand years. This was a revelation for us, as our received ideas of "the old country" had been drab scenes from American films that depicted the shtetlekh and derfer (Yiddish "towns" and "villages") of Eastern Europe as dreary, shabby, depressing. In village after village, in story upon story, we find testimonies to a loving devotion to the land that echoes throughout the yizkor memory books, which are monuments to Jewish life in Europe before the Shoah. We have been deeply moved by the memories and reminiscences of those who survived, because they reveal a side to our grandparents and great-grandparents that has largely been cut out of our collective memory. The denial of this aspect of our common history has left many Jews like us, especially those who work with plants, to wonder about our relationship with and to the natural world. With this book we hope to further close this gap in our common Eastern European history.

In the pages to come we tell the larger story of the folk healers of Eastern Europe, both Jews and their neighbors, in all their diversity; we profile some of their most helpful plant allies (both those you might expect and some surprises). While we continue to center our research on Ashkenazi Jewry, we return to the rich brocade of healers, particularly women healers, from the various cultures of the region, highlighting the central role they have played in bringing life and health to their communities, keeping their families and their neighbors hale and in balance. In the plant section we expand upon the Ashkenazi Jewish (and common Eastern European) materia medica, paying close attention to the plants' paths of transmission. Etymology is a very useful (albeit blunt) instrument for telling the story of healing plants and their place in the collective folk culture of the region. And whenever possible, we include recipes we have discovered that, in many cases, are still being relied upon by the surviving Jewish communities of the former Pale.

We'd like to reiterate that when we take care of each other, we take care of ourselves, and, by extension, the world around us. For most of our common history, this sentiment has been understood and passed down. We feel this belief must be restored to our world. Since time immemorial, plants themselves have *never* discriminated, not among peoples, not by age, not by gender, not by ethnicity, not by religion, nor demanded remuneration for their healing powers. Plants have given generously of themselves to help our world thrive, and we humans would do well to follow their example.

We believe that plants bring diverse peoples together, no matter the time or place. If we could be as generous and magnanimous as the plants, and moreover, this beautiful planet, then our world could find some peace. Even though neither of us was raised with nor has ever practiced Judaism, our ancestry is Ashkenazi. Therefore, we have tried as much as possible to tell the stories of our forebears and their neighbors through as sympathetic a lens as possible. Again, we feel we must emphasize that we are concerned with the pre-Shoah history of Eastern Europe and the peoples living within the former administrative territory known as the Pale of Settlement. The question of what it means to be Jewish is a complex one, and the question of the degree to which Jews, particularly Ashkenazim, are to be considered as "native" to the lands of Eastern Europe as their non-Jewish neighbors even more so.

We hold that the place and its plants make the people, and hence the communities of the Pale who have drawn strength and health from the plants that have surrounded them can be defined as much by their healing practices as by their language, religion, or "ethnicity," if not more so. The female or male folk healer—whether Jewish opshprekherin, Slavic znakharka/znachorka ("one who knows"), Slavic šeptuxa ("whisperer"), Tatar fałdżiej ("diviner"), Lithuanian użkalbėjimas ("exorcist"), one who heals with divination, plants, and charms, one who is skilled at diagnosing and curing the evil eye, and one whose practice is most devoted to caring for women and children—is the defining figure of Eastern European folk medicine.

What is this world that we call the Pale of Settlement? This is that stretch of territory, the North Eurasian plain, where Yiddish-speaking Ashkenazi Jews (and some Sephardim) have lived in communities large and small for a thousand years.

As for the land itself? Variously called the Polish Plain, the Russian Plain, the Sarmatic Plain, it extends from the Vistula River eastward, and from the Baltic Sea south- and eastward, all the way down to the Black Sea. We're going to concentrate on three broad sub-regions where we have found the strongest evidence of shared healing cultures among Eastern European Jews and their neighbors: in the land the Jews call Lite (more or less modern Lithuania, most of Latvia, northeastern Poland, and northern Belarus); what Julian Talko-Hryncewicz called Ruś Południowa (Southern Rus' or Ruthenia: modern southeastern Poland and western Ukraine); and Bessarabia, after the lands once known as Basarab, where Romania, Moldova, Hungary, and Bukovina all come together. In Lite, before the war, we find Ashkenazi Jews, Karaim Jews, Lipka Tatars, Lithuanians, Latvians, Estonians, Poles, and Belarusians. In Southern Rus' (Ruthenia), in the late nineteenth century, the population consisted of Ashkenazi Jews, Ukrainians, Hutsuls or Rusyns, and Poles, as well as smaller numbers of Tatars, Armenians, and Greeks. In the south, in Bessarabia, the historic populations have included Romanians, Moldovans, Roma, Ukrainians, Magyars, Ashkenazi and Sephardi Jews, and Christian Gagauz Turks.

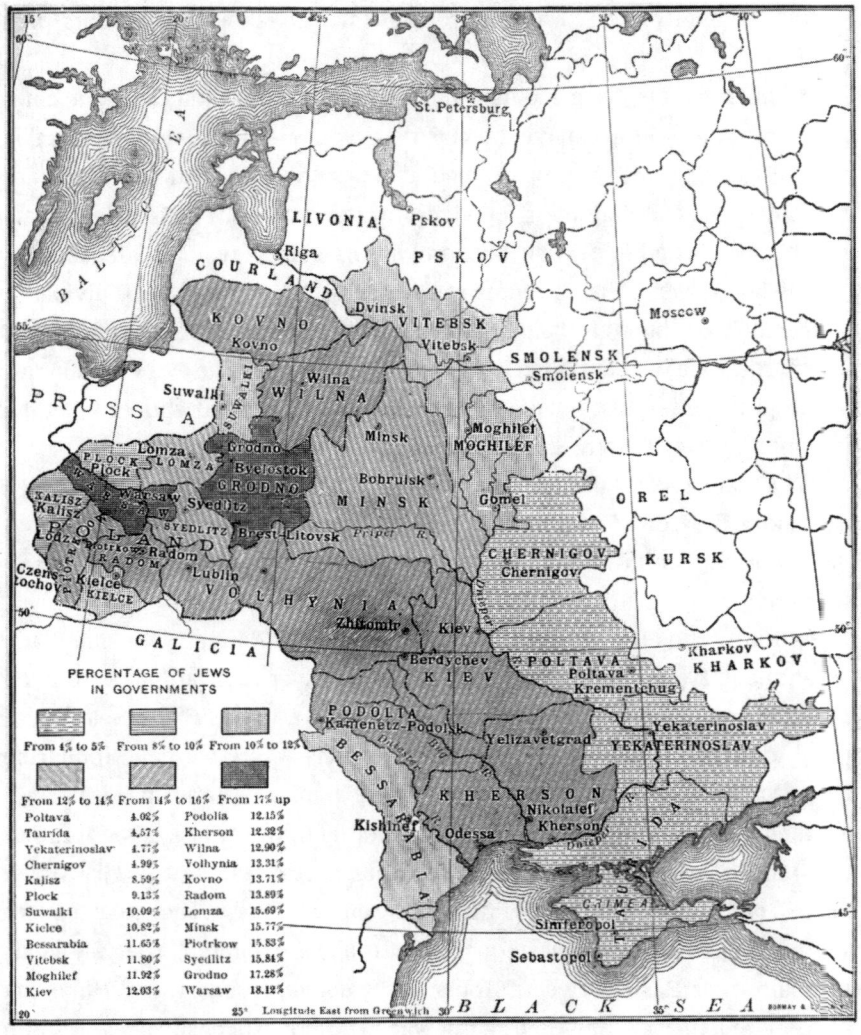

The Pale of Settlement in 1901, showing Jewish inhabitants as a percentage of the overall population. Adapted from the *Jewish Encyclopedia*, New York: Funk & Wagnalls, 1905.

We want to stress that we're not historians, either of large-scale population movements, or of the broader political history of Eastern Europe, to say nothing of Jews and Judaism. But it's difficult to disentangle ourselves from this history, as much as we'd like to, so the problem of what to call this part of Eurasia remains. Why is this important? Because we're looking to native plants and the cultures of healing that they have knit together over the centuries. Eastern Europe is a land of cold winters, hot summers, fertile soil, flat plains, swollen rivers, endless steppes; and regional histories have defined it according to whichever state formations have prevailed at one time or another, from Kievan Rus' or the Polish-Lithuanian Commonwealth to the Russian Empire and the USSR. Our focus is on Ashkenazi Jews and their communal lives with their neighbors, so we're going to identify, for the sake of clarity, emphasis, and convenience, this territory, this plant world, by the name it was given in the late nineteenth century: the Pale of Settlement, or Pale for short.

Suffice it to say, the Pale, before the Second World War, had gone through several political ruptures: mostly part of the Russian Empire before the First World War, in the 1920s and 1930s it was divided among the Soviet Union, Lithuania, Latvia, Estonia, Czechoslovakia, and Poland (now we would include independent Belarus, Ukraine, and Moldova).

But the Pale (and its surrounding environs) is an enormous territory; we can't cover all of it. We've focused our recovery of this common history on those parts of the Pale where it was most richly and diversely shared—the region's tapestry as documented in fleeting keyhole glimpses a century and more ago by Talko-Hryncewicz and others: the regions of Polesia, Volhynia, Galicia, and Podolia—the most densely populated, which contained the region's greatest diversity of faiths, languages, ethnic groupings, and so on.

As a snapshot, in the late nineteenth century, in the northern reaches of the Pale (Polesia, Lithuania), Poles, Lithuanians, Ashkenazi Jews, Lipka Tatars, Belarusians, and Karaim Jews lived together. In the center regions, in Galicia and its environs, lived Jews, Poles, Rusyns, and Ukrainians. A bit further east, in Volhynia and Podolia, there were Ukrainians, Poles, Jews, and even Armenians, Greeks, and Germans. To the south, along the Dniester River from Bukovina and Moldova down to the Black Sea, lived more Jews, Ukrainians, Russians, Greeks, Romanians, Tatars, Gagauz, and Roma.

We can't entirely avoid human geography, even within the timeless realm of plants and their gifts. The Pale and broader Eastern Europe have been the homeland of the Balts and the Slavs for at least several thousand years, and likely longer, at least according to the historical linguistic evidence. As for

Jews, Tatars, Roma, and so on—their arrival can be dated, because the documentary evidence indicates when they appeared in the various medieval kingdoms: the Jews in the tenth century or so (accelerating quite a bit later, at the close of the Middle Ages), and the Tatars in the fourteenth century, around the same time the Roma begin to appear in the historical record.

Or to be somewhat more specific, we focus largely but not exclusively on the following historical communities. First, we center our attention on Jews: Jews have lived in Eastern Europe for at least a millennium. The largest population of Eastern European Jews, the Ashkenazim, originated, as most people know, somewhere along the Rhine River in Germany (known in Hebrew as Ashkenaz), and they took their dialect of German, which evolved into Yiddish, with them. They mostly went east to the Polish lands, which consisted of a huge span of Eastern Europe. After 1492, when Jews were expelled from Spain and later Portugal (known in Hebrew as Sepharad), many Sephardim migrated to the Ottoman Empire, which extended, as late as the seventeenth century, well into Podolia. While we generally regard all of Eastern European Jewry as Ashkenazi, significant numbers of Sephardim did live in the Pale, particularly in Bessarabia, along with members of other Jewish communities from throughout the Russian Empire, such as the Bukharan Jews of central Asia, mountain Jews from the Caucasus, and Georgian Jews, and of course, the Karaim Jews of Lite, Ruthenia, and Crimea.

Next, we spend some time with the Tatars, which in our work refers to three very specific populations who share a common place (central Asia) and a common ancestral language (Turkic) of origin: Lipka Tatars, Crimean Tatars, and Karaim Jews. We most often encounter the Polish-Lithuanian Lipka Tatars (from their name for Lite). This population is descended from Tatars who were, like the Jews, invited by the Polish-Lithuanian crown to settle their lands in the late Middle Ages. The larger part of the Lipka Tatar community has been centered around what is now Lithuania, northeastern Poland, and northern Belarus. Many Lipka Tatars assimilated not only into the ethnic Polish community, but into the ranks of the Polish nobility. They continued (and continue) to profess Islam, although by the nineteenth and twentieth centuries most Tatars had become monoglot Polish speakers, and their religious leaders often knew no Arabic. Lipka Tatars lived in smaller communities throughout Ruthenia.

Crimean Tatars remain a large community in and around the Crimean penin-
sula on the Black Sea. Like all Turkic peoples in the region, they are descended
from several broad waves of migration and invasion, dating from the tenth or
eleventh century, up until the end of the eighteenth, when Russian imperial
expansion erased the various Tatar khanates. They are distinct from Lipka
Tatars.

Then there are the Karaim: a very small community of Turkic Karaite Jews,
who, unlike their Lipka Tatar neighbors, continued to maintain their Turkic
language (Karaim) practically until the present day (their language is endan-
gered). Their remaining communities are centered in Lite (in Trakai, Lithuania,
historically at the center of a mixed community of Karaim Jews, Lipka Tatars,
Ashkenazi Jews, Poles, Lithuanians, and Belarusians) and Galicia (in Halych,
Ukraine, historically at the center of a mixed community of Ashkenazi Jews,
Poles, Rusyns, Ukrainians, and some Lipka Tatars). Like Lipka and Crimean
Tatars, the Karaim have close historical ties to Crimea, specifically to the
Karaite Jewish community there.

In addition, we devote some attention to Turkic communities further to the
south, in Bessarabia: the Gagauz, an Orthodox Christian Turkish community
living in Moldova, Ukraine, and Romania; and the Turkish populations of
Ottoman and post-Ottoman Bosnia, Macedonia, and Bulgaria.

How do we disentangle this multicultural knot (to mix some more met-
aphors)? As readers of *Ashkenazi Herbalism* may recall, Deatra found that
Natalia Osadcha-Janata's 1952 monograph *Herbs Used in Ukrainian Folk
Medicine* was in fact a *hidden* herbal, documenting plant medicinal traditions
in predominantly Jewish communities of Ukraine just prior to the Second
World War.

With this knowledge, we were able to look more closely at a vast and
relatively underexamined body of published research spanning the mid-nineteenth to mid-twentieth century (thank you to Marek Tuszewicki, whose
A Frog Under the Tongue [*Żaba pod językiem*] provided us a roadmap).

The most important of these newly analyzed sources has been Julian
Talko-Hryncewicz's *Zarysy lecznictwa ludowego na Rusi południowej* (Sketches
of Folk Healing in Southern Ruthenia; Kraków, 1893). Talko-Hryncewicz
(1850–1936) was a Polish anthropologist and ethnographer of Lithuanian

descent who compiled a study of folk medicine in what was then the Russian Empire, specifically, the regions of Subcarpathian Ruthenia, Volhynia, Galicia, and Podolia—a significant geographic overlap with the region investigated by S. An-sky and the Jewish Ethnographic Program before the First World War, and the YIVO ethnographic research program and the Soviet ethnopharmacological surveys of the interwar period. Unlike the latter expeditions, two of which were explicitly devoted to documenting Jewish folk culture, Talko-Hryncewicz openly acknowledged that he and his colleagues were exploring a highly diverse region, and in his introduction, he basically affirms (if not confirms) our own thesis regarding the woven roots of the Pale:

> Let us take a closer look at the ways in which natural and medical beliefs came to Ruthenia: Superstitions common among other peoples could have been brought by these same peoples who had settled there centuries prior [. . .] or they could have been borrowed subsequently from neighboring peoples utterly transformed, more or less. [. . .] We know that even a homogeneous people has more foreign influences in its language, customs, and beliefs along its borderlands than at its center. [. . .]

> From Germany to Russia and the entire Slavic region, many medicines commonly used today have been passed on, such as lubricating the gums of teething children with blood dripped from a coxcomb, treating consumption with birch sap, etc. The influence of the old empiricism was also transformed under the influence of religious ideas, as we see in the famous cure for jaundice, which is to stare at the color yellow, generally yellow flowers or metal of the same color; and in Germany, whence this superstition passed to the Slavs, it was also advised to stare at a yellow cup or yellow patina.

> The influence of Byzantine civilization on the eastern borders of Russia in Ukraine is pervasive, and leaves its mark on superstitions and folk beliefs; around Chełm, or throughout Galicia, in these beliefs we see the mutual influence of two clashing ecclesiastical civilizations, eastern and western. The constant relations that contemporary peoples maintain among them contribute much to the transmission of beliefs and superstitions, both eastern and western. Natural and medical beliefs, which in their origin resemble those of the Far East, apart from those transmitted to Russia deep in antiquity, might have passed to Russia by another route that has not yet been closed.

> Roma, in their nomadic life, carry many superstitions from one people to another, being the sowers of Indian beliefs, which, according to [one]

hypothesis [. . .], is even more probable when we take into account their Indian origin. Of the numerous beliefs in Rus' that betray Indian origin, I will cite a few examples:

The superstition about the danger of reptile bites must have passed to Ruthenia from India, where even today there are many kinds of snakes whose bite can be fatal; from there must also come the belief that such snakes once existed among us. This statement is further proven by some beliefs concerning snakes or by the invocation of healing from the bite of a reptile, in which [one scholar] found words of the Sanskrit language, such as: "Sarp nutes Sirkiwajen, Nutes sarp sirkiwajen, Sirkiwajen nutes Sarp."

We can see the same influence in the treatment of certain diseases by means of writing, which is practiced in Ruthenia, especially by the Tatars. For example, in case of colds, they order the sick person to swallow a piece of paper rolled into a ball bearing the inscription 'Abrakadabra.' This word, according to many authors, is said to be pronounced in India today during certain ritual customs and is supposed to cure crowds of people from the malignant colds prevailing there.

[. . .] Probably not a few beliefs, both Eastern and medieval, were spread throughout Ruthenia by Jews from Germany who settled there, and today German and Czech colonists, who have settled in Volhynia and who move from one place to another, also spreading various superstitions, contribute even more to this. In this same way, Moravian, Slovak, Serbian, and German beliefs have spread across a much larger area and for a very long time by trading Slovaks wrongly called "Hungarians." In order to make a modest living, they traverse the vast expanses of southern Ruthenia with a box on their backs, and sometimes they spend their whole lives wandering beyond their home country, selling fancies and giving advice, medicines, love potions, elixirs of youth or long life, distributing various remedies and cures for diseases, and at the same time spreading among the people the strangest natural and medical beliefs.

It was gratifying to learn that considering Eastern European folk healing as a syncretic system was a common consensus in Polish scholarly circles more than a century ago. Why then was there no follow-up? Again, we've discussed this in *Ashkenazi Herbalism* and elsewhere: Folk medicinal traditions, particularly Jewish folk medicinal traditions, have been subjected to a seemingly endless series of erasures: the erasure of folk wisdom from Jewish historiography since the Haskalah, the Jewish Enlightenment; the erasure of women's knowledge from male-dominated cultural history; the erasure of the Jewish presence in the Pale from both landscape and memory; and on and on. As we can see, it is not only Jewish folk wisdom that is erased: the region's tapestry has been unraveled ever since. Who today remembers that in Lite the Tatars were revered above all healers, and that people would walk half a day just to be treated by the Tatar fałdżej? (In the Pale two types of Tatar healers were consulted: the fałdżej worked with divination and amulets to tell fortunes, while the siufkacz would blow sacred smoke, often from burnt amulets, onto the patient.) Who even knows that the Gagauz introduced a rich tradition of Turkish and Middle Eastern folk medicine to Bessarabia, and were strongly influenced in turn by their Moldovan, Ukrainian, and Jewish neighbors? Even today, the obvious importance of the Roma—as Talko-Hryncewicz attests—to folk medicine, particularly veterinary medicine, is barely known, and scarcely documented.

On this last point, even Talko-Hryncewicz inadvertently obscures. The charm quoted earlier ("Sarp nutes Sirkiwajen"), "of the Sanskrit language," is possibly derived from Romani. Rulikowski provides us some context: It was recorded in the late nineteenth century in the shtetl of Horodnica (now Horodnytsija, Ukraine), from a "starozakonny" ("Old Testament," i.e., Jewish) informant named Boruch, or Burcio, a wood trader renowned throughout the region for his skill at curing snakebites, and the charm was specifically intended to "order" (banish) the effects of a nonpoisonous snakebite. Burcio did not know the meaning of the words he used but said he had learned them from his father, a brakarz, or quality-control inspector. What are the shadowy communal links that would have carried this knowledge with the Roma into the Jewish and ethnically mixed communities of the Pale?

In this work, we continue to stitch together, as best we can, the threads of this lost or nearly lost knowledge from these vanished or nearly vanished peoples (and their surviving neighbors). We have relied primarily on the ethnographic literature of the late nineteenth and early twentieth centuries, mostly in Russian, Polish, Ukrainian, German, and Yiddish, so as to document healing modalities and healers in the region we refer to as the Pale. We have continued to retrace the history of particularly Jewish medicine as documented in the written record, especially in the early modern (seventeenth- and eighteenth-century) treatises on health and healing by Tobias ha-Kohen and Issachar bar Teller, a Jewish healer of seventeenth-century Prague. We have also drawn on the literature of both the Jewish memory books (yizkor bikher) and the interwar Yiddish-language scholarship in ethnography and folklore undertaken by YIVO and other organizations. When necessary, we have consulted the extensive contemporary scholarship in ethnopharmacology and ethnobotany in the region, which documents plant remedies and practices still applied by these populations today, including the remnants of Lite's Jewish and Tatar communities.

In the time we've spent working on this book and talking about some of our discoveries, we have been humbled by how little we know and how rich were the traditions that have been lost, liquidated, or left behind. Even the literature that remains is only a tiny fraction of the knowledge that once was. Already in the latter half of the nineteenth century, researchers recognized that much of the traditional knowledge of the region—not only that of smaller assimilated populations of Lipka Tatars and Karaim, but also that of Poles, Ukrainians, Lithuanians, and Jews—was fast disappearing. We've done the best we could with this book, and we're still making our way through the vast richness of this ancestral knowledge—with more to come, kinnahera, as our grandmothers used to say, to ward off the evil eye (from Yiddish kayn ayn hoyre, "no evil eye").

We have tried to give a balanced account of the Pale and its shared traditions. There is simply less evidence for some aspects of this common culture of healing than we would like to have had: as we've said, Roma folk culture is poorly documented, even more so than some other cultures. Many of the sources we have consulted focus on plant medicine among the Roma of the British Isles. We can confidently state that the Roma renown for herbal veterinary medicine, especially their knowledge of and skill in employing the widest array of healing plants, accompanied them throughout Eastern Europe (Lipka Tatars of the Pale enjoyed a similar, albeit more local, reputation). We have noted shared beliefs found among some Roma and Jewish communities of Eastern Europe regarding the supernatural property of the elder ("devil's tree" in Yiddish, "devil's wood" in Romani) and the importance of the red thread in healing magic.

It is amazing how, within a couple of years, our research took us from the question of whether there were any plants other than, say, dill, or garlic, in the Ashkenazi medicine cabinet, or did such a cabinet exist at all, to: Were there any plants they and their neighbors didn't rely upon? Among kitchen plants, local wild forage, nonnative and likely imported herbs, and commerce and trade, how are regional cultures of healing put together? How are they a common project? These are huge questions, and we've only just begun to attempt to answer how Ashkenazim and their neighbors evolved this common culture.

First come the plants, obviously. Most of the common plant materia medica native to Eastern Europe is broadly distributed across Eurasia. There are some marginal instances—such as sanicle and rosemary in the monographs to come.

So who do we think brought what, and is this even a legitimate question?

Plants and plant healing traditions of western Europe were known and employed to the east, but a number of plants, remedies, and beliefs were likely brought eastward from the German lands. Although Germans certainly settled widely throughout Eastern Europe, their absence in many parts of the region where Western-derived modalities were common (particularly that "old empiricism" traceable back to Galen and Dioscorides, and carried through the Middle Ages by figures such as Hildegard von Bingen, the twelfth-century abbess whose medical writings discussed many healing plants) suggests that it was their erstwhile neighbors, the ancestors of the Ashkenazim, who likely brought with them plants, remedies, and beliefs that they had shared with Germans.

We should emphasize that plants are quite capable of migrating on their own, so when we make assumptions or draw tentative conclusions as to their provenance, we must use comparisons and etymology to guide us. Most saliently, *Acorus calamus*, a reed native to South and East Asia, which grows on the shores of the Black Sea, is known among Slavs (Poles and Ukrainians) as "Tatar herb" (it is also, in some Ukrainian dialects, called "Jewish flatbread"). It's reasonable to infer that people in the region understood this plant to have been introduced by the Tatar migrations. Or take rosemary, another Near Eastern plant that grows wild around the Mediterranean, and in the Crimea: its common Eastern European name—cf. Polish *rozmarin*—is clearly derived from Latin, and hence likely reached the Pale via Latin-speaking western Europe. And so on.

Knowledge travels with people. In the towns and villages of Eastern Europe, Ashkenazi (and Sephardi) Jews, with their high literacy levels (at least among the men), were able to draw upon classical Western and Eastern medical traditions: books of segules and refues, mystical literature, and of course widely distributed works such as ha-Kohen's *Ma'aseh Tuviyah* attest to the retention and spread of this knowledge (Galenic, Dioscoridean, Maimonidean, Paracelsian, to name a few) among the Jewish communities of the Pale.

Other immigrants brought traditions with them as well. Tatars and Gagauz (and Karaim Jews) brought plant, medical, and healing knowledge from several directions: Gagauz, who came to the Pale from Asia Minor, provide a direct link to the ancient folk traditions of Turkey. Tatars, who arrived in the Pale from the Crimea to the south, and also from the east of Russia, were the deliverers of several traditions: Islamic medicine, Siberian shamanic healing, as well as echoes of traditional Chinese medicine. Roma also brought with them healing traditions, likely derived in part from Unani and Ayurvedic medicine.

What of the healers themselves? Healers and healing were sometimes gendered, sometimes not. Depending on which point in history you regard, the village healer of a typical settlement somewhere in the Pale might be a practical kabbalist, a fałdżej, a znakhar or znachor, a šeptuxa, or a Lithuanian užkalbėjimas or Jewish opshprekher. Women healers throughout Eastern Europe and across many languages were known to all as "babas" or "bobes." Healers had specific skills, which may or may not have combined with other competencies (bonesetting, bloodletting, cupping, eye-licking, snakebite curing); midwives delivered children, but also provided prenatal, perinatal, postnatal, and pediatric care. Women healers were—and still are—almost universally acknowledged as more adept at plant work, whether by cultivation or forage. Both male and female healers were imbued with "magical" or supernatural powers.

Which brings us to the shaman.

Our research for this book has led us to identify the shamanic figure as one of the characteristic healers of the entire Pale, regardless of language, religion, ethnicity, or even gender: viz, the healer who communicates with the spirit world via trance, divination, charms, incantations, ritual, and other intercessions to provide magical medical assistance. Most, particularly the women, work with plants, but some do not. Some are settled, and some wander.

Anthropologists since the nineteenth century have centered shamanic cultures across the sub-Arctic (northern Eurasia and North America), pointing to ceremonies and beliefs common to both sides of the Bering Strait as evidence.

The Pale of Settlement is in many ways a typological continuation of this shamanic cultural belt, with its population mixture of peoples originating in northern Eurasia across the region (e.g., Tatars, of course, but also Estonians, Finns, Sami, and even the ancestors of the Hungarians, or Magyars).

It's significant that the Yiddish name for the magico-religious healer who cures with plants, divination, and charms is opshprekherin/opshprekher, "one who 'speaks away'" (op + shprekher). The name is morphologically similar to the German *Absprechen*, "to arrange, agree, deny," but the meaning is quite different. It's much more similar, both in form and meaning, to the name for the Lithuanian healer, the užkalbėjimas, "one who 'speaks upward/outward'" (už + kalbėjimas), evidence of much closer contact in matters of supernatural apotropaic healing ("speaking away") between Ashkenazi Jews and Lithuanians, and a possible trace of a common immersion in the broader shamanic culture of northern Eurasia.

The communal healing culture that flourished in the Pale, we posit, was a blend of written medical traditions, carried down from the Greco-Roman-Arabic civilizations, mostly by literate (male) Jews; the native plant traditions of the region (passed down by the inhabitants of the longest standing, the Slavs and the Balts); the reliance on sympathetic magic and charms, divination, incantations, and exorcism by healers of both genders who were clearly operating within the shamanic tradition; as well as a universal belief in the evil eye, particularly as a harmful supernatural force most likely to be directed at mothers and children. A long tradition of cultivating healing plants in monastery gardens (as distinct from foraging them in the wild) was a heritage common in central and Eastern Europe; the earliest Polish herbals, such as Szymon Syreniusz's, follow in the footsteps of Hildegard von Bingen.

What about what the two of us have gotten used to calling "the woo"? It's impossible to research the world of plant healing without running up against the supernatural again and again—it is most assuredly a key component of the common culture of healing in Eastern Europe. Those Tatars—revered above all healers in Lite—were particularly renowned for their skill in exorcising evil spirits (djinn and dybbuk). Pouring, whether wax, lead, or tin (along with similar rituals that rely on embers and eggs, etc.), was utterly essential to this shared culture, as both diagnostic tool and remedy guide. The likely origin of this type of divination in the ancient Near East suggests to us that it may well have been introduced to the region by its Jews—such techniques are deeply rooted throughout the Jewish diaspora, including among such distant populations as the Baghdadi Jews of India. So, too, is the common belief in the evil eye, be it the beyz-oyg (Yiddish), ayn hore (Hebrew), urok (Polish), sglaz (Russian), zgłaz (Lipka Tatar), k'oźukm'ak (Karaim), bloga akis (Lithuanian), nazar (Gagauz), nagaza (Romani), or others. We can't understand the history of healing in the Pale without accepting magical medicine—all the more difficult when such healing has invariably been denigrated as "quackery."

Which is to underscore another important point: Healing is a serious business. We're rediscovering and recovering treatments that could heal a patient or, if misused, might kill them. Nothing in this book should be taken for advisory or validated. It is the unearthing of a shared and ancient tradition of folk medicine based on the natural world of plants and other healing substances, as well as the super- or preternatural world of magic. It's a beautiful world, and we love spending time in it, but it must be traversed with great care.

It's a lost world of small settlements, villages, towns, and hamlets, generally located along rivers and at crossroads, sometimes nestled against hillsides or surrounded by forests, many with populations of one thousand or fewer souls. A world without hospitals, clinics, or even pharmacies. A world where people relied on their neighbors for care and aid to deliver their babies, cure their ailments, remove their afflictions (whether physical, psychological, or magical), or offer palliative care and mourning to help them at the end of their lives. Most vanished from this world is the diversity of community: in this lost continent, Jew and Gentile, Tatar and Lithuanian, Slav and Greek, Roma and Armenian, and on and on, lived, got sick, got better, bore children, and died, side by side.

Even though the Pale has been regarded as something of a backwater, a realm of superstitious peasants, it's also a world where healers provided their patients with remedies from all corners of the globe: quinine, soap bark, and tobacco from the Americas, and ginger, nutmeg, cardamom, and cinnamon from the East. The legendary spice routes ran straight through the Pale, at the crossroads of east and west, Europe and Asia, and every local market likely had an herb or spice merchant who could provide the ingredients for the most complex and subtle formulations, for the Pale has long received every type of plant. But in the end, much of the herbal medicine was delivered to the table: many of the most important healing plants among the peoples of the Pale are kitchen plants: dill, parsley, onion, garlic, oregano.

In our discussion of plants and their healing properties and applications, we will sometimes refer to official medicine, although we are excavating remedies provided by folk healers rather than medical professionals. Sometimes the only way to determine the terminus post quem, the date after which a plant can be assumed part of the regional materia medica, is to track its standing in the earlier written record, which, in the case of Russia, particularly in the seventeenth and eighteenth centuries (and into the nineteenth), is in the official state herbals (travniki) and pharmacopiae. (This method was useful in sketching out the story of rosemary in the Pale.)

But of course many mysteries remain. As we said earlier, local plant names are often both fascinating and highly suggestive. How smooth is the path from philology to ethnobotany and ethnopharmacology? Why are some plants called "remedy" (refue) or "charm" (segule) in Yiddish? What about plants whose Slavic name(s) include the appellative "Tatar" (e.g., "Tatar soap" for soapwort) or "Jew" (e.g., *Physalis alkekengi*, "Jew cherry")? Where are the missing links between Hebrew, Aramaic, Arabic, or Greek plant names known in the Mishna and their modern Yiddish counterparts (e.g., rosemary)? How much differentiation was there in healthcare? What do we do about a common culture of healing, a continuum of healing, running from the Baltic to Black Seas, with Ashkenazi Jews as the only common denominator (along with the plants)?

And the plant realm itself. As in *Ashkenazi Herbalism*, we have been forced by limitations of space to restrict our lengthier studies to approximately two dozen plants; all the plants deserve a book in their own right. We have assembled a list of more than eighty plants that are an essential materia medica for the entire region. We hope to be able to provide a fuller survey in the future, as well as further sketch out the past and present of intercommunal healing in what was once the Pale, particularly along its margins (northeastern, southeastern, and central Europe, as well as across Russia into central Asia).

Other conundrums we're still trying to explore: How traceable are the extensive plant links between South Asia and Eastern Europe? To what degree did the Roma, Tatars, Armenians, Georgians, and other peoples along these routes spread Persian Unani and Indian Ayurvedic healing knowledge throughout the region? (Talko-Hryncewicz considered this same question more than 130 years ago.) What are the links between traditional Chinese medicine and the healing cultures of the Pale (e.g., "bankes," or cupping)? Did imported plants and spices arrive in the Pale overland from the Caucasus and central Asia or by sea via Alexandria, Hamburg, Odessa, and other ports, or both directions? How extensive and ongoing were the healing connections between western and Eastern Europe over the centuries? If given enough time (and strength—shkoyach), we hope to keep exploring these connections, answering these questions, and remapping this world.

THE PLANTS

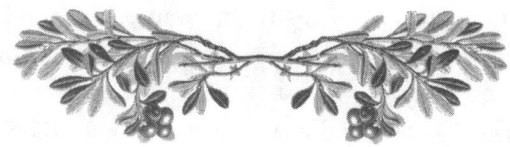

FOR THIS PROJECT, WE RELIED ON a specific set of criteria to help with the selection of each plant in the monographs section. First and foremost was a plant's appearance in Mordkhe Schaechter's *Plant Names in Yiddish*, which itself lists over 1,500 plants. Mordkhe Schaechter was the leading Yiddish lexicographer of our day. He relied upon the published corpus of Yiddish literature, as well as a legion of native-speaker informants (frustratingly, *Plant Names in Yiddish* does not provide enough information about these informants and where they were from). If an entry in that book featured a uniquely Yiddish name—not obviously derived from languages other than Latin or Hebrew—it was given the highest priority for our selection process. For example, this is particularly true for five plants known under variations of the Hebrew word *refue*, "remedy." They are rosemary (*Salvia rosmarinus*), hedge mustard (*Sisymbrium officinale*), kidney vetch (*Anthyllis vulneraria*), sanicle (*Sanicula europaea*), and bearberry (*Arctostaphylos uva-ursi*).

A brief note on the Yiddish refuahdiker "medicinal": it is equivalent to the Latin *officinalis*, which in binomial taxonomy generally refers to plants that, during the Middle Ages, would have been kept in the (monastery) officina, where medicines were stored.

In some cases, a plant's Yiddish or Hebrew name is redolent of woman-centered divinity: just as the Yiddish name we found in Schaechter for calendula ("segule-rosh-koydeshl") seems to acknowledge the women's holiday of rosh kodesh, we learned that, for ha-Kohen's early modern readers, linden was known as the Asherah tree, after the ancient Semitic mother-goddess.

The monographs ahead represent detailed explorations into how an herb might have been understood by many different peoples of the region over several centuries. Unlike our first book, *Ashkenazi Herbalism*, this research depended almost exclusively on Eastern European sources. One of the most important of these is a Polish ethnobotanical survey published in the late nineteenth century. As with our first book, the close examination of a little-known or -studied document yielded significant and unexpected findings, and so can be considered another "hidden herbal." Because this particular publication centered on late-nineteenth-century locales in Poland—and what would later become Ukraine, Lithuania, and Belarus—the demographics we collected on the towns and villages named in the study have been gleaned from 1897, or thereabouts, census data.

In the monographs that follow, we first identify a given town by its name in the work cited, along with its Yiddish and modern official names, and Jewish population, if relevant. For towns cited by Talko-Hryncewicz, the name will be in his Polish. For towns cited by Natalia Osadcha-Janata in her *Herbs Used in Ukrainian Folk Medicine*, we use the Yiddish place-names cited in *Ashkenazi Herbalism*. Please refer to the table in the appendix (p. 305) for more detail.

Because our perspective is necessarily centered on Ashkenazim, another of our selection criteria was that a plant's healing application be recorded in a locale with a significant Ashkenazi Jewish population at the turn of the twentieth century. There are a few exceptions, such as when the locale, as in regions such as Berdychiv or Zhytomyr, was generally amidst surrounding settlements with high percentages of Ashkenazi Jewish populations.

Other significant sources we looked to while preparing the plant monographs include Issachar bar Teller's Yiddish-language *Be'er mayim hcyim* (Wellspring of Living Waters), a medical advice book published in Prague in the mid-seventeenth century; ha-Kohen's Hebrew-language *Ma'aseh Tuviyah*, first published in Venice at the turn of the eighteenth century and regularly reprinted well into the twentieth century for Jewish folk healers of the Pale (and their modern traditional descendants: the latest edition of *Ma'aseh Tuviyah* was reprinted in 1977); many yizkor memory books offering a surprising trove of medicinal plant and folk healing information, not to mention all the hidden gems of historical and cultural information absent from the mainstream literature that discusses the former shtetls; *Mentshn, flantsn un refues: algemeyre shmuesn* by C. H. (Khone) Garber, an Eastern European immigrant to South America prior to the Second World War who published a Yiddish guide to medicinal plants in Buenos Aires in the mid-1940s; and a trio of Lithuanian master's theses (by Austina Kvederavičiūtė, Ruhangiz Manafova, and Kristina Ratkevičiūtė) that document plant medicines among contemporary healers of Lithuania—its surviving Jews and Tatars, and Lithuanians who acknowledge the shared wisdom of their Jewish neighbors before the war. Kvederavičiūtė's 2019 thesis focuses exclusively on contemporary Jewish plant healers of Lithuania; Manafova's 2014 thesis focuses on Tatar and Azerbaijani healers of Lithuania; Ratkevičiūtė's 2018 thesis profiles traditional healers (almost entirely women) of the Lithuanian town of Kaišiadorys and its environs, the oldest of whom were raised in a region that had been majority Jewish before the war, in a community wherein neighborly transmission of plant knowledge was a significant component of the local culture of healing.

One of the most interesting discoveries in this trio of unpublished master's theses is that Jewish folk healers focus their treatments more acutely on digestive health, as opposed to their Muslim counterparts who are more concerned with respiratory support. This revelation reflects the older Eastern European Jewish herbal sources, such as ha-Kohen and Teller, and also seems to gel with the (traumatic) legacy of growing up in Ashkenazi households, where several generations of Jewish children were endlessly threatened with enemas, castor oil, and a constant refrain of "Did you make?"—all part of the unwritten remedy book to ensure good (digestive) health, a long-standing focus of Jewish medicine.

These contemporary Lithuanian empirical studies reaffirm a fact that resurfaces again and again: most folk healers were and remain women. This has been true throughout most of our own research—in both the Ukrainian and Polish surveys we foraged—and for other researchers who examine similar folk healing practices. We have also continued to survey the contemporary literature on Eastern European folk medicine, relying on works that broadly cover Polish, Ukrainian, Lithuanian, and Russian plant healing (see "A Note on Our Sources," p. 299).

Personal experience in my own body and conversations with friends and family have also informed these monographs. Some stories, like my grandmother's tale about her sister's infection being cured by an opshprekher in South Philadelphia in the late 1910s, are included in the monographs (see *Daucus carota*, p. 81) whereas others, while relevant to folk healing, are not completely plant-related but fascinate nonetheless. One of these concerns my discovery in the last few years that my grandfather owned and used his own set of bankes (cups) for his respiratory health. Another is the way my mother used to treat bumps on the head by pressing the flat side of a butter knife onto the swelling. This is a common but little-known healing method among Ashkenazim and can probably be traced back to the use of iron as a curative and protective substance.

It was extremely difficult to decide which twenty-five plants to cover in the monographs. Because we wanted to reveal how extensive plant medicinal knowledge was in the region, we've also included a shorter "kitchen herbal"—a collection of "minigraphs" devoted to the healing plants most common in the Ashkenazi (and Eastern European) kitchen, furnishing their names in all relevant languages, and, wherever possible, we offer a brief annotation on the more interesting aspects of the plant's healing applications.

We contemplated organizing these monographs by type or application: kitchen plants (horseradish, carrot), wild plants (calendula, kidney vetch), "practical" plants (madder, linden, flax, hemp, soapwort), and the like. But so many plants have so many amazing applications that we decided the least complicated approach was to put them in binomial alphabetical order. (Although, because the stories we tell in our *Daucus carota* monograph are so emotionally charged, we considered leading with this plant.)

We cannot reiterate enough that plants are complex beings with lives both separate and intermingled with our human world. They've been here far longer than us and have developed beneficent ways to coexist on this planet that we humans would do well to learn from.

ACORUS CALAMUS | SWEET FLAG

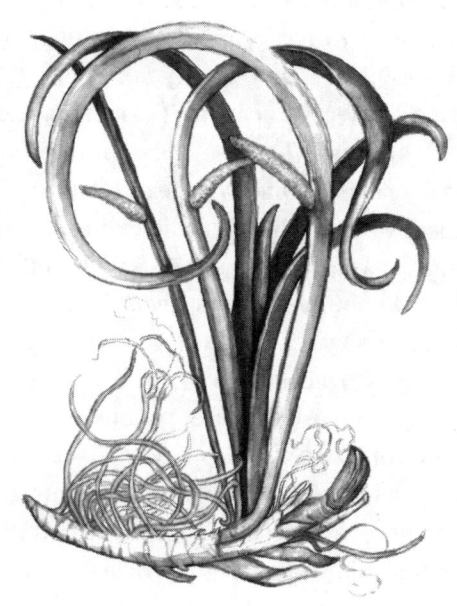

FAMILY Acoraceae

YIDDISH שאַווער (shaver); Schaechter also lists the following transliterated names: (d)zhaver, shover, shever, shaber, shavan, shuvares, ayer, kalmes, kolmes, kvitshers, fayfelekh, lepekhe, lepak

POLISH Tatarak zwyczajny, tatarak wonny, tatarak pospolity, agier, ajer, cypr, kalmus, łabuzie, plaskoć, pluszcz, pluszczaj, sasyna, sowar, tatar, tatarczuch, tatarski korzeń, palma, trzcina, szuwar, bazuny, bluszcz, gałga, gałgan, jasyna, kalamus, kalmusz, kłącz, lepecha, lepiech, lepiecha, łabzie, łącz, łobuzie, panny, panny na rzece, panny w rzece, sacyna, szczar, szczwar, talerz, tatarcuch, tatarcuk, tatarcze ziele, tatarczok, tatarczuk, tatarsky korzeny, taterz, źdźbło

UKRAINIAN   Аїр (Aïr), татарське зілля (tatars'ke zillja), лепеха (lepexa), шувар (šuvar), агир (ahyr), агір (ahir), аєр (aer), аїр (aïr), аїрний корінь (aïrnyj korin'), аляр (aljar), арник (arnyk), вишера (vyšera), гав'яр (hav'jar), гаїр (haïr), гайвір (hajvir), галки (halky), галяр (haljar), гогорудза (gogorudza), ір (ir), ірник (irnyk), ірниця (irnycja), ірячник (irjačnyk), йор (jor), кальмус (kal'mus), канки (kanky), катерина (kateryna), кияхи (kyjaxy), коломня (kolomnja), косатень (kosaten'), косатник (kosatnyk), коситеня татарове (kosytenja tatarove), коситень (kosyten'), кувшинки (kušvynky), лепех (lepex), лепеха (lepexa), лепеха вонюча (lepexa vonjuča), лепеха жидівська (lepexa žydivs'ka), лепеха-різак (lepexa rizak), лепеша (lepeša), лепешник (lepešnyk), лепешня (lepešnja), лепешняк (lepešnjak), лепиха вонюча (lepixa vonjuča), лепіх (lepix), лепішник (lepišnyk), лепішняк (lepišnjak), липих (lypyx), липниха (lypnyxa), липуха (lypuxa), ліпаха (lipaxa), лір (lir), лопух (lopux), осока (osoka), осока пахуча (osoka paxuča), осока широка (osoka široka), острий бур'ян (ostryj bur'jan), падиволос (padyvolos), паи)-хурка (pa[i]xurka), півники жаб'ячі (pivnyky žab'jači), піщалка (piščalka), плишник (plyšnyk), плющай (pljuščaj), рамник (ramnyk), ревінь (revin'), різак (rizak), рогіз (ro'hiz), сасина (sasyna), саш (saš), саш білий (saš bilyj), сашина (sašyna), сашина біла (sašyna bila), сівар (sivar), смичка (smyčka), тартараки (tartaraky), татара (tatara), татарак (tatarak), татар-зілля (tatar-zillja), татаринник (tatarynnyk), татариння (tatarynnja), татарка (tatarka), татарник (tatarnyk), татарове зілля (tatarove zillja), татарське вонюче зілля (tatars'ke vonjuče zillja), татарське зілля(є) (tatars'ke zillja[e]), татарський корінь (tatars'kyj korin'), татарче зілля (tatarče zillja), тетерник (teternyk), тросник (trosnyk), троща (troščа), цар-зілля (car-zillja), царське зілле (cars'ke zille), шабальник (šabal'nyk), шавар (šavar), шалана (šalana), шаш (šaš), швар (švar), шивар (šyvar), шивар зелений (šyvar zelenyj), широка трава (šyroka trava), шівар (šivar), шовар(ник) (šovar[nyk]), шувар (šuvar), шувар звичайний (šuvar zvyčajnyj), шувар татарський (šuvar tatars'ky), шуварник (šuvarnyk), шувор (šuvor), щувар (šuvar), явгір (javhir), явер (javer), яве(і)ровий корінь (jave[i]rovyj korin'), яв'єр (jav'er), явір (javir), явор (javor), ягір (jahir), яр (jar), ярус (jarus)

BELARUSIAN   яер (jaer), плюшнік (pljušnik), явар (javar), aip (air), аер (aer), ірны корань (irny koran'), шувар (šuvar), ярай (jaraj)

THE PLANTS

LITHUANIAN Balinis ajeras, kaliamas

RUSSIAN Аир обыкновенный (Air obyknovennyj), аир болотный (air bolotnyj), аир тростниковый (air trostnikovyj), ирный корень (irnyj koren), гавиар (gaviar), игир (igir), ир (ir), касатик (kasatik), касатник (kasatnik), косатик (kosatik), лепёха (lepëxa), лепёшник (lepëšnik), пищалка (piščalka), татарский сабельник (tatarskij sabel'nik), татарское зелье (tatarskoe zel'e), явр (javr)

GERMAN Kalmus, Kalmes, Kalmser, Gelbe Gilge, Gewöhnlicher Kalmus, Kaninchenwurz, Kaninchenwurzel, Karremanswurz, Karremanswurzel, Schwertheu, Magenbrand, Magenwurz, Nagenwurz, Ackerwurz, Würtzriedt, Gewürzkalmus, Rotting, Zehrwurz, Deutscher Ingwer

HEBREW קנה (kaneh)

TATAR Кылычүлән (Kylyčùlän), кылыч уты (kylyč ùty), кылыч үләне (kylyč ùläne), җир тамыры (žyr tamyry), җиртамыр (žirtamyr)

Like St. John's wort or garlic, *Acorus calamus* could have an entire volume devoted to its history with humans. In brief, calamus is a reed-like aquatic plant with stylized curved shoots and a cylindrical rhizome emitting many rootlets; it grows in watery conditions and can be distinguished from plants with a similar appearance by what Maude Grieve calls its "curious, agreeable scent," especially the root, which is sought for its medicinal powers.

Grieve, the early twentieth-century British herbalist and author of the standard reference work *A Modern Herbal*, identified many of its common names in English—sweet flag, sweet root, sweet rush, sweet cane, gladdon, sweet myrtle, myrtle grass, myrtle sedge, and cinnamon sedge—but this admirable English litany is dwarfed by the plant's extensive catalog of designations in the former Pale of Settlement.

All historical botanical sources agree that calamus is indigenous to India. The ancient Greeks considered its best medicinals to be derived from its "orange tawny" roots, which had the most knots, splintered when broken into pieces, and were sticky, astringent, and somewhat pungent when chewed. Dioscorides found that calamus helped with urination, edemas, coughs, and promoting menstruation, and was an effective sitz bath for women. It also contributed its aroma to incense and fragrances.

The etymological record suggests that calamus arrived in the lands of the Pale of Settlement as an imported plant, perhaps via trade or travelers; the fabled roots of this plant spread quickly in fresh water. It may have also arrived in Eastern Europe through military conquest; in the Middle Ages, according to the Russian scholar V. V. Teljat'ev, Tatars brought calamus to Russia, believing its roots could purify water sources they came across. Thus, traveling on horseback, they would carry pieces of fresh root to toss into any water they encountered, thereby making it safe to drink without the risk of becoming sick.

Calamus is absent from the materia medica of the twelfth-century German herbalist, abbess, and polymath Hildegard von Bingen, simply because the plant is not attested in Germany until 1588, a number of centuries after the abbess's death.

There is some question as to which plant the Jewish polymath-philosopher Maimonides, a twelfth-century near-contemporary of Hildegard, refers to when he writes about Greek akoron, but the record shows that calamus made its way into the Yiddish-language medical literature almost immediately after its attestation in Germany: in a section of his remedy book devoted to treating plague, Issachar bar Teller, who lived and worked in Prague, advised readers to avoid constipation, and one of his recommendations involved chewing on a bit of preserved kalmus after breakfast, before leaving home for the day.

By the time the physician Tobias ha-Kohen documented calamus in the early eighteenth century, in his book *Ma'aseh Tuviyah* (The Work of Tobias), there was no doubt that *Acorus calamus* was the herb he identified in Greek as akurus, in Latin as kalamus aromatikus, in Turkish as aigir, and in Mishnaic Hebrew as kaneh. Scholars such as Moldenke and Moldenke claim that *kaneh* is a Biblical catchall term for any reed plant, while others associate it with calamus, a plant that was carried along the spice routes as an essential ingredient in the anointing oils prescribed in the Torah. Another assertion holds that calamus's psychogenic properties suggest it was also relied upon to enhance ritual observances.

Etymology is a very important tool for understanding calamus's role in Eastern European plant medicine. Mordkhe Schaechter, in his book *Plant*

Names in Yiddish, gives us a clue as to how important the herb was in the former Pale. He recorded at least a dozen regional names for calamus, some derived from Slavic, others from Turkish, and some uniquely Yiddish, such as kvitsners or feyfelekh, not to mention zhaver. Shuvares, another Yiddish name for the reed, almost seems like a deliberate play on the name of the Jewish holiday Shavuos, and it is not surprising that calamus was often the herbal star of that observance. In the yizkor memory books of both Ostrovtsah (Ostrowiec Świetokrzyski) and Sokolov-Podl'ask (Sokołów Podlaski), both in Poland, survivors remembered with great tenderness how the plant was gathered from the banks of the river and strewn upon the floors of homes during the holiday itself, lending its sweet scent to the early spring celebrations.

Polish American author Sophie Knab also recounts this tradition during the days of the Pentecost in Poland in older times:

> *The second most important greenery to be collected for the home on this holiday was the fragrant sweet flag, known in Latin as Acorus calamus. In Polish it is known as tatarek pospolity, ajer and kalmus. Growing in wet, marshy areas near rivers and streams it was placed in vases on a home altar or in the corners of the main room of the cottage. There was a saying: "Zielone świątki tatarek w kątki" (the green holidays-calamus in the corners). The most preferred method of having sweet flag in the house was to cut or chop it into smaller pieces and scatter it on the floors of the house. Whether on a humble, hard-packed cottage floor or the wooden floor of a manor house, the sweet-smelling herb (which many say smells like cinnamon) was indispensable. In the mid-nineteenth century Polish ethnographer Oskar Kolberg described it thus: "On the day (Pentecost) they sweep the porch and the front of the house and sprinkle the place with calamus."*

This recalls Maude Grieve, who writes that the plant was formerly scattered across the floors of churches during festivals and often in private houses—she also affirms that it was the Tatars who introduced calamus to Poland.

In the nineteenth-century Polish ethnobotanical literature, calamus appears in over a dozen folk remedies and has carried a number of regional appellations depending on where it was known to healers. Near Kyiv, it was called haviar; in western Galicia, szuwar (cf. Yiddish *shuvares*, mentioned earlier); in Po_tava it was reported as ir (cf. *air*); and in Zwiahel (Yiddish Zvil, in the late nineteenth century 55 percent Jewish; now Zviahel', Ukraine), it was called tatarka and tatarskie ziele, or "Tatar herb." In some Ukrainian communities, calamus was known as lepexa žydivs'ka, "Jewish flatbread" (both Slavs and Yiddish-speaking Jews might also call calamus "lepex" or "lepexa").

In the town of Olszana (Yiddish Olshan or Vilshana, in the late nineteenth century 20 percent Jewish; now Vil'šany, Ukraine), a complex formula that included calamus and several other herbs bore a striking resemblance to the fabulous trianke (see Trianke monograph, p. 207) and was given to induce menstruation.

One regional superstition encountered in eastern Galicia at this time maintained that children were prone to attacks by "rusalki," malevolent water creatures who targeted young victims during Pentecost. For protection against rusalki, it was customary to scatter calamus and burdock on the floors of dwellings. In this prophylactic remedy against supernatural forces, we hear an echo of the Polish custom Knab describes. It was also common to cover cradles with wormwood to safeguard vulnerable children.

Childhood wasting diseases, including consumption or tuberculosis, were a grave concern at the turn of the twentieth century. Folk healers often gave baths to young patients because it was believed that the disease could be drawn out of the body this way. Magical means often accompanied these remedies—for example, if one bathed a young child in a decoction of willow branches, the spent water was to be poured into the soil beneath the tree afterward. A bath with a decoction of calamus root was reported as common practice, although no further instructions were recorded.

In Eastern Europe, as recently as a century ago, many people would perform strenuous labor that at times might cause them to have a "detached feeling" in their intestines. Folk healers would offer remedies either internal or external (such as a compress) or an "ordering"—an incantation meant to banish the debilitating condition. Because this type of injury was regarded as similar to some aspects of pregnancy, in the towns of Zwinogródka (Yiddish Zvenigorodka, in the late nineteenth century 38 percent Jewish; now Zvenyhorodka, Ukraine) and Łysianka (Yiddish Lisinka, in the late nineteenth century 40 percent Jewish; now Lysyanka, Ukraine), the zapiekanka (a formula whose name means something like "toast," similar to the trianke formula) was offered to treat this discomfort. The zapiekanka was a vodka infusion of herbs such as galangal, sarsaparilla, bogbean (bobownik), cinnamon, and cloves. In Hussa-kowa (Yiddish Husakov, in the late nineteenth century 30 percent Jewish; now Husakiv, Ukraine) patients would drink buttermilk all day long as a cure. In the village of Jurkow (known in the late nineteenth century as Jurkowszczyzna, in a rural community whose environs were more than 50 percent Jewish; now Yarun', Ukraine), they would cover the crosses with brewed calamus. Close to Jurkow, one folk healer was known for grinding the thinner end of a fulgurite (earth hardened in the shape of a dart by a lightning strike) in vodka; if the liquid turned red, it was taken as a sign that the patient would be cured.

Other abdominal problems were characterized by a lack of appetite, stool retention, stomach pain, or impaired nutrition. The most common herbs given in decoction formulations for nausea, gas, and distention were wormwood, bogbean, and peppermint. In Jurkow, a brew of dried calamus was an option. Other herbs reported as curative teas in that town were those of angelica or elecampane—but only if the root were dug up in the spring—as well as bistort or sorrel, among others.

We note that bogbean, *Menyanthes trifoliata*, was a common remedy for stomach problems among Ashkenazim and their neighbors in the Pale: Berl Glezer, a survivor who grew up in the shtetl of Trashkun (now Troškūnai, Lithuania), recalled the paradise of healing plants that suffused his childhood in his memoir "My Shtetl Trashkun":

The shtetele was like an island surrounded not by the sea but by broad fields and a thick ancient forest. All kinds of beautiful trees grew in the forest— pine, fir, birch, alder, aspen, ash, and oak—and many kinds of mushrooms and berries: blueberries, bog blueberries, raspberries, and red bilberries.

In early spring a mantle of green covered the fields and meadows. Later corn and rye would come up amid sticks of straw. The ears of corn seemed to lift their heads to heaven. A narrow winding stream ran through the meadow. It wasn't deep and you could reach in with your hand to touch every little clean-washed stone lying on the bottom. There was a wider, deeper place that we called the whirlpool. We went swimming there, especially on Friday afternoons.

The stream, known as Yoste, was where the laundry was washed. The wet clothing was spread out in the meadow to dry. While we waited for it to dry, we gathered fallen goose feathers and various plants—one called bronelkes

[Prunella vulgaris, selfheal] for making tea, and one with three little leaves known as bobovnik [Menyanthes trifoliata] that was a stomach ache remedy. Many other healing grasses grew in the meadow among the yellow flowers. Sunrise and sunset could be seen above the high treetops as if over broad seas.

Edemas, or swellings, were generally believed to be caused by drinking too much vodka or too much water, or even by having a cold. Many folk healers treated this condition with herbs they considered diuretic, but there were external remedies as well, such as placing linden leaves over an affected area. Some reported remedies hearkened back to an earlier era, as in Ryżanówka (Yiddish Rizinivka, in the late nineteenth century 33 percent Jewish; now Ryžanivka, Ukraine), where a healer poured dried and ground-up frogs mixed with fat onto the swelling (the importance of frogs in Eastern European folk medicine is worthy of a book in itself). In Smykowce (now Smykivci, Ukraine), just outside Tarnopol, which in the late nineteenth century was a large shtetl that was more than 50 percent Jewish, a tea made from rowan berries was applied. In Zwinogródka, boiled fresh nettles were a simpler method for reducing swelling and cooling the area. Another remedy in the same town called for a tea blend of wormwood, calamus, juniper berries, pepper, and camphor that was to be poured on the sore spot for an extended time. It was also reported that Jewish healers would rely on octane with sea conches dissolved within to rub onto edemas. Another remedy reported from Zwinogródka required a water solution of blue stone, which recalls the story of the folk healer from Eishyshok (present-day Eišiškės, Lithuania) who never went anywhere without his trusted curatives (see *Inula helenium*, p. 97).

Causes for headaches could be varied, and included bad air, cold, or the evil eye. There are many herbs reported by folk healers in the Polish lands of the late nineteenth century to combat this malady, one of which was attested in the town of Nowa-Uszyca (Yiddish Nay-Ushitsah, in the late nineteenth century 56 percent Jewish; now Nova-Ušycja, Ukraine), where calamus was pounded and, as a compress, was applied to the forehead and temples to treat the ache. (Could this be the "Jewish flatbread" of the Ukrainians?)

One superstition of the era held that sleeping or staying in places where animals dwelled could make a person sick. In Russia, it was believed that one could get ringworm from walking or sleeping in areas where wolves roamed, and in Ukraine the condition could be contracted merely by placing one's foot on a spot where a horse had rolled. The many folk cures for this condition included treatments of kerosene, oak gall, onion juice, celandine, or blue stone mixed with a decoction of peas. In Nowa-Uszyca, healers recommended saliva mixed with saponaria or dried and powdered calamus sprinkled on the area to remove the infestation. More magical means could involve transferring the condition from the body to an article of clothing—like a sweaty shirt—and then burying the shirt. Or finding a folk healer like an opshprekherin to banish the infection with a ritual and an incantation.

Calamus was a trusted herb for getting rid of bad breath in the town of Lipowiec (Yiddish Lipovetz, in the late nineteenth century 48 percent Jewish; now Lypovec', Ukraine). The town is thought to have been founded by Lipka Tatars.

In the early twentieth century, the Polish ethnographer Regina Lilienthal, in her ethnographic study *Dziecko żydowskie* (The Jewish Child), wrote that children in Jewish communities in Poland made whistles out of calamus ("tatarak") reeds as part of their games.

Nosal' and Nosal' mention the plant's role in combating cholera, typhus, and Spanish influenza in their twentieth-century official Ukrainian herbal, but calamus was applied more widely in folk healing at that time, particularly in cases of wounds and infections. According to Müller-Dietz, Russian folk medicine also promotes calamus root (whether decoction, tincture, or powder) internally as a stomachicum (particularly in veterinary medicine) and for cystitis.

A yizkor book from Alderney Road, Sussex, quotes an inscription on the matza (tombstone) of Rabbi Saul Berlin of the Great Synagogue of London (1756–1842): "Here lies the great rabbi, famous, wonderful, uprooter of mountains, sweet calamus. . ." This gnomic epitaph is difficult to interpret but, regardless, points to calamus's importance as a healing plant to be associated with magico-religious authority.

Even as late as 1917, nurses in the United States were being trained on the medicinal qualities of herbs. Calamus was described in a nursing textbook of the period as chiefly "a carminative and as such [it] acts well for post-operative and fermentative flatulence."

In contemporary Lithuania, the roots of *Ajeris balinis*, as calamus is called there, are part of the medicinal repertoire of the region's remaining Jewish healers. They look to the plant to address gastrointestinal tract disorders and to treat inflammation of the kidneys, bladder, liver, and gallbladder. The root can also serve as a mouth rinse or strengthen hair roots (recalling the Ukrainian name padyvolos, meaning "hair-fall"). For promoting healthy urination, folk healers simmer one tablespoon of the herb in two cups of boiling water and drink a glass of this tea half an hour before meals, three to four times a day.

Present-day Lipka Tatars of Lithuania rely upon a decoction of the root to maintain good metabolism. They mix the roots with milk and drink this formula to ease anxiety. For strengthening the hair, they rub a decoction of the root into the scalp.

These traditional applications for calamus are in complete agreement with present-day Western herbalists such as Ryn Midura and Katja Swift of Commonwealth Herbs in Boston, Massachusetts. They write of calamus's ability to shift a person from a state of tension to one of "rest and digest," making the herb a good choice as a before-meal digestive bitter. This relaxing quality, German herbalists Peter and Barbara Theiss tell us, has made calamus popular as part of postprandial digestive formulas in France for many years.

Michigan herbalist Jim McDonald has an extensive calamus post on his website herbcraft.org. Aside from describing its physical properties and recounting its well-documented medicinal possibilities, he delves into sweet flag's ability to calm the body, mind, and spirit if just a little bit of the rhizome is chewed. As I write this, sitting in a noisy café, I've just put a small piece of calamus's aromatic root in my mouth and immediately noticed all over again how its flavor is reminiscent of cedar, and that even this tiny sliver can mingle its subtle fragrance with the strong coffee aromas wafting from the roasting machines in the shop's back rooms. Even the enthusiastic group of knitters sitting across from me have been unable to break my concentration today—and I'm not even wearing earbuds.*

---

* The first-person singular is used by Deatra throughout to describe her impressions and experiences in researching and writing this book.

ANTHYLLIS VULNERARIA |
KIDNEY VETCH

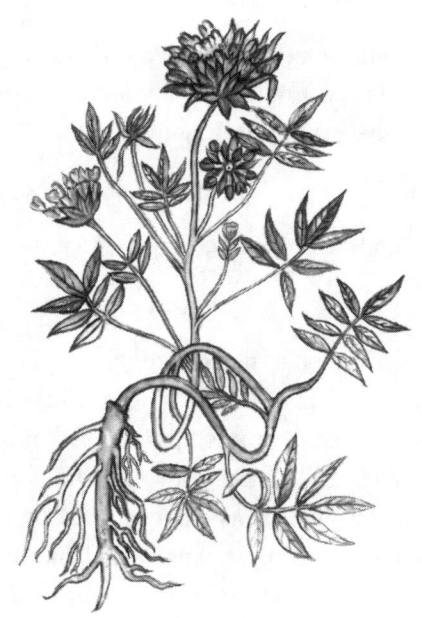

FAMILY   Faboideae

YIDDISH   רפֿואהדיקער וווּנדקלעווער (refuahdiker vundklever)

POLISH   Przelot pospolity, odczyn, oczyna, solnik

UKRAINIAN   Заяча конюшина багатолиста (Zajača konjušyna bahatolysta), заяча конюшина звичайна (zajača konjušyna zvyčajna); болгай комушка (bolhaj komuška), комушка звичайна (komuška zvyčajna), перелет (perelet); валашок жовтий (valašok žovtyj), зайчик (zajčyk), зільник (zil'nyk), зольник (zol'nyk), зольник звичайний (zol'nyk zvyčajnyj), клевер заячий (klever zajačyj), команиця заяч (komanycja zajač), комонина (komonyna), конюшина заяча (konjušyna zajača), коɔівки (korivky), котикоє (kotykoe), лапки котячі (lapky kotjači), опучай (opɹčaj), откосник (otkosnyk), перелет соколій (perelet sokolij), перелета (perɛleta), п'ятисильник (p'jatysyl'nyk), ранник (rannyk), язвенник (jazvennyk͈

LITHUANIAN   Paprastasis perluotis

RUSSIAN   Язвенник обыкновенный (Jazvennyk obyknovennyj), язвеɹник ранозаживляющий (jazvennik ranozaživljajuščij), зольник (zolɹnik), заячий клевер (zajačij klever), желтый заячий клевер (želtyj zajačij klɘver)

SORBIAN   Raniwka

GERMAN   Echter Wundklee, Gemeiner Wundklee, Gewöhnlicher Wund-klee, Tannenklee

As much as we apply our rational methods to its study, the plant world often remains mysterious to us. This is true in a scientific, and even a linguistic sense—sometimes our ancestral words themselves know more than we do about a given plant. Such is the case with *Anthyllis vulneraria*, or kidney vetch, which is one of the five plants—out of many hundreds of entries—specifically designated as a "refue," or remedy plant, in Schaechter's *Plant Names in Yiddish*. Rather than revealing the mystery, a reflection upon its special status as a refue plant deepens it.

Kidney vetch's Yiddish name, refuahdiker vundklever, testifies to its importance in Yiddish-speaking communities of Eastern Europe. Far less common than its Latin cognate *officinalis*, a *refuahdiker* appellation demands closer attention. It calls to us, offering a glimpse of our richly textured history that's been forgotten in recent decades, but which has always been closely interwoven with the green world.

This pea-family herb grows throughout Europe but prefers dry grasslands and rocky environments up to an altitude of approximately one thousand feet. It has a creeping yet upright body, and can grow anywhere from two inches to a foot and a half in height. Pinnate leaves sport leaflets that are mostly smooth on top with silky hairs on the underside. From July through October, yellow spherical flower heads appear in the majority of subspecies, but one variety offers petals with bright red tips, a detail that suggests blood and hence a doctrine of signatures explanation for the plant's species appellation.

Kidney vetch is not really covered in the history of Jewish medicine. What little documentation is available on the role of kidney vetch in the plant medicine of the Pale and Eastern Europe is somewhat confusing—even the ancient sources raise more questions than they answer: Dioscorides mentions two types of Anthyllis, neither of which seems to describe today's kidney vetch. Dioscorides does state that the root of Anthyllis can help with difficult urination, soften uterine inflammations, and treat injuries, and he also calls attention to the variety of Anthyllis "that resembles ground pine, and in addition to its other benefits, also helps epileptics when drunk in an oxymel." Remarkably, the plant is not mentioned by many of the standard sources we've relied upon for comparative-historical research, whether old (Maimonides, Maude Grieve) or new (Sophie Knab, Igor Zevin).

For wounds or other physical afflictions, kidney vetch hardly figures at all in the plant medicinal history of the Pale of Settlement, as some ethnobotanists such as the Polish scholar Adam Fischer have noted. In the mid-nineteenth century, Russian folk healers might rely on the plant to treat rabies or the bite of a rabid dog. We were intrigued to learn (from Annenkov) that in Grodno, Belarus, kidney vetch was a remedy to treat the matted hair affliction common in Poland that was known as the Plica Polonica, the Polish plait (known in Polish as kołtun, in Yiddish as kaltine). Ha-Kohen may have been the first to document this affliction (see *Salvia rosmarinus*, p. 163).

Yiddish vundklever, "wound clover," is derived from German, and also reveals a bit about the plant's story as a healing agent for traumatic injuries. According to Fischer, in the 1930s, folk healers in the town of Oszmiana, Poland (Yiddish Oshmene, before the war the Jewish population was just under 50 percent; now Ašmjany, Belarus), prescribed an infusion of kidney vetch to treat anxiety.

In German-speaking lands, kidney vetch has so many common regional names that it's impossible to ignore just how significant this plant has been in central European folk medicine. The *Handwörterbuch des deutschen Aberglaubens* (Dictionary of German Superstition) tells us that there the plant's main affinity is its wound-healing abilities, but it has also been relied upon to allay coughs—and even more curiously, kidney vetch, also known as wound-wort, when placed in the cradle, is believed to provide magical protection for babies from being verschreiend (bewitched), as indicated by one of the plant's regional monikers, Schreiklee ("scream-clover"), attested in the Sude-ten German communities of Bohemia a century ago. The name and the notion were borrowed from their Slavic neighbors, who referred to this plant as a bewitching plant (Beschreikraut), which explains the Czech name for kidney vetch, úročník, from urok, "evil eye." Throughout this part of central Europe, kidney vetch was employed to prevent cattle and other livestock from being harmed through bewitchment (or to ensure they gave good milk). Calves would take a decoction of kidney vetch to drink; goslings received a fumigation of its burning leaves.

A bit further east, according to German ethnobotanist Heinrich Marzell, in the highlands of Moravia, nineteenth-century shepherds along the Polish border would put kidney vetch and centaury in their sheepfolds on Saint John's Eve (June 23) to protect herds from bewitchment. In Poland, near Kraków, Fischer tells us that the herb was similarly given to cows for the same protection.

As attested in the late-nineteenth-century Polish ethnobotanical surveys, kidney vetch is not profiled as a medicinal plant but is mentioned only as a protector of widows against intrusive apparitions. A widowed woman would fumigate herself with this herb as a safeguard before going to sleep. In twentieth-century Ruthenia (western Ukraine), according to Varxol', the plant's power against the evil eye is commemorated in its local name, vročnik (from Ukrainian vrok, "evil eye," similar to the Czech).

Where there was a bewitchment, so were witches. We'll note in passing that much of the historical period we're discussing, from ha-Kohen onward, coincides with the era of the European witch hunts (Ma'aseh Tuviyah was published just over a decade after the Salem witch trials in Massachusetts). Historian Michael Ostling tells us that while this cruel mania was never as widespread a phenomenon in Eastern Europe (whether in the Polish-Lithuarian Commonwealth or Russia) as it was to the West, a number of records have come down to us documenting the accusations leveled at "witches" (in Russia, it was not uncommon for Tatar healers to be accused of witchcraft). In at least one trial, kidney vetch was admitted into evidence, presumably for its ability to ward off evil. The Polish folk names for kidney vetch, odczyn and oczyna, meaning "acting against," underscore this apotropaic quality.

Such supernatural associations suggest to us that in Eastern Europe's Jewish communities, a refuahdiker "magical medicinal" plant would have been one sought out by opshprekherins to explicitly protect from the evil eye or other supernatural afflictions. We see a bright trace of this in traditional Romanian pediatric folk medicine: the flowering tips of kidney vetch were given as a tea to treat fright (so often caused by the evil eye) in children.

Kidney vetch does figure in twentieth-century Eastern European plant healing. In 1927 Jan Muszyński, the pioneering Polish ethnobotanist of the interwar period, photographed three women selling herbs at the Saint John's Eve market of Vilna: two older women hold bunches of *Nymphaea alba* and *Mertha piperita*; the younger woman in the middle holds a sprig of kidney vetch, which Muszyński recorded as a local treatment for kołtuns (the Plica Polonica) and (unspecified) eye ailments. In Ukrainian folk medicine, according to Grodzins'kyj, kidney vetch is known to have soothing, binding, diuretic, tonic, and wound-healing properties. An infusion of the herb is drunk for insomnia, stomach ulcers, kidney and bladder diseases, diabetes, maladies caused by overexertion, and as a tonic after a debilitating illness. Children are given an infusion for fright or for epileptic attacks, recalling the fright remedy also found in Romanian pediatric folk medicine. In the form of a compress or lotion, the infusion will treat wounds, ulcers, or bee stings, or dissolve benign tumors. As a mouth rinse, it can heal inflammation. Chopped fresh kidney vetch grass is applied to boils and wounds to speed their healing.

These somewhat chimerical findings regarding the place of this refuahdiker plant in herbal medicine (among animals and humans, and in various parts of Europe) can be frustrating for a researcher determined to furnish concrete answers regarding its place in communal healing. But perhaps this plant's enduring mystery can be a lesson for us to patiently permit some unknowns to remain so. After all, in this era of relentless scientific progress, a little mystery is somewhat underrated and a highly uncommon quality for beings both great and small.

ARCTOSTAPHYLOS UVA-URSI |
BEARBERRY

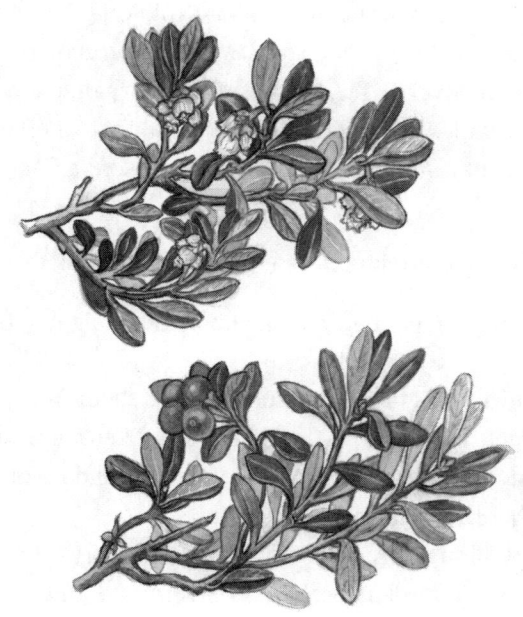

FAMILY Ericaceae

YIDDISH רפֿואהדיקע בערן–יאַגדע (refuahdike bern-yagde)

POLISH Borowka, tołokniak jeżówka

UKRAINIAN Мучниця звичайна (Mučnycja zvyčajna), мученик (mučenyk), ведмежа ягода (vedmeža jahoda)

BELARUSIAN Талакнянка звычайная (Talaknjanka zvyčajnaja), талакнянкі звычайнай (talaknjanki zvyčajnaj), мядзведжыя вушкі (mjadzvedžyja vuški), мядзведжая ягада (mjadzvedžaja jahada), мучальнік (mučal'nik), мучанні́к (mučannik), мучанні́ца (mučannica), мучы́нні́к (mučynnik), талачанні́к (talačannik), мучан (mučan), мучані́нні́к (mučaničnik), талаконні́к (talakonnik)

LITHUANIAN Miltinė meškauogė, arkliauoge, kiauluoge

RUSSIAN Толокнянка обыкновенная (Toloknjanka obyknovennaja), медвежья ягода (medvež'ja jagoda), медвежье ушко (medvež'e uško), медвежьи ушки (medvež'i uški), медвежий виноград (medvežij vinograd), костянка-толокнянка (kostjanka-toloknjanka), толоконко (tolokonko), мучница (mučnica), толокница (toloknica), толоконка боровая (tolokonka borovaja)

GERMAN Echte Bärentraube, Jackaspapuk, Jakaslapuk

FINNISH Sianmarja ("pig berry"), sianpuolukka ("pig cranberry")

Arctostaphylos uva-ursi is very difficult to write about in the context of the Pale of Settlement, especially as it relates to Ashkenazim: the traces of its medicinal presence are scattered, scarce, serpentine, and far more shrouded in mystery than other herbal tales of the region.

What initially piqued my curiosity about bearberry—one of the plant's English names—was Mordkhe Schaechter's entry in *Plant Names in Yiddish*: רפֿואהדיקע בערן–יאַגדע, "refuahdike bern-yagde," or refuahdiker bearberry.

But of course the interesting question is: Why is bearberry, a plant with leathery evergreen leaves, small drooping clusters of flowers, and small bright-red berries, one of Schaechter's five refuahdiker plants, out of the hundreds and hundreds of plants profiled in his life's work?

If this weren't enticing enough, as soon as I consulted ha-Kohen for his connections with this plant, I began to realize that this was a puzzle with more than a few pieces missing.

In the section of *Ma'aseh Tuviyah* devoted to children's health, ha-Kohen expatiates upon something unusual for him: witchcraft. He begins his discussion by identifying two terms, both of which describe what he and other physicians of his era considered the possible causes of a specific childhood disease. The terms ha-Kohen offers are in the languages of Sepharad and Ashkenaz

(Spanish/Ladino/Judezmo and German/Yiddish): embushada and benumien, "enchanted, bewitched" (cf. Spanish *embrujada* and German *benommen*). Ha-Kohen offers his readers technical terminology in his multilingual glosses, this time for the cause: little worms that grow in the flesh of the shoulders and arms, known to ha-Kohen "in the language of France" as krinunish (cf. French *crinons, cridons,* or *cirons,* terms current in early modern medical science for parasites believed to cause itching and discomfort in children, derived from Latin *crinis* "hair"), in "the language of Sepharad" as loysh ishpinikash (los ispinikos? cf. Spanish *las espinillas*), and "in the language of Ashkenaz" as dia mitesir (cf. German *die Mitesser,* "blackheads"), and describes the disease itself as a failure to thrive and, we are told, one sometimes accompanied by a worm-like parasite (*Mitesser,* literally "with-eater") that infests the upper body.

At the time of the composition of *Ma'aseh Tuviyah,* the practice of sorcery was cause for controversy between followers of Galen's ancient medicinal opinions and those promoted by the adherents of the newer alchemical techniques introduced by Paracelsus. Schooled in both these traditions, ha-Kohen writes that the childhood affliction might very well have been brought on by "a mere glance, by an evil eye, by the poisonous breath of a menstruating woman, or even from the infant's mother herself."

Ha-Kohen mentions that religious songs or passages from the Tanakh were recommended by the sages for combating an evil eye or the other deleterious effects of witchcraft. But it's the plants he calls on to provide succor to a suffering child. In this case, what's really interesting about his remedies is that they are so much more magical in nature than other aspects of his medical work. For example, to eradicate the effects of witchcraft from an infant suffering from an infection, he advises pulverizing the desiccated placenta from the birth of a first child and giving this dust to the ailing baby to ingest, either in a liquid or in mother's milk. In another recipe he invokes the magical number three wherein a horseshoe is seared in fire, then "softened" in vinegar three times, and the steam created by this procedure is used to fumigate the sick child against any baleful influences. To me, both of these methods evoke images of women healers and their ancient, unwritten ways.

The most compelling remedies, however, involve the plants, and here ha-Kohen offers two suggestions regarding bearberry. The first is a tea of uva ursi and "paradise grass," which was to be ground up and given as an infusion to the patient to drink in small quantities. A second prescription was much more magical, and it involved creating an amulet by shaping a placenta into a sac and placing inside it the highly protective flowers of *Hyper cum perforatum*—known in Yiddish as sheydim shits, "protection from demons"—along with uva ursi berries and snapdragon seeds, or "grass." Ha-Kohen does not go into detail about what to do with this amulet, but rather for the sake of brevity, vaguely mentions that there are many such remedies to be found in books. (One of the many sources of frustration when approaching ha-Kohen is wrestling with his lack of a bibliography.)

Again, for me, this remedy conjures the figure of the opshprekherin, the wise bobe who intoned incantations and "knew hundreds of ways to cure a patient," as Abraham Rekhtman tells us, an estimation based upon his experiences on the An-sky Jewish ethnographic expeditions, while visiting the older women folk healers who were sought out for their expertise in every town and village in the Pale of Settlement. In fact, in the last part of this section ha-Kohen briefly mentions three remedies associated with "the women," including a medicinal bath made with willow leaves, the flowers of aquilegia (columbine), snapdragon ("paradise leaves"), adiantum (maidenhair fern), and St. John's wort. Most telling are two brief sentences that reveal that "the women make incense from asafoetida . . . or ammoniacum" (a gum-resin exuded from several perennial herb species in the genus Ferula in the umbel family, related to asafoetida), presumably to purify the body of an ailing child.

By the nineteenth century, in Zwinogródka and other towns in the Polish lands, bearberry was a remedy of choice for those with bladder stones. This application is much more in keeping with Western herbalism's understanding of the plant, and Maude Grieve corroborates this for us by explaining that bearberry's diuretic action can be ascribed to the presence of the glycoside arbutin, which, when absorbed into the body and excreted via the kidneys, remains chemically unaltered: by retaining its original chemical state, the compound has an antiseptic effect on the urinary mucous membranes. It is this action in the body that has, for millennia, made bearberry leaves a reliable herb for folk healers wishing to address inflammatory conditions of the urinary tract, urethritis, cystitis, and so on.

In the Soviet Union in the late twentieth century, the plant's Russian names, medvež'e uško ("bear's ear") and medvež'ja jagoda ("bear berry"), were meant to warn anyone curious enough to taste them that these fruits are only suitable for bears. Soviet Russian plant medicinal prescriptions include a leaf brew to treat inflammation of the urinary tract. Like the folk healers of Ruthenia in the late nineteenth century, Russian herbalists, according to Zevin, had found this same decoction can relieve the pain of bladder stones and gravel attributed to urolithiasis. The plant has other applications in Russian official medicine, including treating gynecological infections, problems in the gastrointestinal tract, and cardiac insufficiency, to name just a few. In Russian folk medicine, bearberry is sought out for relief of bronchitis, asthma, and colds.

Contemporary Lithuanian Jewish folk healers look to bearberry as a tea that helps calm inflammation in the urinary tract and bladder, inhibits pain in the urethra, and serves as an antibacterial.

To clear up a bout of cystitis, I have worked with a tea of bearberry leaves mixed with corn silk powder to relieve pain and dispel urinary tract infections. The astringent and antiseptic qualities of bearberry combined with the demulcent corn silk prove very helpful for this condition.

After this cursory delve into the riddle that Schaechter's Yiddish name presents, uva-ursi's refue connection to the Yiddish-speaking communities of the Pale remains somewhat mysterious, which is in keeping with its association with magical medicine. But perhaps, like so many of the universe's secrets, bearberry's true power is not in being compartmentalized, but rather in its ambiguity?

ARMORACIA RUSTICANA | HORSERADISH

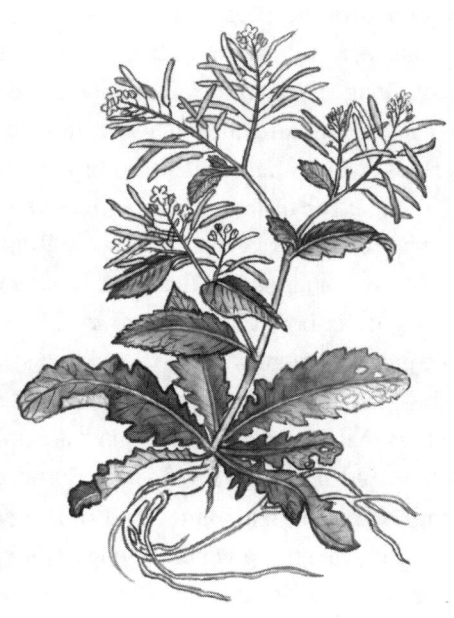

FAMILY Brassicaceae

YIDDISH כרײן, חריין‎ (khrayn)

POLISH Chrzan pospolity, warzęcha, warzucha

UKRAINIAN Хрін звичайний (Xrin zvyčajnyj)

BELARUSIAN Хрэн звычайны (Xren zvyčajny)

LITHUANIAN Valgomasis krienas

RUSSIAN Хрен обыкновенный (Xren obyknovennyj), хрен деревенский (xren derevenskij)

GERMAN   Meerrettich, Kren

GAGAUZ   Ren kökü

HEBREW   חזרת הגינה (khazeret haginah)

Horseradish is a perennial in the Brassicaceae family (which also includes mustard, broccoli, cabbage, radish, and wasabi); it has a fleshy stout root with large leaves at its base, long stems, and small white flowers; it has been cultivated as both a vegetable and a medicament for millennia. Names for this plant have been various, which makes identifying horseradish in the older plant literature a challenge: for instance, Dioscorides refers to it as Persian mustard (persicon sinapi or sinapi persicum). To the Romans it was known as armoracia. By the early Renaissance, the plant was sometimes known as raphanus. Linnaeus first described it as *Cochlearia armoracia*; subsequently it was assigned to the genus Armoracia.

This is going to be a lengthy and involved monograph, so buckle up.

Maude Grieve writes that the origins of this plant are unknown but repeats the speculation that horseradish is native to Eastern Europe, possibly the Pannonian plain of Hungary. Its English name itself, horseradish, continues to serve as a site of etymological struggle: some believe the name to have been "rebracketed" from "coarse" radish (cf. *napron* > *apron*), while others posit it was a false friend translation from German *Meerrettich* ("sea radish") > "mare radish" (mistaking German *Meer*, "sea," for German *Mähre*, "old mare").

Cochlearia armoracia is one of many synonyms for *Armoracia rusticana*, demonstrating that horseradish falls within the same genus as the renowned "scurvy grass," *Cochlearia officinalis*, a medicinal plant that was taken on long sea voyages to prevent scurvy, and which was also found beneficial as a stimulant, mild laxative, diuretic, and as a treatment for paralysis and rheumatism.

In her long entry on the healing plant, Grieve speculates that horseradish was one of the five maror, bitter herbs that Jews are to eat during Pesach, along with coriander, horehound, lettuce, and nettle. Having no background in religious observances, I can't comment on her accuracy, but I'm not sure that her list is correct, at least not in terms of modern seders in the United States. Besides, it's worth noting that many biblical scholars continue to debate whether horseradish (or other plants) was among the original maror prescribed in the Mishna (*Armoracia rusticana* is not native to the Near East).

In the twelfth century, the abbess Hildegard wrote of the German "merrich" as being warm and only "soft" for a short time in the spring, during which it was to be eaten for strengthening "the greenness" of good humors. To consume it later in the season would risk further drying out a lean and dry patient (which is reminiscent of a vata dosha type in the Ayurvedic tradition). With galangal, she writes, horseradish helps fortify the heart, and, in warm wine or warm water, it soothes pain in the lungs.

While horseradish figures not at all in Teller's Yiddish-language remedy book, ha-Kohen offers two Mishnaic names for the herb, תמכא (tamcha) and עדל (edl), referring to it as "maror of the Ashkenazim" (as opposed to the maror of the Torah), and calling it by its Yiddish name חרין (khrayn), borrowed from the Slavic. For ha-Kohen, khrayn was part of a treatment for scurvy along with all other well-known "anti-scorbutic" plants, including watercress, nasturtium, chelidonium, clover, sorrel, mustard, orange peel, ginger, juniper berries, pine oil, and *Veronica beccabunga* (brooklime), to name just a few. Some of these plants are today understood to contain high levels of vitamin C, the lack of which was intuited rather than known as a cause of scurvy among sailors over the centuries.

By the late nineteenth century, plant medicine in the ethnically mixed communities of Ruthenia described in Talko-Hryncewicz's ethnobotanical surveys was highly dependent upon chrzan (Polish "horseradish").

In the towns of Zbaraż (Yiddish Zbarazh, in the late nineteenth century about 47 percent Jewish; now Zbaraž, Ukraine) and Zwinogródka, horseradish was among the herbs given to young women in the early stages of pregnancy to stimulate "delayed" menstruation. This was clearly a remedy of long standing among Ashkenazim: scholar Michelle Klein notes that two early Yiddish-language remedy books (from the late fifteenth and early seventeenth centuries) advised eating horseradish on an empty stomach to effect this result. The Polish surveys also noted that in Zwinogródka, eating an onion cooked in vinegar was another common approach, especially among Jewish women.

In the late nineteenth-century Pale, to relieve a runny or stuffy nose, it was very common to grate horseradish and sniff the shavings. A similar remedy was to place grated horseradish on a cloth before applying to the chest, back, and legs to clear up congestion. The only sympathetic remedy for this condition was reported from the town of Jurkow: it required the afflicted to blow their nose in an attractive rag, and then leave it at the crossroads for someone else to pick up, thereby transferring the cold to the unsuspecting stranger

Coughing was considered one of the most common symptoms of disease in the Pale, and if it lasted longer than a very short while, consumption—or tuberculosis—was suspected. Milder medicines were prescribed for colds than for consumption. Many home cough remedies were reported in Talko-Hryncewicz's surveys, including well-known current favorites, such as mullein. In Podolia, eating horseradish plain or with honey was a popular curative. In this region, a tea made with moistened fresh linden leaves was also much loved. In the town of Złotopol (Yiddish Zlatopol, in the late nineteenth century 79 percent Jewish; now Zlatopil', Ukraine), taking resin (in an unspecified preparation) that leaked from a cherry tree was advised. This is very close to one of my favorite ways of calming a dry cough: I either take a bit of wild cherry bark as a lozenge or make a tea from a few chips and sip it to soothe a persistent hack.

According to Talko-Hryncewicz's surveys, another popular method for treating coughs was to drink a concoction containing a moisturizing fat, such as sugar in olive oil, or to swallow raw eggs. Jews of the region were known to take milk with melted butter, which is very similar to a remedy provided by a bobe, or folk midwife, in Korosten, Ukraine, as recorded in Pauline Wergeroff's *Memoirs of a Grandmother*. Another remedy, the guggle-muggle, at its base a honey mixture, is very common in many Jewish households.

Also reported in the Polish surveys was a remedy that was considered more sympathetic or magical; it required mashing a raw onion and applying the goo to the wrists and soles of the feet. This is a variation of a well-known and effective cure for colds, where sliced onions are placed on the soles of the feet and then covered with socks before going to sleep.

For difficult breathing caused by coughs of all types, one remedy cited in the Polish surveys called for putting a mustard or horseradish compress on the neck and the chest, with the addition of two or three leeches to take blood from the neck.

The Polish surveys also noted that folk healers weren't as precise in their diagnostics as official medicine at the time, particularly in cases of heart trouble. If the patients of the era presented multiple symptoms, such as difficult breathing, chest pains, nausea, or coughing, folk healers often understood these outward signs as digestive complaints. In addition, many who suffered from these afflictions concealed their symptoms. Talko-Hryncewicz suggests that folk healers did not have sufficient knowledge of cardiovascular function and therefore had fewer remedies to properly treat an abnormal condition. In Zwinogródka, for example, a healer offered a decoction of motherwort to help with breathing (which is not a common application in Western herbalism) and to calm a racing heartbeat (which is). In Jurkow, a tea of *Physalis alkekengi* ("Jew cherry") was given to someone suffering from heart pain. But in general, along with hot or cold compresses, it was common to apply plasters of horseradish to the chest for shortness of breath.

In Poland, a "kolka" (generally translated as "colic") was described as any deep or piercing pain in the chest or more often in the abdomen, and it was a disorder common throughout central and Eastern Europe. Many home remedies were applied to combat a kolka, including some rather unusual ones, such as in Machnówka (Yiddish Makhnovka, in the late nineteenth century 46 percent Jewish; now Maxnivka, Ukraine), near Berdychiv, where folk healers washed picture frames, windows, and benches, then poured the dirty water through a hole made in the bench (for this purpose?) to ingest for pain relief. In Zwinogródka, where fresh leaves of horseradish were a remedy for a kolka, wet or dry cupping was employed for pain relief; in Podolia, the ground roots of the plant were mixed with vinegar and rye flour and applied as a plaster to address this ailment.

Bladder stones were treated by eating horseradish in the town of Bohaczówka, near Zwinogródka (now Bahačivka, Ukraine; a village that in the late nineteenth century adjoined a significant Jewish agricultural colony), where pollution in the local river (the Sasowa) was thought to be the cause of this apparently common affliction.

If one suffered from headaches, they were believed to have been caused by a number of things, including bad air or the evil eye. There were dozens of remedies to treat this malady, the majority of which were plant-derived, and which are similar to contemporary herbal recommendations, such as drinking teas made with rosemary, betony, or lemon balm. Applying the fresh leaves of cabbage or horseradish to the forehead and temples was a common method among healers in and around Zwinogródka. They would also prescribe wet compresses with lavender or nigella seeds soaked in vinegar. It was far more common to inhale snuff or horseradish, or make a raw dough mustard plaster to apply to the neck. Leech therapy and bloodletting were also used to treat this malady. In addition, sympathetic medicine might also cure a headache. In the town of Włodzimierz (Yiddish Ludmir, in the late nineteenth century 73 percent Jewish; now Volodymyr, Ukraine; home of the famed female rebbe Hane Rokhl Verbermakher, the "Maiden of Ludmir"), it was believed that not combing one's hair was an effective cure for headache, and, for this, cultivating a kaltine might have been a solution.

At times in the Pale, if people became immobilized, whether from fainting, paralysis, or even sunstroke, the first course of action was to shock the stricken victim back into consciousness. Techniques varied, but the least harsh method required moving the person into fresh air and loosening their clothing. Squeezing the hand or the little finger was also reported as a common approach. Plant remedies included placing powdered field mustard seed under the nose to jolt the victim awake. It was also common to apply white mustard seed or grated horseradish plasters (placement details not indicated); different pre-made preparations were easily available for purchase at pharmacies, such as spirits or camphor or other strong-smelling substances.

The Polish surveys identified a disease known in the region by a long list of local names that included the Yiddish kaduches, or fever. In the Radomyśl district (Yiddish Rademishl, in the late nineteenth century 69 percent Jewish; now Radomyšl', Ukraine) near Zhytomyr, people would leave out an offering of honey to keep wandering spirits from infecting their children with fevers.

Dozens of herbal curatives, including horseradish, were employed by both parents and folk healers to treat fever. In Podolia, horseradish (preparation not specified) was applied to the stomach in cases of elevated temperature. In Zwinogródka, a mixture of claviceps ("sporysz") and horseradish was placed on the navel three times a day. Another treatment was to eat three pieces of horseradish each day. In the towns of Smykowce, Tarnopol (Yiddish Tarnopol, in the late nineteenth century over 50 percent Jewish; now Ternopil', Ukraine), Zbaraż, and Załuże (now Zalužžja, Ukraine, part of Zbaraż), black coffee was mixed with grated horseradish or the juice of its root and drunk as a remedy.

When contagion was suspected, according to the Polish surveys, upon visiting a sick person it was common for Jews and the landed gentry to not swallow their saliva but to spit frequently in order to avoid contracting infection. One very common sympathetic prophylactic was to carry garlic in a pouch on the chest. Well known among Jews when a person first became sick was to give sudorifics (sweat-promoting medications or plants), practice bloodletting, or apply cupping in an attempt to stop the progression of illness. It was further reported that both Jews and the landed gentry covered themselves to keep warm, whereas other communities would ignore these symptoms and sleep on the hearth, sometimes even going barefoot on damp and cool ground in the belief that this would cure the fever.

When I was quite young, I overheard a family story about my great-grandfather (from Tarnogród, Poland, very close to the Galician and Ruthenian towns surveyed by Talko-Hryncewicz), who had been poisoned in the old country, leaving behind a widow and four children. At the time, I didn't understand how this might possibly happen or what it meant, but in reviewing the Polish surveys, I see that this situation wasn't as uncommon as one might expect. In the Pale, most poisonings were thought to be the act of "unfriendly people," and, unsurprisingly, many disturbing beliefs and practices were associated with treating such cases. First and foremost, it was necessary to remove the toxin from the victim: emetics were furnished for this purpose. These varied from extremely unappetizing substances to strong-tasting or strong-smelling plants. Horseradish's powerful fresh root was an antidote of choice for many cases of poisoning, and in the Podolia region, it was a trusted home remedy.

The surveys also mention scurvy as a possible affliction, although Talko-Hryncewicz notes that it was less prevalent than it had been in earlier times. The cause, people believed, was drinking spoiled juice, and one remedy in the town of Zwinogródka and the region in general was to counter the effects of scurvy by drinking horseradish root boiled in beer.

Like other ethnographic literature of this era, the Polish surveys were not free from the stain of racism. One passage alleges that Jewish tavern-keepers of the Pale encouraged their (non-Jewish) customers to drink more alcohol by putting tobacco leaves on the tables and advising drinkers to eat horseradish (presumably the same way bars today provide complimentary salty treats such as peanuts or pretzels). In the Pale, the landed gentry who owned the breweries and distilleries would only award tavern concessions to the region's Jews, who were often resented by their neighbors for this near-monopoly.

For hemorrhages of all kinds, internal or external, folk healers employed magical remedies, such as banishing incantations, but relied even more on plant preparations. Some herbs reported for staunching hemoptysis—bleeding or blood-stained mucus from the mouth, originating in the respiratory tract— were scarlet pimpernel, centaury, and European blackberry, each taken as a tea. A horseradish plaster was a common remedy throughout the region for hemorrhages of any kind.

In Podolia, to prevent frostbite, fresh horseradish leaves were rubbed on potentially exposed areas.

For rheumatic pain, various therapies were offered by folk healers in the Pale. For example, Lipka Tatars called for animal substances such as warm dog dung to be applied to rheumatic body parts. Talko-Hryncewicz notes that in Russia, both Russians and Jews relied upon fat from wild animals such as boars, badgers, bears, or birds for rheumatism, stating that such remedies stemmed from "the influence of old empiric medicine," that is, the ancient Greek and Roman sources.

Other healers simply applied warmth or encouraged sweating out rheumatic pain, even during the hot summer months. Some of the more unusual methods to treat rheumatism involved insects. A folk healer in Zwinogródka made "ant spirits" by luring ants into a pot of honey, and when the vessel was filled with them, pouring vodka or other spirits into the container to make a healing drink, presumably straining out the ants before serving. In some eastern Galician villages, the pot of macerating ants, still unstrained, was buried for nine days so that the liquid would become more potent.

Karaim traditional healers, according to Zajączkowski, also depended on ants as a refue: for internal pains in the chest, the patient was to boil and brew live ants and let the decoction stand for three days, before drinking a half a glass at a time.

Overall, however, the most widely reported remedies for rheumatic pain were plant-related. In the towns of Ryżanówka, Steblów (Yiddish Steblev, in the late nineteenth century 25 percent Jewish; now Stebliv, Ukraine), Lityń (Yiddish Litin, in the late nineteenth century 41 percent Jewish; now Lityn, Ukraine), and Dmytrze (now Dmytre, Ukraine), just outside Lviv, healers beat the painful areas with a broom of fresh nettle stalks. This is the exact remedy I was told about by a Latvian survivor of the Shoah who lived in Los Angeles: known as urtification, it is an ancient method of treating such pain. Rubbing aching joints with horseradish was also reported as a common therapy throughout the region.

In those days in the Pale, eye pain was thought to be caused by a number of things, such as tainted blood, too much sun exposure, or by working in a hot kitchen (where many women and girls spent much of their day). To prevent eye pain, it was common practice to have young girls wear earrings or pieces of protective coral around their necks. Taking snuff tobacco as a prophylactic—probably a more male-dominated curative—was not unusual. A few other plant preparations to guard against eye pain were reported in the Polish surveys, one of which was given by a folk healer in the district of Płoskirow (Yiddish Proskurov, in the late nineteenth century 60 percent Jewish; now Xmel'nyc'kyj, Ukraine), consisting of a back compress of grated horseradish mixed with vinegar.

Methods for improving eyesight were varied and complex. In Zwinogródka, one technique reported was to place the innards of the gudgeon fish into a bottle that was left in the sun to extract a fatty yellow oil to be used as a compress and applied (unspecified location of application). According to Talko-Hryncewicz, this was a method especially preferred by the Jews of the town for those suffering from poor eyesight or cataracts in their later years. Healers in Zwinogródka also relied on eye drops of juice squeezed from rue, or recommended sniffing lavender or mallow roots. But it was especially common to sniff horseradish.

For protecting teeth from decay, strengthening gums, or preventing bad breath, horseradish was one of the more beneficial plants of the Pale. In Radomyśl, the root was cut into small pieces and placed in a bottle of beer that was warmed in the oven for twelve hours before the resulting solution was taken as a mouth rinse, three times a day.

Many people in the Pale also believed that tooth decay and toothache were caused by worms eating the tooth. In addition, pain was associated with different phases of the moon, particularly the new moon, which had the power, along with certain banishing incantations, to relieve toothache. In the town of Rudakovka (Russia), it was thought that if you chewed something a mouse had gnawed, this would strengthen your teeth. In the towns of Zbaraż and Załuże, eating bread that had been previously sampled by a mouse would keep your teeth from hurting. (We discussed this in greater detail in *Ashkenazi Herbalism.*)

The plants that were called upon to relieve this (often excruciating) pain varied, and many of those documented in the Polish surveys are no longer employed in contemporary herbalism because they're considered too toxic— or are even illegal to sell or distribute. Horseradish, however, was favored by a number of healers interviewed, and in Zwinogródka one practitioner offered patients a mouth rinse formula that called for a piece of tar wood (unspecified tree species) to be boiled in vinegar while the patient simultaneously rubbed horseradish on the elbow and hand on the side of the body opposite the site of tooth pain. In the Kamienec region (Yiddish Kamenits, in the late nineteenth century around 30 percent Jewish; now Kam'janec'-Podil's'kyj, Ukrraine), horseradish was applied directly onto the tooth along with cow parsnip (*Heracleum sphondylium*), a plant also known as "borscht"—or באָרשטש (borshtsh) in Yiddish—because it was formerly picked for making the soup. (Polish "barszcz" refers to any sour soup.) In the towns of Dorożów (Yiddish Dorozuv, in the late nineteenth century around 13 percent Jewish; now Verenij Doroživ, Ukraine) and Sidzina (Poland), horseradish root was directly applied to an aching tooth. In the town of Lipowiec, grated horseradish was applied to the pulse of the wrist on the opposite side of the body from the aching tooth. In the Czehryń district (Yiddish Cherin, in the late nineteenth century 30 percent Jewish; now Čyhyryn, Ukraine), grated horseradish root was placed on the pulse of the wrist on the same side of the body as the toothache while, simultaneously, a clove of cleaned garlic was placed in the ear (also on the same side).

These cross-body applications stand out to me—they must have been based upon magical beliefs, but I wonder if this technique was also connected with subtle physiological actions healers had observed about the connections between the nervous system and tooth pain.

In *Ashkenazi Herbalism*, we examined the rituals around dental health that were performed by opshphrekherins, drawing from the memories of the town of Eishyshok, in present-day Lithuania. In the Polish lands of the late nineteenth century, incantations were a common, almost uniform treatment, varying only slightly in wording from town to town. In Zwinogródka, a translation of a curious Yiddish charm addressed to the moon, the heavens, and the earth was recorded as follows:

> Lovely moon, you are lovely in heaven, and you are dead on earth, when you three come together, the sick person's teeth shall ache.

In the town of Sarny (Yiddish Sarny, in the early twentieth century 47 percent Jewish; now Sarny, Ukraine), halfway between Kyiv and Lublin, a Shoah survivor recalled how toothaches and other ailments were treated by bobes and midwives:

> Like many other towns of the same time, even with us, we did not lack for "Bobbehs"—midwives. Many made use of superstitious medicaments. If a malaise covered the face, or an inflammation—either Miriam Kapszuk or Shifra of Pohost would come, take out some flax and a candle, light the candle and warm up the inflammation, and along with this whisper formulations to ward off the evil eye. If a child fell out of a tree and fractured his leg, the horse would be harnessed to the wagon, and they would ride off to summon the potter. The latter would then massage the leg, and cover it, and put it into a wood splint tied with cords.

> If someone felt something in his teeth—he would apply a poultice of garlic dipped in pepper, bathe the tooth in 90% whiskey, and wrap the affected cheek in a warm dressing. If the bones ached—the body would be rubbed with turpentine, drink raspberry juice with two or three glasses of hot tea, wrap oneself in several blankets, and sweat it out. If sharp stabbing pains were felt in the hips or back—a mustard plaster would be applied, or bloodletting?, or remedies of this sort, cupping, or imbibing special drinks in which the roots of medicinal herbs had been steeped.

> The expert in all of these remedies was the lady, Shifra of Pohost (Murawinsky). But even with all this, the dedicated, hard-working widow was not able

to support her children, because this work that she did, was mostly for the mitzvah involved.

This story is just one more example of how healthcare, and care in general, was a communal affair, offered without charge by the healer for the benefit of their community, to restore harmony and health. These remedies for alleviating the very common afflictions of tooth decay and gum disease remind us of how much physical and spiritual suffering people of the Pale experienced through-out their everyday lives, and how hopeful and comforting the presence of folk healers must have been in these tightly knit communities.

In addition to medicinal applications, grated horseradish root was commonly added to drinking water to make it more salutary.

Author Sophie Knab writes that horseradish, one of Poland's oldest condiments and medicines, having been cultivated there since the twelfth century, was "practically like pepper," which was an exotic spice that, because it was imported, was in general more difficult to come by than chrzan. She recounts many of the plant's curative abilities: a remedy for scurvy, a compress for headaches and for hoarseness, and, mixed with fat, as an ointment against rheumatism. She also describes a custom from around Rzeszów, Galicia: Polish families there celebrate Easter Sunday with a breakfast meal known as the święconka, and eat horseradish "in memory of Jesus Christ who was offered bitter vinegar to drink when he suffered on the cross." This recalls ha-Kohen's reference to horseradish, "the maror of the Ashkenazim," and attests to a shared association of this powerful plant with the most important holidays of Christianity and Judaism.

In the interwar Soviet surveys, horseradish was documented as part of a folk healer's formulary for relieving chest pains caused by heart disease in the town of Bohslov (now Bohuslav), Ukraine.

And there the trail of horseradish in the former Pale fades, until we arrive in present-day Lithuania, where contemporary Jewish folk healers have reported working with the root to improve appetite and increase stomach acidity.

A bit further south, in Moldova, Kvilinkova reports that contemporary Gagauz Turkish healers rely on horseradish root as a remedy for lower back pain; they make a tincture of the leaf of the plant ("hren yapraa") to soothe pains in the leg joints.

In my own work with this plant, I have found that grating the root and inhaling the suffused air surrounding the shavings can clear up stuffiness from colds or allergies. I've also made my own version of Rosemary Gladstar's famous "fire cider." This amazing medicine can easily be curated to individual taste and taken by the spoonful, with honey if needed, or included in recipes to add a tart balancing effect or savory component to salad dressings. To make your own fire cider, you need any combination of these strong herbs:

Sliced onion

Sliced garlic

Grated or sliced horseradish root

Sliced or grated ginger

Jalapeño or other hot pepper

Lemon slices

Place these in a large jar, and cover with apple cider vinegar. To keep the vinegar from eroding the lid of the jar, you can put a piece of thin plastic (I cut a small square from one of those plastic produce bags from the grocery store) between the lid and the jar before closing the lid tightly. Allow the mixture to infuse for at least four weeks. Strain out the plant material and put it in soups or other dishes as desired for added depth of flavor (or compost). The remaining liquid can be taken as medicine at the first sign of a cold. For more fire cider ideas and recipes, see *Fire Cider!: 101 Zesty Recipes for Health-Boosting Remedies Made with Apple Cider Vinegar* by Rosemary Gladstar.

CALENDULA OFFICINALIS | CALENDULA

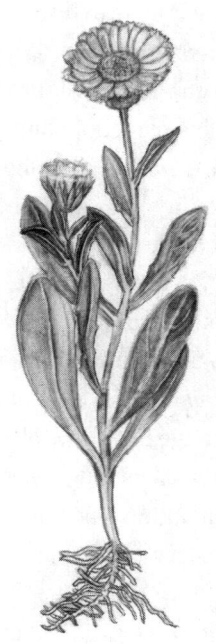

FAMILY   Asteraceae

YIDDISH   סגולה–ראש–חודשל (sgule-reshkhoydeshl), רינגלבלומ (ringlblum)

POLISH   Nagietek lekarski, pazurki, miesięcznica, paznokietki

UKRAINIAN   Нагідки лікарські (Nahidky likars'ki), нюхтики (njuxtyky)

LITHUANIAN   Vaistinė medetka, nadatka, nagatka

RUSSIAN   Календула лекарственная (Kalendula lekarstvennyj), ноготки лекарственные (nogotki lekarstvenneye)

GERMAN   Ringelblume, Garten-Ringelblume

GAGAUZ   Salkım çiçää, ruja

Mordkhe Schaechter's *Plant Names in Yiddish* can be read as a portal into a shadowy and secret herbal past, but those interested in the traditional knowledge of ancestral folk healers will have to bring a magnifying glass, flashlight, and roadmap to decipher the mysterious hieroglyphs left behind by the healers who came before us. Out of the hundreds of plants cataloged in Schaechter's work, the distinctly Yiddish plant appellations (i.e., names that express a uniquely native semantic reality, rather than loan-translations or internationalisms), offer us the most exciting clues as to their importance for Ashkenazi folk healers prior to the Second World War.

But only one plant, out of the hundreds that Schaechter discusses, is identified as a segule (charm) plant, a term that in the context of folk medicine can be interpreted as a magical charm or magical remedy.

The full Yiddish name for calendula, a plant with alternate, oblong leaves and flowers that gather into orange or yellow blossoms, is ‏סגולה–ראש–חודשל‎, or sgule-reshkhoydeshl, which translates roughly as "the little magical beginning of the month plant." This designation has a number of possible explanations, but none fully resolves the mystery of what at first glance seems to be a rather straightforward medicinal plant.

If we remove the Yiddish prefix *sgule*, what remains is *rosh khodesh*, a minor Jewish holiday that marks the end of one month and the beginning of the next in the lunar Hebrew calendar. This is likely why this holiday is associated with women. The name calendula, from the Latin for "calendar," reminds us of the flower's appearance at the turn of every month; in Italy at the beginning of the twentieth century, the plant was known as il fiore d'ogni mese, "the flower of each month." Polish country folk over the years always knew of the plant as "the country clock." These designations run somewhat parallel to the Yiddish, yet none hint at any possible magical qualities, as does the invocation of the sgule. For what it's worth, Ringelblume (cf. English *ringlets*), the plant's German name, is also one of its Yiddish names.

Calendula's ancient medicinal applications seem murky. Dioscorides doesn't include the plant in his materia medica; Maimonides discusses a plant (buknūr maryam, "Mary's incense") that may or may not be calendula (a maror plant, it might also be horehound). Curiously, Hildegard writes of calendula as an antidote for poisons, and she recommends the plant, crushed with lard, as a means of softening and removing crusts on the scalp. Ha-Kohen reports extensively on similar uncomfortable conditions, but if he recommended calendula as a curative, its presence in his work is quite obscured. Avicenna describes various species of the genus Calendula as aromatic vermifuges, and attests that the species *Calendula officinalis* is a sternutatory (sneeze inducer); he also warns that overindulgence may bring on miscarriage (interesting, given how often Hovorka and Kronfeld inform us that in Eastern Europe calendula is called upon to prevent miscarriage—as we will discuss later).

Fascinatingly, in the Polish lands over the centuries, according to Knab, calendula was employed to banish the evil eye, possibly linked to the sgule plant's magical standing among Yiddish speakers. In those regions, calendula was also believed to ward off fevers and remove warts; fried in butter with comfrey, its sauce created a healing salve for wounds and swollen glands; a tea that settled the digestion and supported the heart was infused from the dried flower petals. Polish folk medicine also recommends the herb's juice to bring on menses, which hearkens back to the ancient Hebrew holy day allusion to women's monthly concerns.

The synonymous pot marigold can also be found in more recent herbal documentation in the lands of Eastern Europe. For example, in Polish kitchens of the past, calendula was relied upon to lend butter, cheese, bread, and cake a warm, vibrant golden color. It was also a component of formulas for dyeing hair and fabric. Before the Second World War, calendula was an important ingredient in folk medicine throughout Poland. In Zwinogródka and in the resort town of Zakopane, calendula, along with other plant remedies, was cooked in water or sweet milk to be taken to rebuff insomnia. Out of the several calendula folk remedies reported in the Polish surveys, at least one was recorded to address general uterine complaints. In cases such as these, a calendula tea was provided—again, in a faint echo of the association of the plant with women's "monthlies." This tea was also a remedy for sores in general. According to Wereńko, folk healers of Lepel', Belarus (Yiddish Lieplie, in the late nineteenth century 50 percent Jewish) would offer a vodka infusion of "szapran" (saffron) or calendula flowers, obtained from a pharmacy, to induce menstruation. Apparently, according to Kašinskij, calendula's color meant that some spice traders would use it to adulterate saffron. According to Fischer, calendula also served as a vulnerary and ulcerative ointment (around Kraków), and in a decoction against burns in Zakopane, and, in Tarnobrzeg, against eye diseases.

In Polish official herbal medicine of the mid-twentieth century, per Biegański, calendula was valued for its stimulant, antiputrefactive, diaphoretic, blood-cleaning, and diuretic powers. Infusions of the plant and its flowers were recommended against enlargement and hardening of the liver and spleen, scrofula, and to promote healthy menstruation.

Calendula has been an effective folk treatment in Poland against mental disturbances, such as anxiety (as well as insomnia). This trust in calendula as a spirit lifter is also found among the Roma of western Europe: in the words of Juliette de Baïracli Levy, who spent many years living among and learning from Roma healers, its "flowers make a cup of good Gypsy cheer, which relieves mental depression." In the Belarusian town of Putilkovchi, near Minsk, Wereńko tells us that nineteenth-century folk recommendations advised drinking a calendula tea against "agitation."

A bit further north, according to Krebel, Estonians of the mid-nineteenth century treated childhood coughs with a blend of calendula flowers and mullein mixed with butter; for sore nipples among nursing mothers, they prepared an ointment of calendula flowers and sour cream, which was also used for treating skin rashes. In late nineteenth-century Latvia, according to Alksnis, an infusion of calendula flowers served as a folk remedy for diarrhea.

In Minsk gubernija in the 1880s, Sicinskij reports that akušerki (certified midwives) treated newborn children suffering from rashes in a bath of a calendula and celandine infusion. Similarly, in Romanian pediatric folk medicine, children plagued by insomnia (likely due to fright) were given calendula baths.

In present-day Lithuania, calendula has been reported by Jewish herbalists as one of their most valued remedies. They collect the flowers during the blooming season and find them helpful for the external treatment of superficial wounds and for minor inflammation of the skin and oral mucosa, such as sore throats, bleeding gums, and mouth ulcers. For sore throats caused by tonsilitis, they boil one tablespoon of calendula flowers in a glass of water for fifteen minutes on low heat, then strain and cool before rinsing with the warm decoction every two hours. This recipe is almost identical to the one author Sophie Knab recommends for healing wounds.

Most thrilling of all, these modern Jewish healers report medicinal pot marigold as a treatment *specific* to women's health issues. In comparison, Lithuanian Muslim healers (Lipka Tatars and Azerbaijanis) report this plant to be helpful in treating sore throats caused by tonsilitis; they also mix calendula with other herbs to reduce stomach acidity (see *Matricaria chamomilla*, p. 105).

Afflictions of the heart and digestion are often correlated with nervous disturbances, and contemporary Lipka Tatar remedies may be a legacy of the renown in which the fałdżejs of past centuries were held for their skill at treating mental illness.

Tatar healers, both fałdżejs (who relied on divination) and siufkaczes (who would cure their patients by "blowing" divine embers and ash across them), could and did treat mental illness. The YIVO researchers (in this instance, E. Sosnovik) documented this reputation in the interwar period:

> *Fifteen kilometers from the shtetl of Nay-Pohost there lives a Tatar (kedar). People (the majority Christians) go to him in cases of madness or some other nervous disease. He does not receive any payment, he only requests that the lung and liver of a sheep be brought to him; these he keeps. Bread should also be given to him. He whispers* [Yiddish sheptshet] *to them; they are not to eat. He waves the lungs and liver in circles around the patient. Heard from a second* [informant]*: one patient with an "open stomach," mistaken for a nervous patient, went to a nearby Tatar. The latter "bled" the little finger of his hand; he did not take any money.*

The siufkacz, in particular, specialized in removing the mental affliction by blowing on the patient. In one early nineteenth-century account, Polish memoirist Stanisław Morawski reminisced about a young medical professional from Vilna named Fortunat Jurewicz who lost his senses due to a broken heart: "His own medical acumen was worthless! For six months he suffered. When nothing else would help, a neighbor, a Tatar from Trakai, famous for his secret of treating 'fixations,' was brought in. He fumigated the room, read passages from the Koran, and Jurewicz, having been blown on (with smoke), returned to his senses and made a complete recovery."

The Tatar skill at treating psychic disturbances is also singled out for attention in standard reference works of the nineteenth century. The Polish *Słownik geograficzny* of 1883, a gazetteer-encyclopedia that covers the towns and villages of the Polish lands of the late nineteenth century in exacting detail, informs the reader that the dozen or so Muslim Lipka Tatar families of Kowalówka, Poland, "practice farming, gardening, tanning, dyeing, and treating mental confusion."

In Juvkivci, near Šepetiv, Ukraine, the local Tatars were also known for their skills at farming and treating the mentally ill, "and in this respect it is observed that they have a great number of patients who travel to them from the most distant parts of the country. Their method of treatment, which they have kept for many generations, is secret; they say that their ancestors brought it from their ancient homeland in the east."

Talko-Hryncewicz devotes some attention to this reputation in his survey:

> The treatment of the insane in Ruthenia remains mostly in the hands of the Tatars, who in this respect enjoy a well-earned and deserved fame, and to whom the people ["lud"] bring the deranged even from distant regions. In Ukraine, widely known Tatar psychiatrists practice in Bohuslav [near Kaniv] and around Šmila [now Smila, near Cherkasy]. The method of treatment among them all is similar: the patient is to swallow sheets of paper with inscriptions, and then is tormented and tortured in various ways. They [Tatar healers] shake the patient every which way, bounce them in rickety carts, beat them with whips, and so on. Healer-psychiatrists who rely on similar treatments are also to be found in Lithuania, such as Aleksandrowicz and his three sons in Birštonas. They are also to be found in Crimea.

The specifically Muslim confessional reputation for psychic healing is widespread throughout Eastern and southeastern Europe. Scholar Safet Hadži Muhamedović has provided a thorough account of the role of Muslim healers in psychological care in multi-confessional Bosnia. That the psychic healer in many regions of Eastern or southeastern Europe was either a Muslim or Jewish "kedar" is a fascinating phenomenon worthy of a great deal more attention than we have been able to apply here: for instance, the most common term for magical amulets found among the Lipka Tatars is *chamaił* (ultimately from Arabic *ḥamala*, "to carry"; cf. Turkish *hamail*). While Muslim healers across Eastern Europe also refer to amulets as nuska or muska, the specifically Lipka Tatar term is all the more striking given that their one-time Ashkenazi Jewish neighbors, according to scholar Marek Tuszewicki, knew their healing amulets as hamaylesn.

Other Turkic healers of Eastern Europe, the Gagauz of Moldova, rely, according to Kvilinkova, on a calendula decoction to soothe inflammation and cirrhosis of the liver.

Contemporary Lithuanian healers from the formerly majority-Jewish region of Kaišiadorys rely on calendula flower infusions to treat inflammation of the mouth, throat, intestines, and urinary tract, as well as in a mouth or throat rinse. Calendula baths are a treatment for women's health issues, and calendula flower ointments are held to heal scars. In modern ethnic Lithuanian folk medicine, according to Vasiliauskas, calendula is relied upon to treat stomach and intestinal growths, as well as inflammations of the mouth and throat. Calendula juice is recommended for wounds, ulcers, and bruises. Zevin tells us that in Russian folk medicine, calendula is employed to delay menstruation and alleviate painful menstruation.

To be honest, it's taken me years to overcome my aversion to calendula's sticky residue and sharp acrid scent. These days, though, I can happily report that calendula lends its brilliant presence to our garden for most of the spring. When the flower heads dry, they transform into loosely held clutches of curved, curiously knobby seeds, which when allowed to scatter will bloom again in the spring. In modern Hebrew, calendula is known as "cat's nails," which describes these seeds very well.

In contemporary Western herbalism, calendula is a favored plant for skin products, and in my own practice, I find it lends a magical vibrancy to salves, and especially lip balms, that has proven remarkable at preventing chapped lips year-round.

CANNABIS SATIVA | CANNABIS

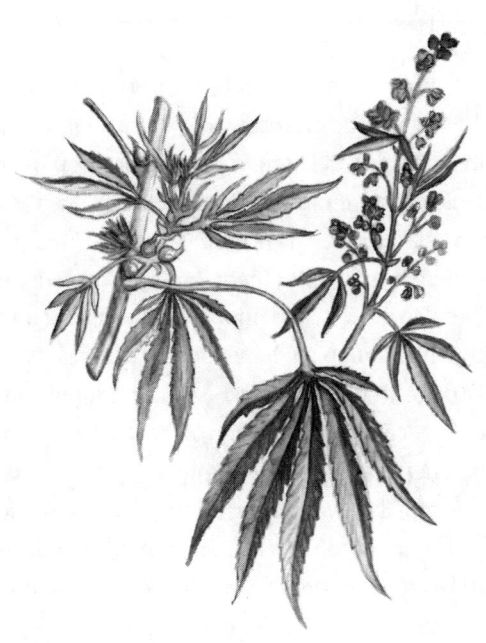

FAMILY Cannabaceae

YIDDISH הַאנעף (hanef), קאנאָפליעס (kanoplies)

POLISH Konopie

UKRAINIAN Коноплі (Konopoli)

BELARUSIAN Каноплі (Kanopli)

LITHUANIAN Kanapė

RUSSIAN Конопля (Konoplja)

GERMAN Hanf

HEBREW   קָנֶה בֹּשֶׂם (kaneh bosm), כנבוס (khanebus)

TATAR   Киндер (Kinder)

GAGAUZ   Kenevir otu

When I was in my teens, before cannabis's constituents were teased out and intensified, the father of a good friend would supply his daughter with weed, and she and I would get high and listen to records or jump the fence of the local country club to sit on the manicured green of the golf course or walk to the convenience store to get snacks. Even then, I felt that this plant was not very concerned with my recreational enjoyment, but peer pressure nagged. I eventually made a lot of friends who insisted upon my sharing the indulgence, and so I continued to engage with cannabis whenever the occasion arose. It wasn't until I graduated from college that I started to pay more attention to my intuition, and it was then that I became truly aware of how uncomfortable I felt being high. Decades later, when I tried the newfangled legal plant to see what all the fuss over dispensary cannabis was about, I immediately sensed that there was something deeply "off" about the entity I encountered, a difference I attribute to the business model of the now-legal cannabis industry to develop and market strains that accentuate the plant's psychogenic actions. But this isn't going to be a diatribe against human engagement with cannabis. It's my own contemplation of an entity that has been maligned, outlawed, used, abused, and now highly (no pun intended) modified and commodified—none of which sits well with me, but not everyone has the same experience with plants.

For the ancient Greeks, cannabis was useful for braiding strong ropes (from here on, *hemp* will refer to the textile), even though it was "malodorous"; according to Dioscorides, the buds of the female plant soothed "the organ of generation" (a poetic euphemism) when eaten in large quantities. Even the juice, extracted when green, was helpful for earaches. The Greek historian Herodotus observed that Scythians, an Iranian people who lived in what is now Ukraine over two millennia ago, would intoxicate themselves by gathering in tents where they would burn cannabis.

According to Meyerhof, Maimonides erroneously ascribes "banğ," the Arabic name for *Cannabis sativa var. indica,* to another plant, likely henbane, which for me adds to the plant's mystique. With an unmistakable scent, distinctive and sharply cut leaves, and separate male and female genders, it seems difficult to mistake cannabis for any other plant.

Issachar bar Teller, on the other hand, wrote of cannabis seeds as part of a formula to bring on delayed menses. Throughout his book, Teller gives his Yiddish-language audience hints as to his kind nature, and even though it's apparent that assisting those in need is his deepest concern, he consistently reveals his deference to powers greater than ourselves when he ends this recipe thus: "I could write a great deal about these things, but I fear the Lord."

In another remedy that required burning cannabis, one meant to combat plague, Teller describes a method of taking the famous theriac (see "Trianke," p. 207), or mithridate, enveloped within a cored onion, then wrapped in either a flax or hemp cloth, which was to be placed on burning embers until the little bundle blazed. Once this was accomplished, one was to remove the first layer of the onion, crushing the remaining bulb and its contents in a mortar, mixing in warm vinegar, and straining the resultant black juice through a cloth before swallowing. This remedy caused a patient to sweat, and reportedly saved countless lives with its sudorific powers.

For his part, ha-Kohen mentions cannabis seed in the context of the reproductive system, reminiscent of Dioscorides's earlier advisory. He provides two names for cannabis in his plant glossary: khanebus, "in the language of the Mishnah," and in Turkish, kiniviar; throughout the text, his spelling is inconsistent.

In the late nineteenth-century Pale of Settlement, *Cannabis sativa*, or konopie as it is called in Polish, was much sought after as a medicinal plant. In the town of Ryżanówka, where at least one eye-licking healer lived, the plant was used to predict future love matches by girls who would make wads of flax or hemp fibers, light the little clumps, and throw them up in the air. If the burning cinders flew upward, it meant a boy liked them; if they dropped to the ground, the boy in question was not a match. While Talko-Hryncewicz and his informants are silent regarding any possible intoxicating effects, we can't help but notice how often the rituals require that the cannabis be burned.

Many rituals around the birthing process were observed by bobes in the shtetls and villages of the Pale. In the town of Łysianka, it was common among

Jews to smear the blood from the umbilical cord on the newborn, immuniz-
ing the baby against the evil eye. In the same town, and in others around
Zwinogródka, folk midwives tied boys' umbilical cords with a hemp thread
made from the male plant, while girls' were tied with thread from the female
plant. This practice ensured fertility as the children matured. Another superstition, common among Jews, Polish gentry, and the Slavic lud (Polish, Ruthenian, or Ukrainian peasants), was to hide away the umbilical cord and its
ligature, to be saved and given to the child when they turned seven. The child
was supposed to now untie the cord, which was held to have some (unex-
plained) effect on their memory. According to the ethnographer Heinz Wlislocki, the Roma of nineteenth-century Hungary would fumigate a sick child
with the smoke from a burnt umbilical cord, called a "divine chain," because
it could bind evil spirits.

In the weeks after childbirth, the mother's recovery was often complicated.
In the town of Płoskirow, several folk remedies were recommended by bobes
for vaginal discharge, including having the patient drink a decoction of the
bark of *Physalis alkekengi*, otherwise known as Jew cherry (see *Prunus padus*,
p. 125). Another remedy for this condition featured the female cannabis plant
in the form of a body fumigation. Cannabis, burned in the form of a hemp cloth
decoction (flax could also be used), was a similar treatment.

Heartburn was considered a temporary discomfort, especially among
people who had eaten too much, and for pregnant women, but it was also
believed that enchantment could bring on the malady, especially if the victim
had dined with the wrong person. In Płoskirow, taking cannabis (method
unspecified) brought relief, as did a teaspoon of poppy seeds.

For treating diarrhea, many home remedies were reported in the Polish
surveys; the most common remedy was to consume a tablespoon of any oil at
hand, be it cannabis, sunflower, castor, or the like, or drink powdered birch
charcoal several times a day.

Quickly raising a healthy cannabis crop was the subject of a lengthy incantation recited by a folk healer from Ryżanówka for banishing "colic." While
we won't attempt to provide an English translation of a Polish transliteration
of the Rusyn language, the charm urges that all the stages of growing cannabis,
from planting to sowing, reaping, and drying, each occur in a single day. The

ailment ("kolka") was defined as any deep or piercing chest pain, but it more often affected the abdomen, in both children and adults.

In Zwinogródka, a folk healer's recipe for easing the pain of bladder stones combined a handful of unwashed cannabis with poplar leaves, which were boiled in milk or water and then applied to the tender area.

Back then, deadly poisonings were common in the Pale (the presumed fate of my own great-grandfather, see *Armoracia rusticana*, p. 51). Poisoners were known as "unfriendly people," and the descriptions of case studies in the literature are extremely unpleasant. Unsurprisingly, most of the antidote remedies are steeped in magic. On the practical side, however, one of the first things folk healers administered when treating poisoning was an emetic. In the town of Nowa-Uszyca, a decoction of the bark of a lilac bush, mixed with equal parts cannabis seed extract, was given to the victim to purge themselves of the toxins.

Infected wounds often became painful abscesses, such as paronychia, which was considered to be exclusive to women. Such wounds were often treated by applying herbs to the infection, lest sepsis or gangrene lead to the loss of a finger, or worse. In Nowa-Uszyca, a folk healer reported one such treatment with steamed poppy seeds or cannabis. It was also common to apply honey to infected skin, which was the remedy Sore Mordkhe-Yoysef, the opshprelherin of Biłgoraj whom we profiled in *Ashkenazi Herbalism*, applied to a patient's erysipelas. Today, honey is well known for its antibacterial qualities, which have been universally understood by folk healers for millennia.

Many skin conditions required the application of healing herbs. In Ryżanówka, the inner bark of the elder was rubbed with cannabis seeds and applied to infected areas. Other remedies were less appetizing: one in Zwinogródka called for chopped or ground-up frogs fried in oil and applied topically. Less unsavory and much more common was a whole-body salt bath for relieving skin ailments.

In the Pale, where it was not unusual to contact ringworm in the late 1800s (see *Acorus calamus*, p. 29), a folk healer in Dorożów, near Lviv, applied hemp seed oil to cure the rash. Another late nineteenth-century herbal source from eastern Germany, cited by Deriker, notes that in Calau, a Sorbian town in Brandenburg, cannabis seeds were eaten in a soup or broth to promote breast milk.

Author Sophie Knab tells of cannabis as part of blossom-gathering rituals held in Poland in the springtime, and also mentions the plant's ability to discourage snakes from lingering in farmers' fields. She writes that oil from cannabis seeds was a remedy for improving digestion. In Moldova, according to Kvilinkova, Gagauz healers also prepare cannabis teas to treat diarrhea. In Romanian pediatric folk medicine of the latter half of the nineteenth century, cannabis seeds (method unspecified) treated skin infections and impetigo. According to Knab, the plant was widely cultivated in Poland not only for its oil but also for its strong hemp fibers that were "retted, dried, and broken on a flax brake . . . the thick inner fibers were spun on a spinning wheel for making sacking or very strong thread. They were often plied together to make rope."

Innumerable yizkor memory books tell stories of shtetl artisans and tradespeople who spun rope from hemp. The An-sky ethnographic expeditions captured a photographic image that perfectly illustrates Knab's description of the process: three men standing around a wheeled contraption literally spinning rope from a wad of fibers that the youngest worker holds while another turns a crank. I remember reading somewhere that hemp grown in the northern hemisphere produces the strongest and longest fiber most suitable for spinning rope and thread. It seems almost implausible that this plant, so ubiquitous and so fundamental for life in the Pale, wasn't also understood for its intoxicating effects, particularly since cannabis as an intoxicant has been attested in the region for more than two thousand years.

Scholar Eddy Portnoy has been instrumental in recovering much of the story of cannabis among world Jewry, pulling back the curtain to reveal what communal history has often concealed. Some of this history can be coy. What do we make of this anecdote from the yizkor of Suwałki, Poland (birthplace of Adam's great-grandmother)? The author recalls some of the early twentieth-century "figurn un geshtaltn" (figures and personages) of the shtetl, among them "Gavriel Slup. Very poor; as tall as a pine tree, with a beard like the fragrant hemp threads (pakules) in which etrogs are packed. He invented a wonderful snuff (shmektabak) that no chemist in the world could duplicate. He used to carry this snuff around from synagogue to synagogue on Yom Kippur, to revive people who had fainted from fasting. He would hand out the snuff dressed in his white robes, with his head covered by his prayer shawl."

Meanwhile, in the New World in the twentieth century, cannabis was acquiring an outlaw reputation. Before it was made illegal throughout the United States in the 1930s, the flowering tops—or buds—of the female plant were part of a nurse's materia medica, which documented them as a reliable sedative that "in small doses relieves pain" and "causes great exhilaration, intoxication, and delirium, followed by a prolonged and deep sleep . . . yet very seldom proved fatal."

Further south, in Argentina, an Ashkenazi émigré cautioned his Yiddish-language readers against the perils of hashish—a concentrated substance made from the resin of female cannabis buds—as a recreational plant. But, he added as an afterthought, in exceptional cases, it might be prescribed to calm convulsions and madness.

DAUCUS CAROTA | CARROT

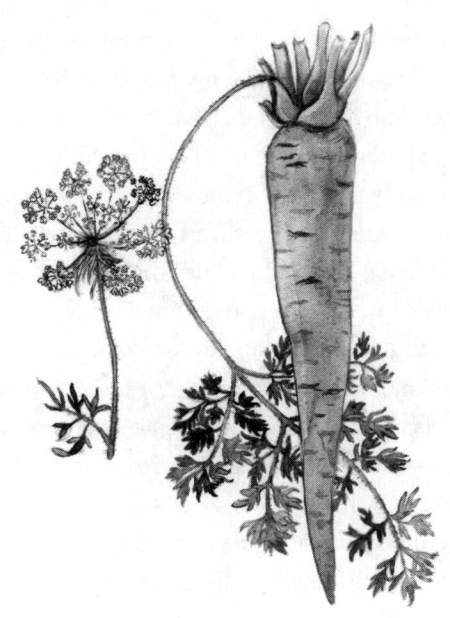

FAMILY Apiaceae

YIDDISH מער (mer), מייער (meyer), שפיצן–שלייערל (shpitsn-shleyerl) (Queen Anne's Lace)

POLISH Marchew zwyczajna

UKRAINIAN Морква звичайна (Morkva zvyčajna), морква дика (morkva dyka)

BELARUSIAN Морква дзікая (Morkva dzikaja)

LITHUANIAN Paprastoji morka

RUSSIAN Морковь дикая (Morkov' dikaja), Морковь обыкновенная (Morkov' obyknovennaja)

GERMAN Möhre, Karotte, Gartenmöhre, Mohrrübe, Gelbe Rübe, Wurzel

HEBREW גזר הגינה (gezer haginah)

Around the turn of the twentieth century, one set of my great-grandparents immigrated to the United States from Kyiv and settled in South Philadelphia. One of my father's cousins told me that my grandmother and her siblings had been taken as toddlers to an "old country" folk healer in the neighborhood who was known as "Leybele the shprekher." This would have been in the 1910s to 1920s. The visits likely involved removing an evil eye. The stories were never fully explained to me (I never heard about Leybele from my grandmother or my great-aunts), so I didn't think much of it until 2022, the year after *Ashkenazi Herbalism* was published (we did briefly mention Leybele's role in my family history in an endnote in that book).

That summer, my aunt sent me a copy of a recording she had made way back in 1981, for a class assignment, when she interviewed her mother (my grandmother), who would have been sixty-three at the time. The prospect of hearing my grandmother's voice again after so many years was comforting, so I dug an antiquated portable CD player and a pair of dusty speakers out of the closet and sat down to listen to the interview. About ten minutes into the recording, to the intermittent clinking of dishes and my aunt's occasional cough, I heard my grandmother reminiscing about her childhood among the row homes and narrow streets in the twenties. Her familiar voice, with that distinctive South Philadelphia accent, quickly brought back to me long-forgotten memories of an earlier time in my own life. But my nostalgic reveries were abruptly interrupted by my aunt's unexpected question about local superstitions, which my grandmother answered with a description of the family visits to Leybele.

An aside: This was the second instance of my grandmother making a direct contribution to our research. The first time, I was sketching out our first book, specifically drafting the section on the wax-pouring divinatory practices of the opshprekherins. After long days of writing, I went looking for something diverting to read, and one evening for some reason lighted upon a paperback novel my grandmother had given me decades ago. I remember her handing it to me and urging me emphatically to read it. This was unusual: my grandmother and I had very different tastes in literature and we never recommended titles to one another. I took the book and over the years faithfully packed it up and brought it with me whenever I moved to a new place, thinking I'd eventually get around to reading it. So that evening, a quarter-century and more later, I started it. By the time I got to page nine, I couldn't believe what I was reading: a detailed description of the pouring ceremony, in vivid detail—only instead of wax, it was lead being melted, and rather than an Ashkenazi woman performing the divination ritual, here was a Baghdadi Jewish grandmother in India trying to rid her granddaughter of a suspected evil eye. The book was *Flowers in the Blood* by Gay Courter, and to me this passage suggests that the pouring ritual is quite ancient and likely has its roots in the East.

Returning to the interview, taped in 1981, I found myself riveted as I listened to my beloved grandmother tell the story of our family consultations with Leybele the shprekher. *Shprekher,* of course, is an abbreviation of *opshprekher,* the healer who works with charms and plants—and other natural substances—to cure the patient of their afflictions. The Yiddish word can be roughly translated as one who exorcises—"speaks away"—sickness through incantations, charms, amulets, and offers medicines to protect against illnesses that might be caused by the evil eye. (For more detailed information on these folk healers, their practices, the evil eye, and related Jewish folk culture and history, please refer to *Ashkenazi Herbalism.*)

Over the centuries, concurrent with the evolution of what we know as modern or "Western" medicine, most Jewish communities relied upon folk medicine—right up until the Second World War—due to familiarity, affordability, availability, accessibility, habit, and preference. We've found that the ancient magical and herbal medicinal practices of the Jewish folk healers of the Pale, the opshprekherins and bobes, were not only deeply rooted in Jewish culture and tradition, but were also more often than not highly similar, if not identical, to the practices of folk healers from neighboring cultures. Rather than representing cases of mere borrowing or imitation, the commonalities (and the distinctive differences we also encounter) strongly suggest that healing in the region of the former Pale of Settlement was and has been a communal affair—thus underscoring the quotation from Zimmels we provided at the beginning of this book, which has been the ongoing inspiration for our work.

As my grandmother's story unfolded on this scratchy digitized recording, I learned that my great-grandparents had taken my aunt Betty (my grandmother's older sister), a toddler at the time, to see Leybele, who, like my great-grandparents, had immigrated to the United States from Ukraine. The visit was to get a consultation about an infection on Betty's chin. This would have been around 1918. The local (Western medical) doctors had already advised the family to take Betty to a surgeon to operate, but my great-grandparents looked to the more familiar healing ways of the "old country," so they went to see Leybele at his practice in the neighborhood, on the corner of 4th and Monroe. They followed the herbal prescription he gave them, and in a very short time, Betty's infection cleared up and she was back to her old self. The wonder in my grandmother's voice is clearly audible as she recounted this tale sixty years later, even through a muffled forty-year-old cassette recording.

I treasure my grandmother's story, not only as family lore but as a precious cultural heirloom that both confirms and affirms so many parts of our collective historical memory that have rarely if ever been recorded or even acknowledged. What little has been deliberately preserved of Eastern European Jewish ancestral folkways has concentrated on aspects of our folk culture that don't include the healing arts, most specifically the medicinal plant knowledge of the Ashkenazim.

This isn't a unique predicament—many peoples and cultures have been forced to painstakingly reconstruct this forgotten piece of their collective past. Even at a time when disappearing folk practices in Eastern Europe were being recorded—a century ago, by the last generation of scholars with the opportunity to explore the totality of Jewish folkways in Eastern Europe—there was an almost total lack of curiosity regarding medicinal plant knowledge on the part of the ethnographers and other social scientists of the time, and consequently, this aspect of history has been nearly erased. And this erasure was made permanent both by the Shoah and the assimilation of the Jewish diaspora who found themselves in new lands where folk medicine was not only discouraged but actively suppressed by modern medicine and its practitioners.

Nevertheless, my grandmother's childhood experiences in the Philadelphia of the late 1910s demonstrates that healers like Leybele were still treating communities of newly arrived immigrants like my great-grandparents and their children. And in fact, since hearing my grandmother's story, I've heard from others who have written about their own families' visits to Leybele.

You might not be surprised to learn that Leybele's remedy for my aunt Betty's infection came from a deep and ancient wellspring of magic and plant medicine that he learned from the generations that came before him. Because my grandmother was a first-generation American, her understanding of timeless healing methods was influenced by her acculturation in the West, which is why she described Betty's treatment (which, according to other stories my cousin Mark has told me of Leybele and our family, possibly involved a ritual that relied upon an egg and an incantation) as "witchcraft." As we describe in *Ashkenazi Herbalism*, this practice was a common and communal combination of curative techniques practiced by traditional healers throughout Eastern Europe, regardless of their religious, ethnic, or cultural affiliations. What is extraordinary is my grandmother's clear recollection of Leybele's remedy, which spared my Aunt Betty from unnecessary surgery. Leybele's prescription consisted of grated carrot; castor oil (*Ricinus communis*), a medicament historically applied topically for common skin complaints; and lemon (*Citrus x limon*), with its cooling astringent effects, combined and applied as a poultice for the swelling and purulence. Overnight, this cataplasm drew out the pus and the infection, and within a few days my Aunt Betty was healed (and she lived into her nineties).

Wild carrot, or *Daucus carota* (Queen Anne's Lace in English), is known in Yiddish as שפּיצן־שלייערל (shpitsn-shlayerl), or "lace veil," and is an herb that folk healers of Eastern Europe continue to apply to an assortment of ailments. Domestic carrot, a cultivar of *Daucus carota spp. sativus*, is known in Yiddish as מייער (mayer) or מער (mer). Although my great-grandparents lived in an urban community, Philadelphia was (and still is) quite ruderal, and while it is possible Leybele prescribed shpitsn-shlayerl, it is more likely they relied upon mer root. We should note that wild carrot resembles other plants in the Apiaceae (or Umbelliferae) family that can be deadly if misidentified.

This linguistic evidence testifies to the importance of *Daucus carota* to Ashkenazi Jewish healers and healing communities. In general, Yiddish plant names either reveal their German roots (so to speak) or their borrowing from a neighboring (generally Slavic) language. In the case of carrot, the name for the domesticated plant, mayer or mer, indicates the former (cf. German *Möhre*). In fact, the common Slavic (and Lithuanian) word for carrot (Russian *morkov'*, Ukrainian *morkva*, Polish *marchew*), is a loan-word from Germanic. The variation in pronunciation of the Yiddish word (mayer versus mer) suggests, perhaps unsurprisingly, that the ancestors of Ashkenazi Jews brought the carrot with them at a very early stage in the development of Yiddish. More interestingly, the terminological distinction between domesticated and wild carrot (mayer/mer and shpitsn-shlayerl) is a linguistic one for Yiddish-speaking Jews in a way that is not the case for their Slavic neighbors. In the absence of so much other information of a nearly vanished community, we find that occasionally linguistic evidence, particularly in the lexicon (what words do they use, and how are these words made?), can help us determine the relative importance, and even the origin or application, of a given plant to the world of the Ashkenazim.

The linguistic evidence supports what would seem to be common sense: that carrots were important to Eastern European Jews (and everyone in the region). A survey of the relevant herbal literature indicates that in Eastern Europe both wild and domesticated carrot have historically provided similar healing efficacy when the root is grated and applied to skin wounds.

In Poland, carrot has long been relied upon medicinally. Wild carrot root is grated and placed on infected skin to draw out the pus. In postwar Poland, carrot juice was still taken as a remedy for jaundice, women's health, and skin infections; it was prescribed in official herbal medicine as a pediatric restorative for anemia, as a vermifuge, and to treat digestive problems among infants. At the turn of the twentieth century, in the Polish lands, carrot had many folk applications. For women's health, to induce menstruation, Jewish girls in Zwinogródka ate onions cooked in vinegar, but they would also eat raw carrots for the same purpose. In the town of Ryżanówka, midwives recommended eating raw carrots for postpartum pain. In the Zwinogródka district, baked carrots were advised for increasing milk production. To treat leucorrhea, the Polish landed gentry in Podolia would commonly drink a "coffee" made from carrots. For any disease characterized by debility and chronic cough, carrots were dried, ground, and then cooked and drunk like coffee with milk. In Płoskirow, broths of carrot were taken to treat diarrhea. In cases of urinary retention, regardless of the cause, be it bladder stones, gonorrhea, or swelling, an extensive array of diuretic herbal remedies was offered. In Zwinogródka, the patient was given plain cooked carrot. Around Humań (Yiddish Uman, in the late nineteenth century 58 percent Jewish; now Uman', Ukraine), eating raw carrots was a recommendation for treating syphilis. For burns, it was common to place grated potatoes, beets, or carrots upon the wound. In the town of Majdanówka, near Zwinogródka (now Majdanivka, Ukraine), dairy butter sprinkled with grated carrots was applied to burns and then reapplied after it dried. In Zwiahel, it was the custom to place grated carrots on a fresh cut, an application that strongly recalls Leybele's practice. This remedy was also generally sought out for treating gangrene. In the Podolia region, folk healers recommended compresses steeped in water in which grated carrots had been soaked as a remedy against eye diseases.

In Russia, where both wild and domesticated carrot are regarded as medicinal, Annenkov's standard botanical dictionary (first published in the late nineteenth century and still consulted today) indicates that "in addition to kitchen use, carrots are also given for worms, either raw or in the form of squeezed juice; externally, they are applied to wounds or even cancer." In modern Russia, the wild root is boiled and mashed before being applied to the infected area; freshly grated domesticated carrot is another topical remedy. In Romanian pediatric folk medicine, the root, leaves, and seeds of carrot are applied externally to treat skin wounds in children, as well as rickets and stomatitis. Incidentally, with regard to rickets, known in the Pale as "the English disease," Karaim healers treated children with a bath of jellied sheep's feet, a remedy they say they learned from their Crimean Tatar relatives.

In their surveys during the 1920s and 1930s, Soviet ethno-pharmacologists recorded carrot serving as a highly prized remedy for many ailments across Ukraine. Then, as now, the herb was both cultivated in gardens and gathered wild in the fields. Many traditional practitioners in the largely Jewish communities profiled in Natalia Osadcha-Janata's *Herbs Used in Ukrainian Folk Medicine* relied upon carrot for women's health concerns and as a remedy for jaundice. Among the Jewish communities of interwar Ukraine, carrot was particularly sought out for children's ailments: Strong teas brewed with the dried plant and root were a remedy against diarrhea in both children and adults. Children with colds were also given plant decoctions of carrot to drink, or in steam baths for their feet. Malnourished children were bathed in a whole-plant decoction, as were newborns suffering from jaundice. Carrots were also reported as benefi-cial for treating children with insomnia, epilepsy, stomach troubles, and rashes. And, of course, across Ukraine, whence my great-grandparents and their lantz-man Leybele the shprekher originated, carrot was well understood as a topical remedy for skin wounds. The descendants of my great-grandparents' Ukrainian neighbors also brought this Old World remedy with them to the New: across the prairie provinces of Canada, Mucz tells us that Ukrainian communities continue to rely upon the ancient plant wisdom of their homeland, treating skin infections with poultices of grated carrot.

But some traditions could not stay for long in the goldene medine (Yiddish for the "land of gold": America). Although Leybele's prescription of grated carrot for a skin infection, particularly for a young child, is entirely in keeping with the communal healing traditions of Eastern Europe, his practice, despite being based on age-old and time-tested wisdom, could not survive. By 1936, Leybele the shprekher was forced by the Philadelphia health authorities to shutter his practice.

By sharing this family story, I hope to inspire more people to seek out and preserve their families' healing traditions. With these and other long-buried or forgotten fragments of knowledge, we hope to show that the plants not only heal physically but have the power to bring communities together, to teach us all how to take care of ourselves, one another, and the rest of the natural world.

GLYCYRRHIZA GLABRA | LICORICE

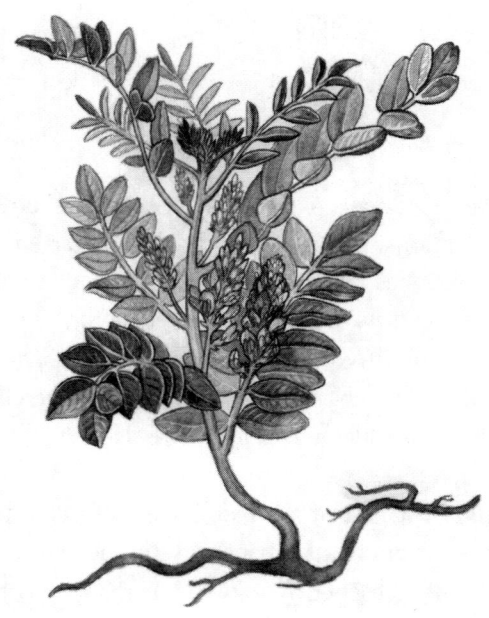

FAMILY Fabaceae

YIDDISH לאַקרעץ (lakrets), זיסהאָלץ (zisholts)

POLISH Lukrecja gładka, słodkie drzewko, lukecrja, lakrycja

UKRAINIAN Солодкий корінь голий (Solodkyj korin' holyj), солодець голий (sololec' holyj), вербець (verbec'), солодка (solodka), солодкий корінь (solodkyj korin'), солодич (solodyč), локриця (lokrycja)

BELARUSIAN Женско биле (Žensko bile)

LITHUANIAN Paprastasis saldymedis

RUSSIAN   Лакрица (Lakrica), солодка голая (solodka golaja), солодка гладкая (solodka gladkaja), лакричник (lakričnik), солодка (solodka), солоцки (solocki), солодижник (solodižnik)

GERMAN   Echtes Süßholz, Süßholz

HEBREW   שוש קירח (shush kirach), ליקוויריצ״א (likviritsiah), ליקוויריציאה (likuiritsiah)

As a medicinal plant, licorice's place in the historical record is very old and, in its various applications, extremely consistent: as far back as the ancient Egyptians, licorice root has been known for its healing qualities, particularly in respiratory health, and its undeniably sweet flavor, which contemporary science has measured as fifty times greater than sugar. Dioscorides recommends licorice root against heartburn and ailments of the chest and liver, as well as disorders of the bladder and kidneys; he also advises it can be applied topically to heal wounds.

Glycyrrhiza glabra is part of a broad lineage of plant healing traditions that span both space—from North Africa and Europe across Asia—and time. Throughout the Fertile Crescent, Loew tells us that it has been known (in, variously, Hebrew, Arabic, Aramaic, Assyrian) as sūs, šūšu, šūša, and the like. It has been valued by Jewish healers for many centuries; Maimonides discusses both licorice root and licorice juice in his work. Asaph ha-Rofe (Asaph the physician), the first "Jewish doctor," who knew the plant by its Assyrian and Greek names, praised the root as rash l'chul ha-refuarot, "the head of all remedies" (from Galen), and recommended it for acute and chronic coughs. Interestingly, Asaph also provided recommendations regarding the less-often-used aerial parts of the plant, preferring עליר (elir), or licorice leaf, to licorice flower.

Licorice is a plant with a penetrating root, erect stem, and pinnate leaves and flowers that form racemes. In modern European languages, the herb's folk name can be rendered in English as sweet root or sweet wood. In Issachar bar Teller's mid-seventeenth-century Yiddish medicinal herb guide, licorice is known as zisholts (cf. German Süßholz, "sweet wood"). Most of the well-known historical herbal literature on licorice focuses on the root's flavor and its ability to help with respiratory complaints, including relief for coughs and asthma. Teller is no exception, recommending "a good potion for the chest and for cough" with the following recipe:

> Take white horehound [Marrubium], Whitlow-wort [Paronychia], maidenhair fern [Adiantum], hyssop [Hyssopus], one handful each; licorice [Glycyrrhiza], anise [Pimpinella], fennel [Foeniculum], coriander [Coriandrum], one loth [corresponds roughly to one spoonful] each; ten figs and five dates. Boil all in one pint of water until one-third of it is consumed [reduced]. Take a good drink of this every morning and evening, and fast for one hour afterward. It is also good for people who suffer from consumption [tuberculosis].

A similar formula elsewhere in Teller features a juice for chest cough and describes how to transform licorice root into a medical implement that delivers sweeter, more palatable doses of medicine:

> Take juice of arrowhead [Sagittaria sagittifolia], juice of common jujube [Zizyphus vulgaris], the juice from the lung of a fox [Lohoch de Pulmone Vulpis], a juice called linctus, which you may find in the apothecary. Mix everything together, the same amount of each. Take a thick piece of licorice [root], scrape it clean, and beat it on its end until it becomes like a brush. Place in the juice and suck on it frequently. It is very beneficial.

Teller also advises that "those who have a cough should not eat salty food, vinegar, raw fruit, or fish, and avoid constipation by having a bowel movement daily." Laxatives are recommended with the caveat that, since coughs are usually due to cold conditions, any medications should be of a warm nature with a sweet taste to promote expectoration, suggesting the addition of licorice to any such formulation. This recommendation is interesting, because it is similar in approach to traditional Chinese medicine's reliance on licorice to harmonize complex formulations.

And "for children who cough," they "should be given crushed candied sugar and crushed licorice mixed into their pap."

Licorice as a remedy to quell a cough was also recommended by ha-Kohen, and his formula is very much like those we find in Teller. Ha-Kohen lists three variant spellings of licorice's Latin name transliterated into Hebrew, along with the Hebrew rendering of the plant's Turkish name, meyan kökü, in his plant glossary. Because ha-Kohen's *Ma'aseh Tuviyah* was published before the refinement of modern plant taxonomy, his multilingual glossary is useful for identifying the plants he refers to in his text. In addition, ha-Kohen recommends licorice as part of a regimen to reduce water retention and to cool the kidneys, especially as a prophylactic against stones.

However, contemporary herbalist Thomas Easley, in his *Modern Herbal Dispensatory: A Medicine-Making Guide,* has warned that

> *although licorice is a safe herb, some cautions are necessary when taking large doses for long periods of time. Licorice should be avoided in cases of high blood pressure or when taking digitalis. It causes retention of water and sodium and excretion of potassium, which can cause water retention, high blood pressure, heart palpitations, or a slowing of the heartbeat. Vertigo (dizziness) and headaches are early symptoms of overuse of licorice. Taking a potassium supplement with licorice can help counteract some of these effects. These side effects are much more likely to occur when using licorice extracts or licorice-derived drugs than when taking whole licorice root. De-glycyrrhizinated licorice is free of adverse effects. Use only under supervision of a qualified herbalist or practitioner in pregnancy.*

Both Teller and ha-Kohen attest to a common store of plant wisdom that Jewish communities of Eastern Europe could draw from. Beyond prescriptive sources such as these, descriptions found in Yiddish-language literature document the root's importance to communal health. Licorice is one of several herbs mentioned in a recently translated mid-nineteenth-century Yiddish tale set in a Hasidic community in Poland. In Jacob Morgenstern's "Bintshe di tsadeykeste" (The Demolished Bathhouse), one of the characters is a female spice merchant who sells licorice cakes [לאַקרעץ־פּלעצל, lakrets-pletsl] along with rhubarb and senna, all well-known aperients. This is pretty intriguing because, as you'll see, these are all components in the fabled trianke (see Trianke monograph, p. 207).

Maude Grieve attests to licorice's ubiquity in Eastern Europe, reporting in her *Modern Herbal*: "*Glycyrrhiza echinata* is native to Hungary, south Russia, and Asia Minor, and it is also the official German species."

Talko-Hryncewicz's ethnobotanical survey of folk medicine in late nineteenth-century Poland and Ukraine corroborates this: *Glycyrrhiza echinata* was the most commonly reported species within the region investigated. In Zbaraż, licorice compresses were placed on the chest to stop bleeding or hemorrhages originating from any number of causes. In Nowa-Uszyca, a water-based solution of licorice was applied to dress fresh wounds. The traditional Russian folk healers known as znakharki recommended taking the juice against coughs. In Russian folk medicine, Zevin tells us, licorice is a treatment for a variety of ailments, including dyspepsia, throat irritations or infections, mucous membrane inflammations, and stomach acid.

In the Jewish diaspora, licorice makes its appearance as a mild laxative in Garber's Yiddish-language materia medica, published in Buenos Aires in 1945. Garber cites both the plant's name in Spanish (Orozu-Regaliz) and in Yiddish (zis-holts) and recommends the root as a tea against colds and sore throats. To bring together the various diasporic strains of licorice's peregrinations from the Near East to Europe and to the New World, linking its ancient and modern names, we note that the plant's Spanish name is clearly borrowed from Arabic (orozu/orozuz < Arabic 'irq sūs, "licorice root").

In the North American diaspora, even the Yiddish writer Isaac Bashevis Singer couldn't resist mentioning licorice root in conjunction with folk healers and their remedies in two of his stories, *The Magician of Lublin* and *The Mirror*. The *YIVO Encyclopedia* also includes licorice in its entry for food and drink by informing readers that lakrits, or licorice root, was boiled in water and served on the Sabbath and at weddings. Even the yizkor books of Vilna and Jadow both contain memories of the medicinal herb.

While some of the Eastern European remedies may seem at odds with the Western record, contemporary research on the herb actually affirms what folk healers in the small villages and towns of the Pale had intuited about *Glycyrrhiza echinata*'s wide-ranging healing abilities.

Aside from its categorization as an adaptogen by contemporary herbalists, botanical researcher Stephen Buhner writes extensively about licorice's ability to resist several bacterial and viral infections, which attests to the herb's excellent actions for healing wounds, thus reaffirming the findings of the Talko-Hryncewicz surveys of the late nineteenth century. It should be reiterated that Buhner and others caution that this plant works best as a synergist, with further caveats warning that prolonged intake of any licorice species can cause harmful effects. Therefore, extensive research must be made and care taken when working with licorice—and all plants—as medicine.

In a specifically antiviral capacity, licorice as a simple can be a powerful topical ally, especially when part of a holistic approach to maintaining overall health. On a very personal note, I've had cold sore (Herpes simplex I) outbreaks since childhood, and over the years was prescribed a few different pharmaceuticals. In the 1970s, one doctor recommended an ointment called Stoxil and directed that the affected area be scraped raw with soap and warm water before application of the product. Needless to say, for a small child—for anyone—this was sheer torture. Years later, the generic compound acyclovir was introduced, in pill and cream forms. Both were somewhat effective, but at significant physical cost. The topical, thankfully, didn't have the immune-suppressing, desiccating, stomach-cramping effects that the pills caused, but unfortunately my healthcare provider almost immediately discontinued the cream from their formulary, and for years I was forced to take the pills whenever I had an outbreak.

For a more gentle healing experience, I'm grateful to herbalist Rosemary Gladstar, who reminds us that paying close attention to our body's unique signals is key to maintaining good health. Rosemary emphasizes that supporting the whole body can lead to profoundly beneficial effects. In the case of herpes outbreaks, she suggests herbal, supplemental, and dietary regimens for preventing and treating not only cold sores and fever blisters but also shingles, herpes zoster, and other forms that the virus can take. One of the key herbs in her recommendations is licorice.

Whenever a cold sore threatens, I pay close attention to what might be causing extra stress in my life and try to adjust my habits accordingly. A daily supplement of 500 mg of L-lysine has been very effective at keeping the virus at bay. If an outbreak does occur, I apply a small amount of licorice tincture to the affected area. Even the hint of an outbreak can be curtailed by this method. The tincture stops the virus immediately, and repeated applications can substantially reduce its duration and the pain and swelling that often accompany it.

To stay supplied with this remedy, I make a simple alcohol extraction in the standard ratio of one gram of dried and cut licorice root to 5 ml of 40 percent (or 80 proof) vodka and macerate the mixture for four weeks in a cool, dark cabinet before straining out the extract, bottling it, and composting the plant matter.

These measurements don't have to be exact for licorice to work its magic. A folk-method version can be just as effective. An easy extraction can be made by putting an amount of the dried and cut root into a clean jar. Cover this with vodka so that there's about an inch of liquid over the plant matter. Let this steep for four weeks in a cool, dark space like a kitchen or bathroom cabinet. Try to shake the container at least once a day to make sure all the herb comes into contact with the alcohol. After four weeks, strain the plant material out. The resulting tincture should be a deep brown color and very sweet to the taste. Don't forget to compost the root that gave its medicine.

For chapped lips, which can often aggravate an outbreak, I make a moisturizing licorice lip balm. To prepare this salve, first infuse a combination of licorice root and calendula flowers in olive oil using a double boiler, but be careful not to let the mixture get to boiling. Continue warming this combination for two to four hours. Then strain the herbs and continue to warm the oil, but this time add small amounts of beeswax to the liquid until it hardens to the consistency of a lip balm or salve. You can test the consistency by dipping the tip of a spoon into the oil and beeswax combination, putting the spoon in the freezer for a minute, then checking the spoon to see if the consistency is to your liking. You can keep adding small amounts of wax pellets and testing after each addition to get the solidity you prefer before pouring the liquid into containers. Once you've got your preferred consistency, add a few drops of vitamin E oil as a preservative. You can also add a few drops of lemon balm essential oil (another herb with antiviral actions) if desired. Then pour the liquid into lip balm tubes or small lidded containers, where it will harden as it cools. It's best to wait until the salve is completely cool and solidified in the containers before putting the lids on, in order to prevent any condensation. Label your finished product with the ingredients and date. This soothing, slightly sweet balm also works well for everyday chapped lips.

INULA HELENIUM | ELECAMPANE

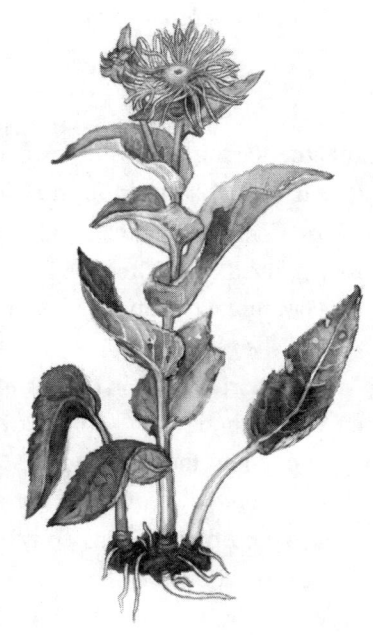

FAMILY Asteraceae

YIDDISH אָמאַן (oman), אַלעַנט (alent)

POLISH Omian wielki, oman dziewosil

UKRAINIAN Оман високий (Oman vysokyy), оман правдивий (oman pravdyvyy), оман справедний (oman spravednyy)

LITHUANIAN Didysis debesylas

RUSSIAN Девясил высокий (Devjasil vysokij), оман (oman), девятисил (devjatisil), девясил (devjasil), дикий подсолнечник (dikij podsolnečnik), дизосил (divosil)

GERMAN Echter Alant, Helenenkraut, Altkraut, Brustalant, Darm-kraut, Darmwurz, Edelwurz, Glockenwurz, Helenenalant, Odinskopf, Schlangenkraut

HEBREW אינולה קאמפאנ"ה (inulah kampaniah), אינול"ה (inulah)

TATAR Андыҙ (Andyz)

Inula, the classical Latin name for the plant, is considered to be a corruption of the Greek *helenion*, which, in its Latinized form *Helenium*, means that the plant's binomial is a tautology. There are a number of legends around the origins of the plant's name, mostly derived from Greek mythology: that it was either the herb Helen of Troy was holding when she was captured by Paris, or that it refers to her tears, or even that she relied upon it as an antidote against poison-ous bites; other lore holds that its origins lie on the island of Helena, where the best elecampanes (a plant with a short shoot and thick roots, alternate leaves, and large flowers) grow. Throughout the Middle Ages, the plant's name was often written as *Enula*. *Elecampane* is a corruption of medieval Latin *Enula campana*, as the Campania region of Italy was considered its homeland. It contains inulin, a prebiotic dietary fiber that herbalist Thomas Easley, in his *Modern Herbal Dispensatory*, reminds us feeds beneficial bacteria in the colon. Current research shows *Inula helenium* is a "biofilm-buster," meaning it has the ability to break up pathogenic mat-like films that aggregate on vulnerable body tissues such as those lining the respiratory tract. So it's no wonder that this herb has had a reputation for relieving lung-related ailments since the ancients.

Dioscorides and Galen both mention the plant's fragrant root, source of its medicine, and both emphasize its curative properties in stimulating urination and menses, alleviating "hip disease" (probably sciatica or lower back pain) and soothing coughs. Hildegard von Bingen cites similar attributes for elecam-pane, while Maimonides looked to the plant as a remedy for urinary conditions such as strangury.

According to Lev and Amar, elecampane has been known to many Jewish healers of the Near East from ancient times, having been cultivated in the region for centuries; it is listed in several materiae medicae found in the Cairo Genizah, and Jews of Iraq and Iran relied on elecampane against bronchitis and phlegm, and as an expectorant and diuretic. Asaph ha-Rofe calls attention to its qualities as a diuretic, antitussive, and emmenagogue, and notes its efficacy against bites, stings, and poisons. Lev and Amar also tell us how Maimonides regarded elecampane as a hot and moist plant, a decoction of which he called "the royal beverage" for its efficacy against the aches and pains of old age, as a tonic for the heart and stomach, and for potency. The seeds could be relied upon to help both the lungs and the brain.

Teller includes the root of elecampane in a powdered mixture, very reminiscent of the trianke, especially in its requirement of several exotic imported herbs. He considered this recipe to be good for the stomach and to fortify the brain. The formula was to be taken as a "generous amount on the tip of a knife," mornings and evenings, and consisted of two loths each of cubeb pepper and the root of elecampane, along with three nutmegs, and blossom nutmeg (mace?), cinnamon, cloves, and fennel flower, one quintal each, in addition to one loth of cardamom and white candied sugar. These were all to be crushed separately, then mixed before taking.

Ha-Kohen refers to "inula" and "kampana" in several contexts in his *Ma'aseh Tuviyah*, including for oral hygiene and strengthening the heart. Elecempane, along with hyssop, scabiosa, coltsfoot, licorice, mallow, iris, dried figs, and Proprietatis and Pectoralis, two alchemical elixirs, is among the remedies recommended by him to alleviate respiratory conditions.

Ha-Kohen's elecampane prescription is closely connected to one of the most interesting entries in *Ma'aseh Tuviyah*, which appears in the section on respiratory health, where he invokes the ancient concept of "the wandering womb." Ha-Kohen held to the age-old belief that an allegedly mobile uterus was responsible for causing a variety of ailments such as asthma or other breathing difficulties.

The concept of the wandering womb is, of course, obsolete today, but in the folk imagination it persisted for centuries and was blamed for many disorders. Even into the twentieth century, the wandering womb, in the traditional medicine of Eastern Europe, continued to lurk as a possible culprit. It might occasionally migrate all the way out to the body's extremities, and because it was commonly held that men as well as women possessed a uterus, complaints associated with the organ could potentially affect anyone.

The Polish scholar Marek Tuszewicki discusses this complex condition and its importance to understanding health in Ashkenazi Jewish culture in his book *A Frog Under the Tongue*; the most common symptoms of the wandering womb were generally abdominal pains and gripe, and a number of herbal remedies were prescribed to counteract the condition, which was "particularly widespread in women." Treatments might include the use of fumigation, compresses, and purgatives.

Amazingly, we can map this belief across the ethnographic surveys of the late nineteenth century: Talko-Hryncewicz documents diagnosis and treatment for wandering wombs in many villages and shtetls in the Pale. For instance, in the town of Zwinogródka, elecampane was the herb of choice for those suffering from the respiratory effects of the wandering womb; it was taken internally as a decoction or externally as either fumigant or lubricant for cough relief. As we can see from ha-Kohen's prescriptions, this suggests a continuing lineage of treatment among Jews and their neighbors in Eastern Europe.

In addition, in the town of Jurkow, folk healers dug up the plant's roots in the spring and prescribed them as a decoction to strengthen and enhance digestion for those with chronic illness brought on by the itinerant uterus. This application implies an intuitive understanding of the herb's prebiotic abilities.

At the time, it was believed that bladder stones were caused by properties of the local drinking water. At one point in the 1890s, in the town of Bohaczówka, along the Sosowa River, six people were found to suffer from this painful condition, whereas no other cases were reported in the surrounding villages. Local folk healers responded by giving their patients decoctions of elecampane to drink to counteract the malady.

During this period, elecampane was frequently called upon to heal skin conditions. Its powdered leaves were also sprinkled on fresh cuts in Jurkow. In Załuże and Zbaraż, an oil ointment prepared with unsalted butter or old lard, blue stone (copper sulfate), and elecampane root was applied to "black pimples," or boils. This remedy recalls a story in Yaffa Eliach's book *There Once Was a World*, in which Bureh der Royfe, a feldsher in Eishyshok, Lithuania, in the early twentieth century, was known always to carry with him his most secret curatives, one of which was a blue stone that he ground into powder for his most popular concoctions (see *Acorus calamus*, p. 29). A related formulation for another skin condition, scabies, was utilized in Nowa-Uszyca, in the form of a salve consisting of blue stone and alchemical compounds of sulfur, soot, and tar.

According to Mucz, a quite similar antidote for the removal of mites can still be found in the Ukrainian communities of western Canada. There they mix lard with powdered sulfur and powdered blue stone, which, if applied regularly, can clear up the infestation within a few weeks.

Scabies was commonly cured with great success in the Pale by drinking decoctions of elecampane or lubricating the affected areas with elecampane root ground with animal fat. In Zwinogródka, one folk healer combined finely chopped elecampane root and crushed ginger with sulfur powder, goat tallow, and cream to rid a patient of the itchy condition. Another technique reported from Zwinogródka called for bathing in a decoction of elecampane; and in Hussakowa, simply washing the body with an elecampane decoction was an effective remedy.

Among Polish folk healers around Kraków between the world wars, according to Fischer, elecampane was a remedy for treating kołtuns, as well as the matted hair of livestock, and an ointment of grated plant root and lard would treat scabies and eczema. In Dziewiętniki (now Dev'jatnyky, Ukraine), decoctions of the roots and leaves of the plant treated rashes, and in Zawoja, Poland, they addressed convulsions resulting in pains in the internal organs brought on by overwork. Around Sieradz, Poland (in the late nineteenth century 31 percent Jewish), elecampane was employed for shortness of breath (this is also attested in the Łowicz district of Poland), coughs, stomach upsets, and scabies. Similarly, contemporary Lithuanian Jewish folk healers look to the plant's roots for respiratory health, to improve expectoration when working with unproductive coughs.

Fischer also tells us that Polish landed gentry (around Vilna) cultivated elecampane as a garden plant; while in Navahrudak (Belarus), a Lipka Tatar town, it was grown as both ornamental and veterinary plant—there, the healers (likely Tatar healers, whose skill at veterinary care for livestock was legendary) would apply its leaves to heal broken bones in cattle, and as part of an ointment to treat skin conditions in horses.

Author Sophie Knab writes that, in Poland, elecampane had been useful as a medication for children and infants suffering from the contagious skin infection impetigo, and that the root when grated into a fat substance alleviated itching or acne, echoing Polish and Ukrainian treatments from the turn of the last century. She also describes how elecampane root was burned to fumigate an area against mosquitoes. In Romanian pediatric folk medicine, a fumigation of elecampane root (iarbă mare, "great herb") has soothed children who cry at night.

Throughout the former Russian Empire (and Soviet Union), folk knowledge of elecampane's strengths is quite comprehensive. The plant's Russian name, devjasil', translates as "nine powers," for its myriad healing abilities. For Yiddish speakers of the Pale, *Inula helenium* had two common names: oman, borrowed from the Slavic, and alent, derived from the German.

According to Zevin, there is documentation of the medicinal plant in the lands of Russia dating back to the seventeenth century, when it acquired a reputation for calming a dry cough, encouraging expectoration, and easing difficult respiration. Much as in the Pale of the late nineteenth century, elecampane today continues to be valued in Russia for its bitter properties that encourage digestive secretions and stimulate the appetite, and thus benefit metabolism.

According to Gammerman and Müller-Dietz, folk healers in Russia turn to elecampane to calm nervous disorders, reduce fevers and catarrhs of the upper respiratory tract, and remedy contagious skin disease via application of parts of the plant (decoctions to wash scabies infections, and leaf plasters against wounds). Traditional healers employ bathing with elecampane root to help with rheumatism and skin diseases.

In nineteenth-century Belarus, according to Demitsch, in Mogilev and Vitebsk, two cities of the Pale with historically large Jewish populations, patients were directed to drink a decoction of elecampane root for stomach and chest afflictions, as well as cholera, and were also prescribed ointments of elecampane and bacon fat against scabies; across Ukraine, brandy macerations or water infusions of the root were taken for various debilities, as well as against syphilis. Most interesting, however, is their association of the plant with both the bringing on of menses and the treatment of heart conditions, and for oral health.

As we've seen, elecampane across the former Pale of Settlement has been a very important plant in animal health as well. According to Bezzenberger, Lithuanian folk healers relied on elecampane (and mullein and St. John's wort) to promote milk production in cows and to protect them from witches. There is a highly intriguing parallel here with veterinary plant medicine among the Pennsylvania Germans in the United States, whom Lick and Brendle tell us have relied on elecampane as an antitussive for their horses.

When I was formally studying herbalism, our class spent as much time with the plants as we could. We tasted fresh and dried herbs, sampled extractions, and contemplated flavors, aromas, textures, and colors. We slept with flowers and leaves and sometimes roots or bark under our pillows. We bathed with fragrant sachets and perfumed our rooms with incense. We planted and watered and pruned and gathered. We foraged and fed ourselves with herbs. In short, it was a very immersive experience.

At one point during my studies, I came down with a cold, and for at least two nights I had one of those coughs that starts with a tickle and ends with insomnia. By the third day, still plagued with an unproductive dry hack, I occasionally caught myself mentally repeating one word over and over: "*elecampane elecampane elecampane. . .*" That evening, while I was getting ready for bed and dreading another sleepless night, elecampane floated through my consciousness again, and it finally dawned on me that the plant had been trying to catch my attention all day. This wasn't an herb we'd studied yet in class, and I had never relied on it before, but I remembered I had a small sample bottle in the house.

I quickly found it and put three droplets of the tincture into a bit of water. The first thing I tasted was the root's cedar-like flavor. Within a few minutes I realized my urge to cough had stopped, and as soon as I got myself into bed, I fell deeply and soundly asleep. Most surprisingly of all, the next morning I had a physical memory of having been gently held all night.

After this experience, I've recommended a few drops of elecampane in a little water whenever someone has a dry, unproductive cough. I never mentioned the mysterious sensation I felt upon waking, but several people have told me they experienced a similar feeling after taking elecampane for a cough before bed.

Since that first encounter, I've grown elecampane here in the Central Valley of Northern California, but the plant gravitates toward the well-watered, shaded areas so its perennial root can survive the crazy summer heat this region is famous for. Every year, elecampane has grown to over six feet tall, even under the old walnut tree, and every time presents us with multiple blooms. By fall, the luminous flowers transform themselves into translucent puffs, a little like their dandelion relations, except these are not round, but the seeds are just as buoyant when the wind catches them.

MATRICARIA CHAMOMILLA |
CHAMOMILE

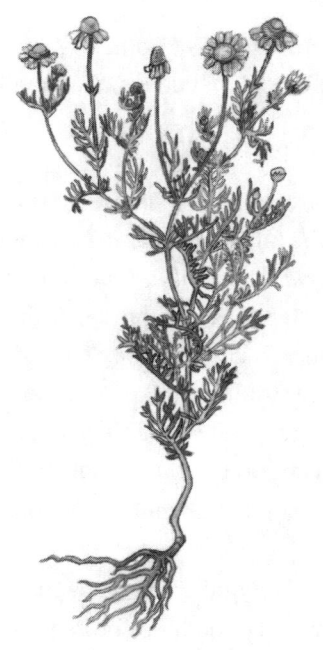

FAMILY   Asteraceae

YIDDISH   געוויינטלעכער ראָמיאַניק (geveyntlekher romianik)

POLISH   Rumianek pospolity, rumianok, rumianeć, rumianok pachuszczyj, korołycia

UKRAINIAN   Ромашка лікарська (Romaška likars'ka) ромен (romen), роман (roman), румянок (rumjanok), романец (romanec), романок (romanok), ромашка аптечна (romaška aptečna), рум'ян (rum'jan), рум'янок (rum'anok), рум'янк (rum'jank)

BELARUSIAN   Рамонак аптэчны (Ramonak aptečny), рамонак абадраны (ramonak abadrany), румонак (rumonak), румянак (rumjanak), рамашка (ramaška), румянка (rumjanka), рамон (ramon), роман (roman), рамонак праўдзівы (ramonak praŭdzivy)

LITHUANIAN   Vaistinė ramunė

RUSSIAN   Ромашка аптечная (Romaška aptečnaja), купальница (kupal'nica), румянка (rumjanka), сосонька (soson'ka)

GERMAN   Echte Kamille

There are two plants called chamomile that are most widely employed in herbal medicine: *Anthemis nobilis* (also known as *Chamaemelum nobile*), or Roman chamomile, and *Matricaria chamomilla* (currently known most generally as *Matricaria recutita*), or German chamomile. Although the two genera are genetically and geographically distinct, they have similar healing qualities—moreover, because they are strikingly alike in appearance (thin taproots, leaves that are pinnate and dissected, and single flowers), they have often been confused in the botanical literature. For the purposes of this monograph, we will use the common name "chamomile" unless our source specifies which plant is being referred to.

As a medicinal plant, chamomile can be traced back at least as far as the ancient Egyptians, who revered the herb for its remedial properties. According to Grieve, the ancients believed in the power of chamomile against ague (understood to be any disease characterized by chills, shivers, and fevers, typically malaria), and so dedicated the plant to their gods.

Curiously, there is some dispute among historians as to whether chamomile was even native to ancient Egypt—the French scholar Max Meyerhof, editor of the standard Western edition of Maimonides, states quite definitively that "*Anthemis nobilis* (Roman chamomile) does not grow in Egypt . . . [rather] the herb is imported and sold in the bazaars by the name of *babūnig* or šiḥ *babūnig*."

Whatever its provenance, chamomile maintained a strong medicinal presence in the ancient world for centuries, finding its way into the healing traditions of a number of cultures, including those of the ancient Near East.

In the twelfth century, the abbess Hildegard recommended German chamomile in a "sauce" (consisting of the plant, mixed with water and lard or oil and wheat) to treat intestinal complaints. The same sauce was consumed by women to "pleasantly and lightly prepare the purgation of inner matter so that menstruation can begin." She also formulated chamomile with cow butter to rub on a painful "stitch" in the side.

It was the sixteenth-century German polymath Joachim Camerarius who gave the plant that he saw growing profusely throughout Rome its first binomial, *Chamaemelum nobile*. Maude Grieve claims that *Anthemis nobilis* was introduced to Germany from Spain in the late Middle Ages. To me, this ambiguity has clad the migratory trajectory of this herb in a cloak of mystery.

Regardless of the timing of Roman chamomile's arrival in Germany, within decades of the plant's new moniker, Teller called upon chamomile no less than eight times in his Yiddish-language remedy book. For those suffering from headaches, under hot conditions, he cautioned against eating too much at night, or consuming foods that produce "vapors," such as onions, garlic, beans, peas, or turnips. In addition, he advised that one should avoid spicy foods or sleeping immediately after eating, especially during the day. For this type of headache, brought on by heat, he recommended that people suffering from pain bathe the head in a tea blend of equal parts chamomile, rue, sage, linden, dill, wormwood, lovage, and hyssop.

For headaches associated with cold conditions, he recommended combining "a handful" each of chamomile, melilot, and arrowhead with one spoonful each of waterlily and poppy heads to promote better rest and sleep. All these ingredients were to be boiled together and the resulting infusion was to be taken as a footbath for a half an hour at night before bed. For a "stitch in the side," a condition understood at the time to result from an excess of bile, chamomile was prescribed as part of a lengthier protocol in the form of an oil applied as a compress to the tender area.

In a section devoted to digestive issues, Teller advised chamomile to help a case of "urgency," or to relieve diarrhea. For stomach cramps and colic, a special clyster (a kind of enema) required that chamomile flowers, poplar, and marshmallow leaves, along with fennel and anise, be boiled and then mixed with fresh butter, olive oil, and a well-beaten egg yolk, then administered warm.

In Teller's time, the spleen was thought to become engorged with unhealthy blood. This caused a person to become melancholic; it might further lead to weight loss due to improperly digested food, which in turn produced poor-quality blood. In such cases, bloodletting was regarded as part of a remedial protocol and was performed through the spleen vessel, or the vena salvatella, located on the left hand between the last two fingers. If the spleen was found to be hardening, chamomile oil was formulated as part of a topical ointment and applied to soften the organ. This remedy could possibly be a vestige of the earlier recommendation by Hildegard for a stitch.

To relieve kidney stones, readers were advised to increase their flow of urine and to thin bodily fluids. Chamomile flowers were part of another clyster recipe administered for this condition. An alternative, less invasive treatment was a bath that included chamomile flowers, linseed, fenugreek, and melilot, all placed in a cloth bag and infused in boiling water. This infusion was added to a bath with water deep enough to immerse the patient up to their navel while placing the bag of herbs on the loins. Before the bath, however, the patient was advised to drink a syrup of maidenhair fern combined with beet water and parsley water.

To soften a boil, chamomile flowers, poplar, melilot, dill, linseed, and fenugreek were boiled as a tea into which a piece of fresh butter and a hunk of hog's fat (the Hebrew obligation "pikuach nefesh," "saving a life," here taking precedence over Jewish kashrut dietary laws) were added to the infusion before it was applied topically to the inflamed infection.

Chamomile was also an important plant for Tobias ha-Kohen, who included it in two clyster formulas. One of these was a water-based, tea-like recipe for stomach pain, and the other, an oil-based mixture for use as a laxative.

My mother once told me that encouraging sweat in a sick person was a well-known Jewish mode of healing. Ha-Kohen was no stranger to this technique (in contemporary herbalism, sweating is considered one of the most effective ways to rid the body of toxins). Ha-Kohen prescribed a method of taking smallish, elongated sacs of herbs that were to be moistened in warm water and then wrung out before being placed at the nape of the neck, the arms, and the feet of the patient, who would then be thoroughly covered with blankets as a guarantee that they would produce a healing sweat within an hour. Among the herbs ha-Kohen mentions specifically for this treatment were sage, rosemary, marjoram, rue, pennyroyal, and chamomile.

Ear pain was also addressed with chamomile extracted in oil, which was to be placed inside the ear. Unfortunately, the rest of ha-Kohen's formulation was much less appetizing, as it also called for a scorpion and worm oil.

Ha-Kohen's work is often difficult to decipher, but in a passage that seems related to Teller's advice on stomach pain and splenic disorders, he incorporated a bit of reverie into his prescription: "How very good is a trip to the markets, gardens, or orchards, in a place with fresh air rather than constant sitting at study, in a dark place." Regardless, he catalogs the likely symptoms of the disease (which he calls "hipukhundriah"): stomach weakness, excess acid, fits of yawning, belching, fainting, heart palpitations, shortness of breath, joint pains, and gas—it's here where ha-Kohen mentions several complex compound formulations popular at the time, such as gum ammoniacum mixed with vinegar or the diagridum, an involved laxative formula taken from Islamic medicine, along with more exotic substances like tacamahac, a resin of plants in the Calophyllum genus, which was often (mis)taken for Balm of Gilead (*Commiphora gileadensis*).

More prosaically, ha-Kohen recommended topical oils including chamomile to relieve pain and to soften swellings. For young children who cried out from colic, he suggested the theriac as a remedy (see "Trianke," p. 207). And if that were too much for them, he called for a tzigil, a warmed brick (cf. German *Ziegel*), to be placed on their stomachs for pain relief.

For toothache as a side-effect of scurvy, chamomile or sambucus flowers could be boiled in milk and given for pain relief.

In the first trimester of pregnancy, writes ha-Kohen, women often suffered from a litany of maladies including vomiting, diarrhea, toothache, headache, dizziness, and nausea. For these complaints, many of his suggestions sound tempting even today—roasted quince mixed with little powdered diarrhodon (a rose-based complex formulation widely employed in early modern medicine for strengthening internal organs and preventing nausea), or aromatic mint water boiled with grains of mastic, cumin, or cinnamon. Symptoms might also be resolved by eating well-baked bread dipped in pomegranate or quince juice, or even some coral dust mixed into a meat broth. Stomach cramps might also be treated with a topical oil of chamomile and rue.

Ha-Kohen again surprises with a recipe calling for butyrospermum oil (shea butter) mixed with chamomile or marshmallow oil as an external remedy for children's stomach pain.

For men's sexual health, ha-Kohen recommended a bandage consisting of rue leaves and chamomile flowers but did not go into detail about its intended placement, instead chastely referring readers to "the many other books that cover this subject."

In Poland in the late nineteenth century, chamomile continued to be a highly regarded medicinal plant with numerous and varied applications. A decoction of *Matricaria chamomilla,* the common chamomile known in that part of Eastern Europe, was one of several plants selected to stimulate menstruation. A complex formulation was given in Olszana, consisting of Roman chamomile, or *Anthemis nobilis,* as one of ten plants (along with *Artemisia vulgaris, Juniperus sabina, Thymus vulgaris, Artemisia abrotanum, Origanum majorana, Salvia rosmarinus, Origanum vulgare, Acorus calamus, Erythrea centaurium,* and *Bryonia*) to be taken four times a day as an emmenagogue. Here we encounter once more an echo of Hildegard's earlier recommendations, calling on German chamomile to gently stimulate menstruation.

In gynecological health, it was common in Podolia to treat leucorrhea in women and girls who were already menstruating with an infusion of chamomile or lemon balm.

Throughout the Pale, many superstitions revolved around the newborn. For instance, it was commonly believed that one should never show an infant to strangers in the first days after its birth, because someone might give it the evil eye, particularly old women. Regarding breastfeeding, Jewish women in the Polish lands were known to nurse babies for up to two years as a way to avoid another pregnancy. In Zwinogródka, Jewish women also believed that boys should be breastfed longer than girls, but for no more than two years, lest their minds become dull. Before nursing bottles were invented, artificial nipples were made from the udders of slaughtered cows. These contraptions could dispense easily digestible foods for the infant, like a pap made from bread soaked in chamomile tea.

The Yiddish name for chamomile, romianik, borrowed from the Ashkenazi Jews' Slavic neighbors, translates as "ruddy." Regina Lilienthal (1877–1924), a prominent ethnographer of Jewish folkways in the Pale, wrote in her 1904 monograph *Dziecko żydowskie* (The Jewish Child) that chamomile was part of the Jewish infant's diet and explained that its name in Yiddish was taken from the Slavic because a ruddy complexion was understood to signify health. Feeding young children this herb must have had the trifecta outcome of calming infants, helping their delicate digestion, and providing the apotropaic effect of good, glowing, rude vitality.

While it's not surprising to find chamomile employed in digestive tract health in the region, one Ukrainian recipe of the late nineteenth century was unusual in that it required the powdered leaves and stems from the plant to be decocted and drunk as an emetic. This exact recipe was also used to treat headaches in Zwinogródka. Chamomile infusions were reported for treating gonorrhea around towns such as Zwinogródka and Walichawłowo (now Vilyavče, near Lviv, Ukraine).

In Zwinogródka, healers sought fresh chamomile for rubbing the body of someone afflicted with fevers caused by an infectious disease. Ashkenazim called this condition kaduches, which is the Yiddish pronunciation of the Hebrew kadakhat, "fevers." The Yiddish term eventually took on the ironic meaning "less than nothing," as in the Yiddish expression "Ikh vel dir geben kaduches": "I'll give you less than nothing" (i.e., a fever).

Elsewhere in the Pale, it was common to wash wounds with a chamomile infusion. In the resort town of Zakopane, Poland, chamomile in the bed was a way to keep flea infestations at bay.

Styes on the eyes were treated with more magical methods. Many treatments required some barley, often counted out in multiples of three, and in Podolia, barley grains were washed with chamomile when they were picked for this purpose. In Nowa-Uszyca, another remedy for eye afflictions called for covering the affected area with cooling pads made of chamomile and mint.

The cause of ringing or pain in the ears was thought to originate from several sources that might include colds, wind blowing in the ears, skin eruptions in the area, worms breeding in the ear itself, insects lodging themselves in the ear, or objects children might insert into their own ears. Folk healers provided as many remedies as there were causes for such situations.

For eliminating ear issues caused by insects, turpentine was a common remedy. In Podolia, clean sheep's wool or raw cotton wool was dipped in olive oil and sprinkled with camphor before being inserted in the ear. In Zwinogródka, a tea of marjoram or mallow (*Malva silvestris*) was the remedy of choice for quieting ringing in the ear. Another common treatment was to blow steam from infused chamomile into the ear.

Chamomile shows up frequently in the yizkor memory books documenting life in Eastern Europe's Jewish communities. In the town of Antopol, Belarus, Jewish healers turned to "popular grasses" such as chamomile, linden, nettles, and the like for "stomach pain and other internal sicknesses."

A more evocative description can be found in the yizkor book of Tsihanovits (Ciechanowiec, Poland), where the descriptions of the landscape take on a dream-like quality in their depiction of the tableau of flora and fauna, including a "grand portal, which lay along the ritshke (brook). Here one could find orchards, forests, and hillsides dabbed in spring with many flowers, among them chamomile."

In the yizkor book for Demblin (Dęblin, Poland), Zalman, the town's folk doctor, is remembered by the author of this memoir as having won the trust of the entire town for his remedies, and that all the residents "wished him eternal life for his goodness and his warm Jewish heart." Zalman was most likely a feldsher who relied on bankes (cupping) and leeches for many of his healing methods. Zalman also drew from a treasure trove of babske refues, "grandmothers' remedies," to heal his community, including applying clean spider webs to fresh wounds to staunch bleeding, and offering chamomile for stomach aches and sour milk for swellings. (Incidentally, my best friend when I was very young was from Ukraine, and her Zaporižže-born mother would dab our summer sunburns with buttermilk, which at the time I thought pretty weird, but its efficacy made enough of an impression that I remember her remedy all these decades later.)

In the shtetl of Rubizhevitch (now Rubjaževičy, Belarus), one memoirist's mother grew dahlias, chamomile, beans, and peas in her garden. The family also built the local tar factory and produced turpentine and pitch for the region, a trade that had been passed down through several generations and inspired his grandmother's nickname, "Fruma the Tar Lady." Incidentally, turpentine was not just a remedy for ear infections in the folk healer's repertoire: the solvent could also be rubbed on as a liniment for aching bones, or taken with sugar cubes as a vermifuge, among its numerous applications.

The yizkor for the town of Gorodets (now Garadzec, Belarus) is a veritable treasure trove of detailed information regarding the many types of Eastern European ancestral folk healers and their practices in the vanished Jewish communities of the region. Chamomile is only one of several herbs inventoried here; it is honored for its ability to bring on a healing sweat when suffering from a cold.

Among the many other recipes, stories, and folk remedies revealed in *The Jewish Book of Flowers,* author and herbalist Naomi Spector shares that in historic Sephardi communities, chamomile tea is drunk to treat a stomach ache, and a traditional Sephardi folk remedy to support a child with a stomach ache is to rub warm oil on the child's abdomen and give them chamomile tea to drink.

In Eishyshok, a town where Tatars, Jews, Lithuanians, Poles, and Belarusians lived in close proximity, one of the healers knew many cures that required chamomile as their key ingredient, including a drink to combat hepatitis, a bath for yeast infections, and an infusion for colds.

In Romanian pediatric folk medicine, chamomile flowers were taken internally to soothe cramping and gas pains in infants, improve respiratory health, and address neurological ailments, including epilepsy. Externally, they were an effective wound treatment, and, in a bath immersion, promoted overall good health in infants.

After the war and across the sea, a Polish Jewish herbalist living in Argentina recorded his knowledge of both German and Roman chamomile. He described the former as an antispasmodic for stomach cramps and a calmative for infant nerves. Externally, he praised the plant as a helpful compress for bruises. He regarded Roman chamomile as less versatile: it would serve as an appetite stimulant, a soother of stomach pain, and a dye for blonde hair.

In present-day Lithuania, surveyed Jewish folk healers reported chamomile and linden as their top choices for traditional medicine. They collect the flowers during the summer months and work with the dried plant alone or in combination with other herbs for a wide variety of treatments or prophylaxes, including eye disease, oral complaints, and disorders of the skin, digestion, or nerves.

More specifically, both Jewish and Muslim (Lipka Tatar and Azerbaijani) folk healers in Lithuania reported chamomile to be helpful in treating indigestion, reducing bloating, and as a carminative. Flower infusions treat restlessness, mild insomnia, and nervous disorders. Externally, applications are for inflammation and irritations of the skin and mucous membranes, including infections of the mouth, gums, and throat. Because of its cooling and disinfecting properties, chamomile is also effective as a compress or rinse for eye inflammation, or as a bath to soothe hemorrhoids. According to Vasiliauskas, traditional folk medicine of ethnic Lithuanians calls upon chamomile teas to treat the digestive tract, cure colds, soothe nerves and skin irritations, relieve pain in wounds, and address sore throats and sinus inflammations.

These applications are also recorded among the contemporary Lithuanian healers from the formerly majority-Jewish region of Kaišiadorys, who rely on chamomile to treat problems of the digestive tract (inflammation, pains, bloating, diarrhea). Chamomile tea may be given to colicky babies. Infusions of chamomile flowers as well as the whole plant serve as an eye wash, topical for wounds, and in a compress for inflammations. Chamomile is held to have a calming effect on children and is good as a rinse for children's mouth or throat inflammations.

Several recipes that call for chamomile are still taken locally by Lithuanian Jewish healers. For coughs, they boil chamomile flowers and one tablespoon of salt in a liter of water. After removing the pot from the heat, they recommend covering the head with a towel before carefully inhaling the steam of this brew.

To stop a runny nose, they put a tablespoon of chamomile flowers into boiling water, then allow the mixture to cool. After removing the plant material, they squeeze the juice from it and drip the liquid into the nose three to four times a day.

For an inflammation of the mouth and throat, these Jewish folk healers make a blend of dried plant materials with two parts three-lobed beggartick, four parts chamomile flowers, two parts linden flowers, and two parts sage leaves. For one serving, they steep two to three tablespoons of this mixture in a glass of boiling water for fifteen minutes, then rinse the mouth and throat with the cooled liquid several times a day.

For a sore throat, chamomile flowers are boiled on low heat for fifteen minutes, then cooled while the plant material is strained out. A throat rinse of the warmed infusion is taken every two hours.

To help a person sleep, the healers steep equal parts peppermint leaves and chamomile flowers in a half-liter of boiling water for ten minutes, after which they strain out the plant material. This tea is taken before bedtime. For children, a simple chamomile tea before bedtime is helpful for sleeping.

Excess stomach acidity is treated with a tea blend composed of equal parts dried peppermint, St. John's wort, calendula, chamomile, cumin, and valerian. From this mixture, they simmer one tablespoon in a cup of boiling water for ten minutes, strain, and take a tablespoon of the brew three times daily before meals.

In addition to recipes from the ancestral lands in and around the Pale, I've found that a warm foot bath infused with chamomile and lavender flowers can be really relaxing before going to sleep. For tired, irritated eyes, dampened chamomile tea bags applied gently for a few minutes can bring cooling and soothing relief.

MELISSA OFFICINALIS | LEMON BALM

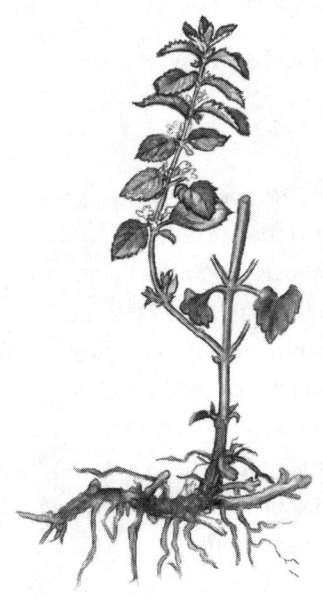

FAMILY Lamiaceae

YIDDISH מעליסע (melise)

POLISH Melisa lekarska

UKRAINIAN Меліса лікарська (Melisa likars'ka), маточник (matočnyk), маточник пчільний (matočnyk pčil'nyj), медунка лікарська (medunka likars'ka), меліса (melisa), ройник звичайний (rojnyk zvyčajnyj), ройовик (rojovyk), бджолина трава (bdžolyna trava), кадило (kadylo), лимонка (lymonka), лимонник (lymonnyk), маточник пчільний (matočnyk pčil'nyj), маточник-роївник (matočnyk-roïnyk), матошник (matošnyk), меді(о)вка (medi(o)vka), медовник (medovnyk), мелиска (melyska), мелісса (melissa), м'ята цитринова (m'jata cytrynova), пчільник (pčil'nyk), пчолина трава (pčolyna trava), роєвник (roevnyk), ройник (roynyk), ройовник (rojovnyk)

LITHUANIAN Vaistinė melisa

RUSSIAN Мелисса лекарственная (Melissa lekarstvennaja)

GERMAN Zitronenmelisse, Melisse

TATAR Милисə (Milisä)

The woman who lived in our house before us was also a gardener. Over the years I've mostly added to her original plantings, and tended to the many volunteers that have meandered onto this patch of ground. In our first years here, I often came upon little clusters of a fragrant plant with opposite and ovate leaves, and small, white or yellowish flowers, sheltering under the wide canopy of the mature walnut tree that's probably shaded the backyard since this house was built almost seventy years ago. I was unfamiliar with this herb but thought its citrusy aroma was a little like lemon-scented furniture polish.

I love the scent of citrus, but I wasn't sure about this variation, so whenever I came across a fresh sprout, I pulled it out. It quickly became obvious that the mystery lemony plant was completely indifferent to my efforts—every time I went out to work in the garden, I'd find new baby sprigs were happily settling in.

Eventually I learned this was lemon balm, and according to at least one source I consulted, it's considered an invasive weed. With this information I gave up trying to get rid of the plant and instead decided to see for myself just what was meant by the alleged botanical bad behavior I'd been warned about.

Twenty years later, there's still a single patch of lemon balm in the shade of the old walnut, a spot I gravitate toward on the hottest days of summer. When I look back on lemon balm's refusal to be pigeonholed as an aggressive interloper, I'm reminded of one of my favorite childhood books, Robert Lawson's *The Story of Ferdinand*, the gentle bull who defied bullfighting stereotypes by refusing to perform in the ring, preferring instead to sniff flowers beneath the cork oak trees.

We have constantly evolving and dynamic relationships with the plants. My initial antagonism toward lemon balm gave way to accepting its presence in the garden. Years later, during my herbal program, I tasted a lemon balm tincture and was not surprised to find that I had no real response to or feeling from it, unlike most of the students in my class who took turns describing experiences that ranged from fantastic to ecstatic, and I wondered if I had somehow built up psychic callouses against this obviously beloved herb. When I confessed that I had no discernible connection with lemon balm, everyone seemed incredulous, possibly horrified. It wasn't until I tried freshly gathered leaves as a tea that I finally felt lemon balm's uplifting, reinvigorating, yet soothing qualities. Herbalist Sajah Popham writes about lemon balm as a cardiotonic, and mentions two more herbs to combine with it to calm an anxious heart: motherwort and linden.

I recount these stories because they're examples of how individual our responses are to plants and other substances. I haven't been immune or resistant to lemon balm's medicinal qualities; I've just become acquainted with them in my own way. In a sense, lemon balm taught me how to appreciate and yield to other beings' differences without jumping to fast conclusions.

Melissa officinalis—lemon balm—is native to southern Europe and has naturalized throughout much of the world. Like most of the mint family, it is square-stemmed, with an easily recognizable lemony scent, and a medicinal history that can be traced back thousands of years. The English word *balm* derives from the ancient Semitic *bosem*, meaning a resinous aromatic substance derived from plants. The binomial, *Melissa officinalis*, refers to the Greek word for bees, who are attracted to the plant's flowers for their honeymaking needs. The species designation, *officinalis*, tells us both that the plant was either of male or female gender (as opposed to *officinale*, which refers to neuter gender) and that it was a recognized medicinal plant in medieval (and later) monasteries and apothecaries.

Lemon balm was highly regarded by the alchemist Paracelsus, who well understood its ability to revive an exhausted person. For many centuries, "Carmelite water," a combined extract of lemon balm, lemon peel, nutmeg, and angelica root, was often found to be helpful for soothing nervous headaches and other neuralgic conditions. According to Maude Grieve, melissa was a plant deemed effective at calming the heart and driving off melancholy. It is also a plant praised for its healing powers in one of the earliest Yiddish-language remedy books known to us, the *Seyfer derekh ets ha-khayim* (printed in 1613, most likely in Poland), whose anonymous author states, "dos kraytekh vos do heyst oyf lateynish melisa | un oyf polnish ptshalnik (pl. pszczelnik) | makht shtark den mogen | un den moyekh un dos herts (The herb called melisa in Latin and ptsalnik in Polish strengthens the stomach and the brain and the heart) "

Is it any wonder then that this is a plant ha-Kohen turned to again and again in his own medical work?

In his section on the heart, ha-Kohen implies that the organ's weakness may be due to an emotional state. Lemon balm is one of the plants he singles out as beneficial to counter this condition. Elsewhere, in a recipe, he calls for either a capon or a rooster with its fat removed to concoct a broth into which he adds several herbs, foremost among them lemon balm, borage, and bugloss, to be taken in spoonfuls several times a day to fortify a weak heart.

In a section that seems to address melancholy and hypochondria, ha-Kohen lists the possible outward symptoms of the malady as indigestion, yawning, belching or coughing, abdominal bloating, constipation or diarrhea, "knock-ing" of the stomach or buttocks, particularly on the left side of the body, inter-mittent grunting, a faint heart, chest pains, organ pains, dizziness, fear and trembling, and convulsions, among others. To strengthen the mind and stom-ach against these predicaments, he reminds readers that plants like mint, rose, parsley, and lemon balm are excellent options, perhaps to be taken as infusions.

Ha-Kohen also apprises readers that the stomach is weaker in the summer (possibly because the body doesn't need to generate as much heat and energy to digest food as during the cold winter months) and recommends waiting nine to ten hours between morning and evening meals, while eating less acidic foods. He also wisely pointed out how very good it is to take a trip to the market or gardens and orchards where there is fresh air to be had, as opposed to constantly sitting or spending too much time in a darkened room.

For the effects of scurvy (known in Yiddish as sharbak), an illness caused by a severe vitamin C deficiency, which can manifest as general debility gum disease, or poor wound healing, among other symptoms, ha-Kohen recommended a formula containing the juice of cabbage, lemon balm, and cochlearia, or scurvy grass. Today we know that all three of these plants contain high levels of vitamin C. During ha-Kohen's time this substance had not yet been isolated, although it was understood that certain plants were capable of alleviating the symptoms of scurvy.

In his chapter on women's health, he writes of cachexia, or the wasting of the body. In the language of Sepharad, ha-Kohen writes, this condition was known as "Abu-dah." For the weakness this disease caused, he advises taking iron in the form of the metal rubbed into good wine or cinnamon water with the addition of pennyroyal, lemon balm, artemisia, angelica roots, and elecampane.

This combination of melissa, artemisia, and pennyroyal appears several times in ha-Kohen's chapter on women's health, including in a decoction to be drunk during a difficult birth; the treatment also required the parturient woman to walk and shout so as to awaken dormant blood in the veins and uterus.

In the Polish lands of the late nineteenth century, leucorrhea was treated by folk healers with a number of plants, including infusions of lemon balm or chamomile or the inhalation of fumes from animal stables, remedies that were all documented in Podolia. One cure well known among the nobility and Orthodox clergy in the Pale of Settlement included eating apples into which clean iron nails had been stuck, a recipe that faintly echoes the recommendation of ha-Kohen (whose family was originally from this region) for combating general weakness.

For indeterminate "uterine diseases," remedies varied. In Płoskirow, aside from taking warm baths, one could also be given a tea made with sparrow's dung that had been ground nine times—a magical number in both Jewish and non-Jewish belief systems of Eastern Europe. In Zwinogródka, an infusion or warm compress of lemon balm was favorable. According to Wereńko, healers in the hamlet of Putilkoviči, Belarus (just outside of the shtetl of Lepel', Yiddish Lieplie, in the late nineteenth century more than 50 percent Jewish), advised drinking an infusion of melissa to induce menstruation.

Nausea, lack of appetite, stool retention, stomach pain, and impaired nutrition were considered symptoms of a single ailment—somewhat reminiscent of ha-Kohen's description of cachexia—in Polish lands in the late nineteenth century. Among the herbal remedies most cited by folk healers to treat this affliction was lemon balm.

Headaches were also a common nervous complaint in the former Pale. In the late 1800s it was believed that the condition was most often caused by a cold or possibly an evil eye. In Zbaraż, it was believed that a change in the weather, especially rain starting, could cause a headache, as could (the acquisition of) wealth. Others believed one should never cut one's hair when suffering from a headache. Another superstition called for immersing the face first while bathing to avoid head pains. Around Perejesław (Yiddish Prejaslov, in the late nineteenth century 39 percent Jewish; now Perejaslav, Ukraine), it was believed that urinating while bathing in a river necessitated an immediate exit from the water lest one's head start to hurt. It was also a common belief that nosebleeds prevented such pains, hearkening back to the ancient notion of bloodletting to maintain health. Among many herbal remedies, melissa, drunk as an infusion, was recommended for treating headaches in the town of Olszana.

In Russian folk medicine, according to Müller-Dietz, lemon balm has been employed as a digestive stimulant and for pain relief. It has also treated heart ailments and (epileptic) seizures, and has served as a remedy for melancholy, anemia, strengthening heart and nervous atony, and to help with urination.

According to Glück, lemon balm extracted in wine or water was also relied upon to treat chronic headaches in the mixed communities (Muslim Turks and Bosniaks, Catholic Croats or Orthodox Serbs, and Sephardim) of nineteenth-century Bosnia and Herzegovina, and had additional effective applications: as an external poultice against scrophula; boiled with chamomile to treat uterine prolapse and back pain; and as a mouthwash against toothache. Healers would also boil young plants in wine for bites (spiders, dogs), stings (scorpions), or intestinal distress. Wine or water extractions of melissa were employed to treat asthma, epilepsy, and heart palpitations.

In contemporary Lithuania, the most common medicinal plants grown are medicinal marigold, calendula, valerian, peppermint, chamomile, and lemon balm. Jewish folk healers surveyed there reported that lemon balm was one of the herbs upon which they rely most heavily. Compared to Muslim folk healers also surveyed in Lithuania, melissa ranked higher in usage among local Jews than Muslims, although both communities reported lemon balm as an important plant in their folk materiae medicae.

For muscle tension ("hipertonija"), contemporary Lithuanian Jewish herbalists mix dried motherwort, lemon balm, and peppermint in equal parts. To make one serving, they put one tablespoon of the mixture into boiling water and let it steep twenty to thirty minutes before drinking.

For nervous conditions, these contemporary Jewish herbalists mix equal parts leaves of dried thyme, peppermint, lemon balm, and oregano. To make a relaxing tea, they put one teaspoon of this blend into a glass of boiling water, turn off the heat, and allow the mixture to steep for ten hours before straining. They recommend taking one tablespoon of this tea three times daily before meals for about a month to soothe anxiety.

PRUNUS PADUS | BIRD CHERRY
[PHYSALIS ALKEKENGI, CORNUS MAS, VIBURNUM LANTANA]

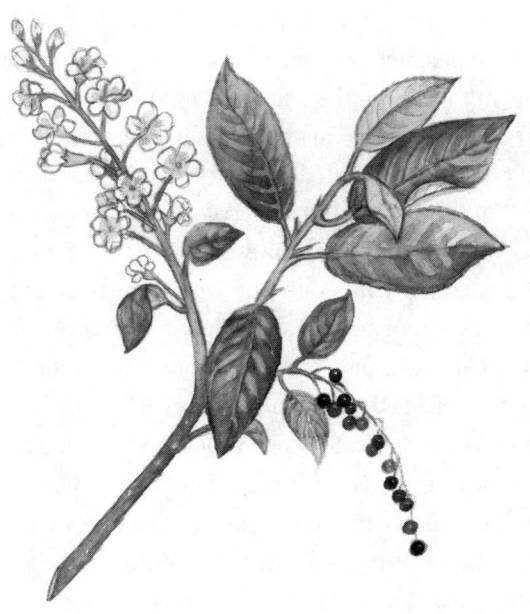

FAMILY   Rosaceae

YIDDISH   פֿייגלקאַרש (fayglkarsh), טשערעמכע (tsheremkhe)

POLISH   Czeremcha zwyczajna, czeremucha, śliwa kocierpka, kocierba, korcipa, korciupa, kotarba, smrodynia

LITHUANIAN   Paprastoji ieva

RUSSIAN   Черёмуха обыкновенная (Čerëmuxa obyknovennaja), черёмуха кистевая (čerëmuxa kistevaja)

GERMAN Gewöhnliche Traubenkirsche, Ahlkirsche, Sumpfkirsche, Elsen-kirsche, Faulbaum

TATAR Шомырт (Šomyrt), гади шомырт (gadi šomyrt)

Various traditional cherry remedies appear in the folk healing literature of the Pale of Settlement at the turn of the last century. Some of these recipes only mention the general term *cherry* (Polish *czeremcha*) with no other modifier, and others are more specific. Whenever possible, we identify a species by its binomial. But before we begin to explore the plant's relationship with humans in Eastern Europe, let's first contrast the two main species of cherry invoked, both of which would have been part of a local folk healer's protocols, and native to the region.

Prunus padus, also known as bird cherry or hackberry, is a small tree with alternate leaves, white flowers, and shiny black drupe berries; it is part of the rose family and is native to temperate Eurasia. *Prunus padus var. padus* is the variety that flourishes throughout Eastern Europe. *Prunus cerasus* has a more complicated botanical backstory, so suffice it to say that both its sour cherry and sweet cherry varieties, which are also somewhat smallish trees in the rose family, bear the more edible fruit we commonly recognize as cherries. They are native to most of Europe, North Africa, and west Asia.

In his day, Dioscorides wrote of *Prunus avium*, the main ancestor of the modern cultivated cherry, *Prunus cerasus*. According to the ancient Greeks, if the fruit were eaten fresh, it could ease the bowels, but if consumed dry, it was known to constipate. For a chronic cough, to stimulate the appetite, to sharpen vision, or to assist those suffering from stones, Dioscorides advised that the gum of the tree be taken in wine.

Maimonides wrote a few lines on the maḥlab plum (or *Prunus mahaleb*), the black cherry tree, but overall does not seem to have devoted attention to the cherry in his medicinal works, which is also true for Hildegard, who wrote of *Physalis alkekengi*, which we discuss shortly.

As for Issachar bar Teller, he refers to cherry only once, in recommending cherry, cooked into a juice and consumed often, as very good for stones. Teller's cherry prescription, perfunctory as it may be, does provide us a glimpse back to early modern applications of Dioscorides's recommendations from a millennium and a half earlier.

Nor does ha-Kohen provide much information on cherry as medicine—but he does include intriguing entries in his glossary for *Physalis alkekengi* and *Cornus mas* (Cornelian cherry), which will also be discussed soon.

In Eastern Europe in the late nineteenth century, both genera (Prunus and Cornus) were part of local plant healing protocols.

In Polish, *Prunus cerasus* is known as wiśnia, "black cherry." According to the surveys we've reviewed, it was common folk medicinal practice in the towns and villages of Ruthenia to stop heavy menstrual bleeding by drinking saffron mixed with a decoction from the peeled bark of seven young cherry sticks. These were to be planed from top to bottom. To induce menstruation, the same formula was brewed, but the bark was peeled from bottom to top. This formula was nearly identical to one reported by folk healers between the world wars in the Ukrainian towns of Barditchev (now Berdychiv), Cherkoss (now Čerkasy), Korosten, Savran, Zwinogródka, Troitsk, Troyaniv, and Vraciivka. Peeling the bark of a healing tree, either up or down, is a recurring ritual in the folkways of Eastern Europe.

For a cough that lasted for a short time—as opposed to a lingering chronic condition that might signal a more serious situation—many herbs were considered. Some of the more common choices were the demulcent linden, marshmallow, or even groats ("kasza"), occasionally cooked with honey. In the towns of Złotopol and Czehryń, tar or sap leaking from the *Prunus cerasus* tree possibly infused in vodka but not specified, was highly reminiscent of Dioscorides's recommendation.

For a catarrh of the stomach, which could manifest with a variety of symptoms including bloating, nausea, lack of appetite, stool retention, stomach pain, and impaired nutrition, herbs were generally the main curative. For abdominal bloating caused by eating fruit, folk healers in the Podolia region recommended eating a cherry pit. For improving appetite, they advised patients to eat freshly dried cherries or a strong tea thereof.

In the late nineteenth century, *Prunus padus*, Polish czeremcha, "bird cherry," was also an ingredient in the folk healer's repertoire, especially for diarrhea. Folk remedies for this condition were borrowed from many sources in Ukraine; for example, a decoction of bird cherry (unspecified part) was a common treatment for the disorder, which again recalls Dioscorides. Another widely sought-out plant in Ukraine for diarrhea was blackberry, in an infused or decocted form, which today is still well known for its efficient astringency to address this condition.

Extreme religious fervor or hysteria is mentioned throughout the litera- ture of the region. In the folk imagination, a frenzied state was attributed to hauntings by evil spirits, or having been bewitched. People who exhibited this behavior are described as being so ecstatic that they caused themselves to spasm (either arms or legs) and even lose consciousness. In the town of Zwiahel, a vodka infusion of bird cherry blossoms was given to calm such a person. This exact remedy is corroborated by the interwar Soviet ethnobotan- ical studies thirty and forty years later.

Many superstitions were also associated with epilepsy. As late as the 1890s, in Poland it was thought that seizures were caused by fear, or that a baby could be born with the condition if its mother were frightened in some way during her pregnancy. There was also a belief that epilepsy was so contagious that it could be caught by looking at a person with the disease. In the town of Zwinogródka, folk healers gave a decoction of the bark and leaves of bird cherry to patients who experienced epileptic seizures.

For skin conditions originating from parasites, such as scabies, a decoc- tion of cherry twigs was one of the remedies reported by a folk healer in Zwinogródka.

Many plants were important treatments for eye ailments. A decoction made from bird cherry twigs was a common remedy in the region; in Nowa-Uszyca, healers provided an infusion of the tree's flowers. Both these remedies again strongly recall the teachings of Dioscorides.

Another method for curing eye disease was to summon the local specialist— called, appropriately, an "eye-licker," for that was what he (and it was gen- erally a man) did—to treat such ailments. These folk healers practiced their trade in every town and village in the Pale, as is attested by many of the yizkor memory books, such as those of Slutsk or Gorodets; Talko-Hryncewicz's eye- licker lived in the town of Ryżanówka.

Between the world wars, bird cherry was investigated as a medicinal plant by Soviet phytopharmacologists. Their findings emphasized its efficacy in ridding humans and other animals of lice. In Ukraine, a decoction of the bark, twigs, leaves, and flowers was applied to affected skin in the towns of Chopovitch (now Chopovyči), Ladizhin (now Ladyžyn), Barditchev, Cherkoss, Zwinogródka, Baturin, Balte (now Balta), Olt-Kosntin (now Starokostjantyniv), and Kresilev (now Krasyliv). This is strongly reminiscent of the Polish studies from the previous century that also focused on the plant's help in curing scabies.

In the Soviet ethnobotanical surveys, it was reported that the tree's bark was used locally for fabric dyes, while its edible berries were made into liqueur, and the berry juice as coloring for wine and spirits; its supple branches were woven into baskets. This last application brings to mind an image from a film documenting pre-war life in the Pale shot by Roman Vishniac (nomen est omen—his last name means "black cherry"). In one of the frames, we see a young Jewish woman in Poland deftly weaving a basket from the twigs of an unidentified tree that may very well have been bird cherry.

Many yizkor memoirists describe cherry, sometimes as treasured food, delicacy, liqueur, or even delicious wine, and other times as a medicine made by mothers and grandmothers. In the town of Gorodets, where survivors remembered their own eye-licker and other folk healers, cherry syrup was a remedy for more serious illnesses, such as measles. And in the shtetl of Mlave (Mława, Poland), "Rifka-Rachel, Wolf Breindels's wife, cooked jams, fermented black berries, cherries, and red forest berries for the entire town as remedies against bellyaches and to promote sweating." In the shtetl of Lubtsh (Ljubča, Belarus), in a litany of mouth-watering recipes, one writer takes a moment to describe "preserves of raspberries ('may there be no need for them!'), cherries, gooseberries, pears, and even of radishes, yes, of radishes, cowberries and whortleberries [. . .] And besides these we must add the big bottles with blackberries, raspberries, and cherries which also served as a medicinal cure."

Contemporary Lithuanian Jewish herbalists also rely on bird cherry—*Prurus padus*—as medicine. In their folk practices, they call on the fruit to relieve diarrhea, reduce intestinal mucosal inflammation, and improve digestion.

My medicinal experience has been with wild cherry as a cough soother. I like to take a small piece of bark like a cough lozenge and observe how simply enjoying the bark's flavor can impart a calm and soothing effect, especially on the cough reflex. I've also brewed a little cherry bark with some honey and sipped this as a tea for similar effect.

Thomas Easley and Rosemary Gladstar both write about *Prunus serctina*, or wild cherry, which is in the same subgenus (*Prunus padus subg. padus*) as Eurasian bird cherry, for its utility as an expectorant for calming coughs. Both also note its ability to improve digestion and promote healthy bowel function; they advise foragers to be mindful of these beautiful trees and only gather cherry's healing bark from already fallen branches.

As promised earlier, there are, along with the taxonomic, a few linguistic oddities we've encountered in looking at cherry healing in the Pale. Three distinct plants have been known as Jew's cherry, although none of them is botanically a cherry, and their ties to any given ethnic group have faded over time. However, we thought it might be worth examining this appellation a little bit more.

Physalis alkekengi, Yiddish כינעזיש לאַמטערל (khinezish lamterl), has many names in English, including winter cherry, Japanese lantern, Chinese lantern, cape gooseberry, strawberry tomato, and ground cherry. In German and French it is known, respectively, as Judenkirsche and Cerise de juif. The species is common across Eurasia, and has been known in traditional medicine both Eastern and Western for centuries (however, it likely originated in the Far East).

Hildegard wrote of this plant's helpfulness in treating cloudy eyes, whereby one was to take a piece of red silk cloth, spread the fruit upon it, and then cover the eyes with the compress before going to sleep. She also advised consuming the fruit for ringing in the ears, stuffiness, and digestive discomforts.

Ha-Kohen mentions a plant called האליקיקאבום (halikikabum), which likely refers to *Physalis alkekengi* (once known as *Physalis halicacabum*). His inclusion of this and other plant remedies from the East (the documentation for this plant in traditional Chinese medicine and Unani medicine dates back to antiquity) demonstrates a general knowledge of many different cultures of medicine.

The plant's suggestive common name "Jew's cherry" is certainly a mystery, and it does raise a question regarding *Physalis alkekengi*'s circuitous journey from its native lands. Does the name refer to those who transported the plant from its place of origin via many trade routes to waiting spice merchants or apothecaries? One possible (and possibly spurious) explanation holds that the lantern portion of the plant bears a strong resemblance to the headgear of medieval European Jews. Whatever the answer, this healing herb deserves to have more attention lavished upon it.

Cornus mas, or dogwood cherry, is a shrub that neither belongs to the rose family nor bears cherries; it is, however, another small tree known in parts of Germany and Switzerland as Judenkirsche, "Jew's cherry." It's also known as Cornelian cherry, and is native to the warmer parts of Europe and Asia; it produces a fruit that resembles a coffee berry containing an ovoid pit.

Schaechter gives the Yiddish name for *Cornus mas* as "דרען" (dren), derived from Slavic (Polish or Ukrainian) *deren*. In the late nineteenth-century Polish surveys, *Cornus mas* was known among folk healers as deren or kizil, a name ostensibly borrowed from Turkic (meaning "red"); the Turkish name for this tree is kızılcık. According to Talko-Hryncewicz, it was common for the Jews of Ruthenia to serve jam made from the fruit as a treatment for fever and as a thirst quencher. He also noted that Jews would pay high prices to procure dren berries.

Zedler's *Universal Lexicon* (1733), an encyclopedia that documents medical knowledge of plants in the early modern era, devotes a long entry to *Cornus mas* and its healing properties. Among other things, Cornelian cherries were known for their cooling, desiccating, and constipating effects, and were deemed effective against dysentery, spitting up blood, and "monthly" problems, as well as in treating elevated temperatures and fevers, which is very reminiscent of the application reported in Jewish communities of the Pale.

Cornelian cherry has a long and varied history as both food and medicine—too much to recount here in detail, but it has been relied upon and enjoyed by many peoples of Europe and elsewhere for centuries.

The backstory of this treat with the curious German name Judenkirsche is another mystery that we hope will be explored further. To begin with, there's evidence that the Cornelian cherry has been planted in Germany since the beginning of the Middle Ages, in (Benedictine) monastery gardens, and in fact, Hildegard, as a Benedictine abbess, recommended the berry against gout and also for digestive troubles. Today wild populations of the tree are found mainly in the south and west of the country, including on the Rhine, near Cologne, and

on the Main River close to Frankfurt, and along the Danube west of Regens-
burg, to name a few locations. All these regions of Germany were formerly
home to the Jews of Ashkenaz, particularly along the Rhine and Main rivers.
Could this possibly explain the plant's striking German name?

Viburnum lantana, the wayfarer or wayfaring tree, is a tree-like shrub native
to central, southern, and western Europe, northwestern Africa, and southwestern Asia. In Schaechter's work, it's known in Yiddish as מעלבוים (melboim), or
in English, flour tree. According to Loew, it is known in Hungarian as zsidó-
cseresznye, "Jew cherry." Is the English name a clue to why Hungarians named
this plant after a people who were also known as "wandering"?

These three stories illustrate how important it can be to follow the linguistic
traces left behind by our herbalist ancestors. Sometimes the most mundane
appellation can be unfolded to reveal the most surprising discoveries.

ROSA CANINA | DOG ROSE

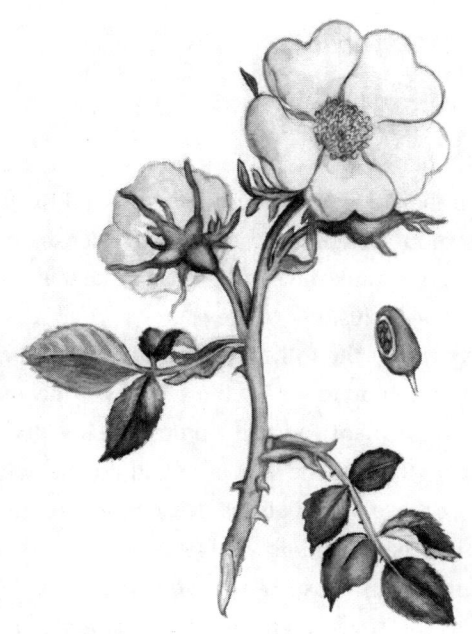

FAMILY Rosaceae

YIDDISH רויז (royz)

POLISH Róża dzika, psia róża, szypszyna

UKRAINIAN Шипшина звичайна (Šypšyna zvyčajna), собача (sobača)

BELARUSIAN Ружа сабачая (Ruža sabačaja), шыпшына сабачая (šypšyna sabačaja), роза (roza), ружа (ruža), шупшына (šupšyna), рожа (roža), шупшыннік (šupšynnik), шыпшына (šypšyna), шыпшыннік (šypšynnik)

LITHUANIAN Paprastasis erškėtis

RUSSIAN   Шиповник собачий (Šipovnik sobačij), роза собачья (roza sobačja), роза канина (roza kanina)

GERMAN   Hundsrose, Heckenrose, Heiderose, Hagrose

TATAR   Эт борыны (Et boryny)

HEBREW   ורד הכלב (vered ha-kelev)

Like so many of the plants we've come to know in our explorations of traditional medicine in the Pale of Settlement, rose—and its entanglement with the peoples of the region—is quite mysterious. In a sense, the tale of rose as a healing entity lingers in a kind of negative space, like that around the smile of the Cheshire Cat, hovering just out of view.

Because the majority of the folk remedies summarized here do not detail the exact species of rose employed by the traditional healers, in this monograph we will refer to the plant generally, unless we specify otherwise.

Rose's healing path through the Pale is a winding one, with many interruptions, and because of these punctuations, it's helpful to look to Dioscorides, for comparison with his seminal knowledge. Nearly two thousand years ago, he identified the white rose (*Rosa sempervirens*) as a large climbing shrub. Today we know it as the "evergreen rose," a perennial species native to the Mediterranean. For the ancient Greek physician, its medicinal portion was its fruit, the rose hip, and when prepared correctly, it was beneficial for checking diarrhea.

Of the rose genus writ large, Dioscorides also wrote about its cooling and contracting qualities, and that if the plant's petals were processed and stored properly, they could be made into ointments for the eyes. Many of his rose remedies remained staples of the European materia medica for centuries: dried roses boiled in wine for relief of headaches, earaches, eye pain, and gum pain—not to mention pains in the anus, uterus, or stomach. Most interesting is Dioscorides's direction for erysipelas: the roses themselves are chopped up without being squeezed, then are plastered directly onto the skin infection.

Nearly a thousand years later, the abbess Hildegard also looked to the rose for eye health and clarity of vision; she observed that the rose leaf was helpful for drawing the pus from a weeping ulcer. Rose was part of a formula for bringing on delayed menses in young women, too. Finally, the abbess empha-sized that the addition of rose to any formulation made that recipe more potent.

Around the same period, Maimonides wrote of the wild rose (*Rosa canina*) as both kitchen and pharmacy herb, from which an astringing sugared preserve could be prepared.

By the time Issachar bar Teller published his remedy book in Yiddish, rose was such a favored ingredient that he includes the herb no less than twenty-five times in his recipes, by far the most common ingredient in his materia medica. Like Dioscorides, and possibly directly influenced by him, Teller found rose's various preparations beneficial for the head. In the case of headache, he was careful to check for any dry conditions that may have caused the discomfort—namely constipation—so before dispensing his medications, he offers a few prophylactic suggestions, such as dietary alterations and bloodletting. For a headache caused by heat, equal parts rose water, rose vinegar, and oil of roses are to be mixed together and then applied lukewarm as a compress to the forehead and temples. For eye weakness, redness, or irritation, rose, once more and in different guises, is a prominently featured ingredient in Teller's treatments. Continuing with maladies of the head, Teller addresses oral health with several formulas that include aromatic and astringent rose, all of which strongly recalls the advice of Dioscorides.

For "redness in the face," Teller describes another condition wherein the body is reacting to an excess of heat. To cool the constitution and an overly ruddy complexion, he suggests adjusting the diet by excluding sharp and salty food and instead eating cooling vegetables, such as sorrel, spinach, and carrot, for example. He also advises an internal cleanse before applying topical med-ications. One such ointment he calls "water for red spots on the face," which included two separate rose preparations to be applied with linen cloths on reddened areas.

If read closely, Teller's description may be a practical remedy for ery-sipelas, because many of his ointment's components are very similar to folk remedies that were later documented in the Pale in the late nineteenth century for treating this skin infection (as we discuss elsewhere in this book).

Teller foregrounds rose in many of his preparations for counteracting diar-rhea in both children and adults, for cramps in the abdomen, for a "stitch in the side," for strengthening the heart, and for women's menstrual health, again recalling the herbalists of centuries past. Also of note in Teller's guide: rose vinegar as part of a regimen for keeping the plague at bay.

Some decades later, ha-Kohen wrote of rose in its many medicinal forms. In his section on healing trees, he identifies rose in four languages, including Yiddish, and writes poetically of gathering the flower and its medicine in gardens. He notes rose's widely known ability to strengthen the organs and gladden the heart, as well as its astringing actions on the stomach and its cooling ability for the liver. Like Dioscorides and Maimonides before him, he distinguishes between the red variety and the white, the former being effective against diarrhea, and the latter serving more as a laxative. He also praises rose's ability to treat "corrupted flesh," and mentions how some species are so aromatic that their scent may waft from afar (whereas others may be much less beckoning).

Ha-Kohen's identification of rose in several languages makes his work challenging to interpret. Both in his glossary and throughout the text of *Ma'aseh Tuviyah*, he uses two different Hebrew words for the plant—*vered* and *shushanah*, as well as the Latin *rosa*, the Yiddish *royz*, and the Turkish *gül*, making it difficult to determine which species or variety he is referencing, or whether the terminology is interchangeable.

To attempt a smidgen of clarity, we've separated out his remedies according to the term used.

Under "rozato," ha-Kohen refers to the diarrhodon, a pre-modern complex medical formula in which rose serves as the main ingredient. This is one of his several recommendations for head pain.

Under "roza," he recommends that the heart be strengthened with rose, again in a diarrhodon formulation, but also with a conserve of roses—possibly in sugar—that includes borage, bugloss, etrog peel, nutmeg, and cinnamon.

Under "shushanah" (from my understanding, in modern Hebrew this word actually refers to the lily, but ha-Kohen includes it as a synonym for rose), he refers to shushanah as, variously, a red rose in a separate chart that focuses on the urinary tract; juiced as a laxative; as part of an enema in the guise of rose honey; a treatment for eye disorders; an aid for oral health while treating scurvy (a disease caused by a deficiency of vitamin C); a balm for an upset stomach characterized by an involuntary hiccough that ha-Kohen identifies in Latin as a singultus, in "the language of Sepharad" as sanglotu, and in Yiddish as shokin (cf. German *schlucken*, "to swallow"); a treatment for melancholia in which the brain is purified with good wine and spices, including roses, mint, parsley, and melissa; as part of several remedies to expel intestinal worms; as an oil infusion to cool the kidneys; as an aid for counteracting undigested food, in a condition he refers to in Yiddish as shtal (cf. German *Stall*, "stall"), that may include diarrhea. For this he calls for oil of roses, along with other herbs such as pomegranate, quince, and barley water.

Before divulging his formulas for podagra (also known as gout), which include several instances of rose, he advises first taking iron bleached in fire, or a burning ceramic tile, upon which should be poured the urine of a young boy, so that its steam might rise and provide relief to the painful gouty area. Soon after prescribing this curious method, ha-Kohen mentions that such a remedy works better for younger men who are accustomed to working and eating and drinking moderately, as opposed (presumably) to a more sedentary scholarly sort. After this editorial aside, ha-Kohen invokes two superstitions that were current at the time: First, we learn that someone who suffers from panaritium (a swollen infected finger, like a felon) and wants to be rid of it should place the afflicted digit into a cat's ear, thereby transferring the infection to the cat. Next we are told of a patient who would cut infected parts of tissue from their feet and stuff them into a hole in an oak tree in the belief that this would cure their gout. But, ha-Kohen assures us, old wives' tales are of no medical value to him.

These passages are interesting today because they show the continuum of healing practices at this time, from the more scientific and "advanced," to the very sympathetic and magical, and everything in between, much of which the contemporary reader may find antiquated, if not a bit wacky.

In the case of podagra, ha-Kohen was also interested in cleansing the body with a good sweat, and this was to be accomplished with a formula that included roses, which was to be taken at night before going to sleep.

The plague was still an enormous health concern at this time (late seventeenth century), and ha-Kohen wrote of fumigation with herbs such as the rotem or retama tree (in Hebrew, רותם), which he also identifies in Latin as juniper (a contested subject among biblical commentators), lign-aloe (Aquilaria), and frankincense (Boswellia). Also beneficial for purifying dangerous plague-rid-den air were rose vinegar and rue vinegar, which may point to rue's apotropaic reputation.

For protecting the eyes of a child, in a case of smallpox, ha-Kohen recom-mended rose water. To soften an abscess, rose honey was mixed with other substances and applied to the area.

Under Hebrew "vered," rose water is part of a protocol for safe bloodlet-ting; rose by this name (as a salve) figures very prominently in ha-Kohen's writings on women's health.

Fragrant rose was also helpful for cleansing the body of the newborn after the expulsion of meconium. To reduce teething pain in an infant, he recom-mends taking quince seed and psyllium (plantain seed), soaked in rose water or water in which mallow has been boiled, and putting this pap into a cloth for the child to suck on.

Aside from distancing himself from idleness and contemplation, abstaining from lying on his back, but rather assiduously studying the Torah, the over-heated male could be cured from the affliction of lust by means of antiperspi-rant remedies. One of ha-Kohen's specially formulated mixtures features seeds of "portulaka" (purslane), "agnus-castus" (Vitex or "chaste tree"), plaintain, and rue, all combined with aromatic rose in sugar.

In the many decades following the publication of Ma'aseh Tuviyah, the path that rose takes through healing in the Pale manifests itself as a mysterious detour, wandering into somewhat uncharted territory. But before we head in that direction, let's recognize the many ways rose has been celebrated in the region. There is no doubt that the plant was, and continues to be, a popular first name; rose is often part of a last name, or a place name; and metaphor-ically and otherwise, rose holds an important position in world literature. In Pokuttja, Ukraine, for instance, in an area that borders Podolia and Bukovina, a Ukrainian song recounts a blooming rose that grew from the drops of blood of a murdered lover (similar motifs occur in folk songs of the British Isles). Aesthetically, rose has been a favorite embroidery pattern throughout the folk cultures of the region, including the Ashkenazim, who decorated Torah man-tles, Pesach towels, and ketubos (marriage contracts) with its intricate image. Rose has also occupied an honored place in the garden, not just in Eastern

Europe, of course, but worldwide; and many cuisines rely on the power of rose to enchant and delight.

In Ashkenazi communities prior to the Second World War, all these qualities were well known and well loved, and were documented in yizkor memory books, in poetry, garden memories, and even a recipe or two, such as this pre-war rose preserve recipe recorded in a letter from a town near the shtetl of Lida, Belarus, by a woman named Frida:

Half pound of roses, removing the petals and then grinding them

Two cups sugar

Two glasses water

Juice from two lemons

Boil the sugar in the water, add cleaned rose petals, and cool until liquid thickens. Add lemon juice and boil for five minutes.

Author Sophie Knab also writes of a similar recipe found in regional Polish cuisines.

So with rose's presence in the Pale firmly rooted, we can now divert our attention to the more "woo" aspects that have been attributed to this herb. As late as the turn of the twentieth century, many people suffered from a skin condition known medically as erysipelas (Greek: "red skin"), but to folk healers in the region, the disease was called rose (Yiddish royz, shoshanah; Polish/Ukrainian roża/roža). Readers of *Ashkenazi Herbalism* may recall one such healer, Sore Mordkhe-Yoysef of Biłgoraj, Poland, who cured a royz by burning a piece of flax and fumigating the infection while intoning a banishing spell and then afterward spreading honey over the area, finally binding it up (with the cloth). This is almost the exact same remedy reported in the late nineteenth-century Polish surveys in the town of Jurkow near Zwiahel. Talko-Hryncewicz documented other local names for this condition, such as a byszycha (likely borrowed from Latin vesica, "blister"). Contemporary medicine treats erysipelas with penicillin and other antibiotics, and understands the disease as a skin infection of the upper dermis, caused by bacteria and characterized by its raised edges and fiery red color. But in the Pale, a royz (or byszycha) was a skin disease that was believed to be caused by bad

air or enchantment; prior to the Second World War, Eastern European traditional healers were highly sought out for the secret magical techniques they
employed to heal this condition.

These magical techniques were among the most likely to leave behind
evidence of a highly syncretic common healing culture. Just as the An-sky
expeditions recorded opshprekherins whose charms against the evil eye were
identical in both form and language to those of their Ukrainian šeptuxa neighbors, so too did Karaim Jewish healers borrow from their Polish znachorka
neighbors: according to Zajączkowski, one Karaim charm for banishing a royz
invoked Lord Jesus walking on the water, and walking through the fields, and
"Lord Jesus held three roses in his hand."

In the early stages of this disease, the Polish surveys of the 1890s reported,
for traditional healers, bloodletting was commonly regarded as effective, but
more often than not, plants were part of the sympathetic healing protocol. In
the town of Zakopane, a red garden rose was burned so that its smoke would
fumigate the infection, which was then covered with soil taken from the base
of the rose bush.

In Lviv, hair snipped from a cat's tail was burned on coals and the smoke
inhaled by the patient. A remedy recorded in Zwinogródka may have been the
most widely used (we have encountered other versions that describe similar
methods for treating this malady), wherein a piece of canvas, likely woven
from linen, was rolled into a tube the width of a pinky. This was lit at one end
and the resulting ash was applied to the diseased skin.

The type of traditional healer who would have performed these healing
rituals is not specifically identified in the Polish surveys. But if you're familiar with our earlier research in *Ashkenazi Herbalism,* you may recognize this
anonymous informant as a baba (Yiddish bobe)—variously known as an opshprekherin, znachorka, znaxarka, or šeptuxa—an older woman who would have
worked with plants and other substances, along with divination, ritual, and
charms and incantations, a familiar figure in the towns and villages of the
Pale. She specialized in treating the royz or any condition that might have been
caused by an evil eye. This was the woman Abraham Rekhtman encountered
during the An-sky Jewish ethnographic surveys, the one who knew "hundreds
of ways to cure a patient," and as we have discovered, the Polish surveys

further reveal many of the ancient forgotten healing practices of these vanished folk healers.

Many of the magical remedies practiced by regional folk healers provide clues to their ancient origins, such as one preventive measure that required washing the face with water prepared with a few drops of the spirit of rose flower, or that of white lily, which was reportedly common practice among the Polish landed gentry. What's significant about this remedy is its allusion to the Hebrew word *shushanah* (which can mean either "rose" or "lily"). The two "interchangeable" flowers applied to this specific disease by local folk healers suggests an association with ha-Kohen's earlier conflation of shushanah for rose.

To prevent the recurrence of a royz, one folk healer required a whole lemon with peel to be taken internally, but the preparation and administration are not provided in the text of the surveys. The specific ingredient of citrus fruit is unusual for this time and place, and it is highly reminiscent of another method (summarized by Marek Tuszewicki) employed by opshprekherins who were known to opbrenen a royz (Yiddish, "burn off a rose") by covering the affected area with something red, such as thick paper or flannel, or another soft fabric, or a sack that had held an etrog. The healer then sprinkled the royz with chalk, white lead, or lye, in order to "draw out the weakness." The technique of covering infected skin with linen or other plant fabric was also employed by the opshprekherin Sore Mordkhe-Yoysef of Biłgoraj, who performed a wax-pouring ritual while murmuring an incantation to banish a "dark rose."

The Polish ethnobotanical surveys record that these methods for treating a royz were very common, and most likely were the preferred prescription for those suffering from this often dangerous condition.

In the town of Zwinogródka, an unnamed healer treating a royz performed a ritual almost identical to that described by ha-Kohen: specifically, his advice to remove an enchantment or an evil eye from a child (see *Arctostaphylos uva-ursi*, p. 45). Two centuries later, Talko-Hryncewicz's unnamed healer acquired a fresh horseshoe that was tossed three times into boiling water; the water was then given to the patient to drink in order to cure the royz. If we recall the causes for this disease as detailed in the Polish surveys, it follows that this particular ritual would be necessary to remove an evil eye, as diagnosed by the folk healer as the cause for the patient's skin condition. The number three is mentioned in many sympathetic remedies because it was (along with the number nine) a powerful magical number for many peoples of the region: Adam's grandmother, whose parents and older sisters came from Pułtusk, Poland, would always ward off an ayn hore by spitting and saying "tfu tfu tfu" (a charm common among both Jews and Lipka Tatars).

Several examples of roses being a specific remedy for cases of erysipelas—along with other diseases—hail from a smattering of settlements. Around Płock, close to Mlave, a town whose Jewish inhabitants documented a great deal of their local folk medicinal traditions, a sick child (illness unspecified) was taken out before sunrise to sit beneath a rose bush. Their escort was to return home without looking back. When they went to retrieve the child, the return home also required not looking back. This was to be performed for three days in a row. Close to the town of Sieradz, field rose and its symbiotic lichens were used to treat a royz. In the early twentieth century, in the town of Chruszczów, near Lublin, the Polish ethnographer Adam Fischer observed that a royz, if slow to heal, could be cured with a fumigation of blessed rose or an application of soil from a rose bush "which has never seen the dead." Fischer also observed that in nearby Turobin (in the late nineteenth century 63 percent Jewish), after "ordering the disease" (banishing it with a charm), folk healers recommended washing patients with a cooled decoction of wild rose (*Rosa canina*) roots.

In the city of Tarnów (Yiddish Tarne, in the late nineteenth century 42 percent Jewish), rose hips, onion, or warm milk were applied to skin ulcers, which may have been another euphemism for erysipelas. In the village of Królówka, near Kraków, part of white rose was mixed with vinegar to treat either erysipelas or burned skin. Folk healers in the mountain resort town of Zakopane treated advanced cases of the disease by covering it with red garden rose. But in Dwory, a settlement close to Oświęcim (Auschwitz), the best medicinal choice for treating erysipelas was rose water.

Polish sources such as Fischer also tell of rose hips for healing a number of ailments, including kidney stones, or how the plant's root was beneficial for curing madness (in the Sieradz region). Healers here also recommended drinking rose hip tea to combat consumption. In the Chełm district, the leaves were applied to swellings in the neck, which might be derived from Hildegard's work.

In Sokołów, Poland, many recipes counseled relying on rose to handle vision health, which strongly suggests a long-standing influence on local folk healing practices from both Dioscorides and Hildegard, not to mention Teller and ha-Kohen. Some examples documented include a simple compress made from juice squeezed from the flower and prepared with wine and applied to cool inflamed eyes. Another recipe for improving weak eyesight called for taking the blossom, along with equal parts cornflower, a bit of cumin, and rosemary, all cut coarsely and macerated in good rye vodka, which was then left in the sun for eight days. The strained liquid would then be gently rubbed onto the eyelids in the morning and evening (care being taken to avoid getting any in the eyes). Rose was heralded for its significant role in counteracting pulmonary consumption, as well as for a "decoction of pale red roses in a plum glaze to give skin diseases and rashes a slow cleansing effect," which possibly referred to cases of erysipelas. In Krzośniewice, Poland, another remedy called for incensing a patient with the plant's leaves to soothe their eye pain.

After the Second World War, in Argentina, rose is recorded by plant healers in the diaspora Ashkenazi community as a stomach astringent, as a support for heart health, and as a wash for eye pain. In contemporary Lithuania, Jewish folk healers recommend taking *Rosa canina* flowers and hips to supplement the diet with vitamins, and as an immune system booster.

It may not seem obvious at first glance, but there's something mysterious about rose's medicinal journey through the Pale, metaphorically transforming itself, or being transformed, along the route, from an aromatic flower to an inflamed skin infection that folk healers treated via magical means. In its metamorphosis, rose's many curative preparations, such as rose vinegar and rose oil, largely disappeared from the ethnographic or medical record, leaving behind something of a fossilized relief depicting a magical healer, be she opshprekherin or znachorka, an ailing patient, a burning cloth, and a beseeching incantation demanding rose's banishment. When and how did this healing transition take place?

A survey of the broader Jewish diaspora can help us trace this winding path. In contrast with the royz affliction of the Pale, herbalist and author Naomi

Spector reminds us that the rose represents health and vitality in Jewish culture as expressed in Jewish languages. For example, the Yiddish phrase "frisn vi a royz" (fresh as a rose) echoes a Sephardi folk song lyric: "tu sos fresca como la rosa."

Spector also notes that popular Sephardi folk songs in Ladino/Judezmo invoke many of the characteristics associated with rose in the Jewish imagination: love, beauty, passion, grief, and longing. To help me through a particularly sad time in my life, an herbalist friend, Naomi Stein, sent me a healing bottle of rose oil she had made from the flowers that grow in her garden.

The rose is also part of holiday, food, and medicinal traditions in Jewish communities across southwest Asia, North Africa, and the Mediterranean. In these communities, rose water and rose syrup are frequently found in their culinary and medicinal practices.

It's hard to ignore roses. At the very least, they're visually captivating. Most of them emanate a distinctive fragrance that conjures itself in the imagination through simple visualization of the velvety flower. And yes, rose's other best-known characteristics are its treacherous thorns, the tiny swords that protect the plant from even its most ardent admirers. You have to respect a plant so confident in its duality.

In our garden, we inherited many rose varieties, and of them all, I tend to gravitate toward the climbing Cécile Brünner. One of my herbal instructors recommended suffusing the plant's pale pink petals in honey, and I've followed this simple recipe ever since. As a jam, or in tea, its delicate scent and flavor can evoke spring even during the coldest, darkest months. To make the rose-infused honey, take fresh petals from the blossoms of a Cécile Brünner climbing rose (one not sprayed with insecticide) and immerse them in a honey of your choice. The mixture will be ready in around a month. You don't have to strain out the petals to enjoy this syrup as a sweetener on foods or in beverages.

RUBIA TINCTORUM | MADDER

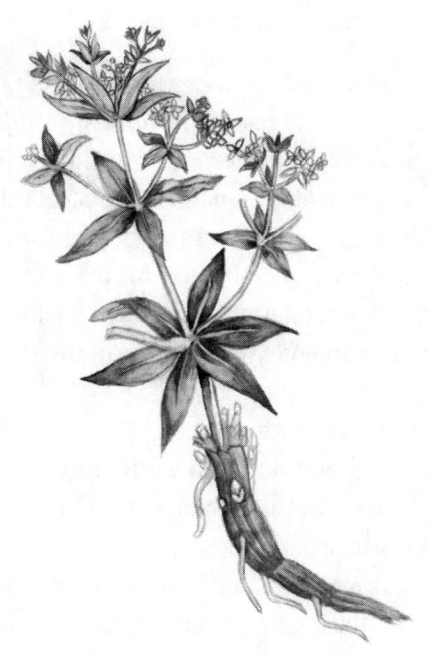

FAMILY   Rubiaceae

YIDDISH   כאַנעפּויעס (khanepoyes)

POLISH   Marzana barwierska, marena, marina, krop, barwica, brocz, czerwone korzenie, czerwony gryk, knap, krap, marzanka, marzann, marzawu, marzanna, marzka, reta

UKRAINIAN   Марена фарбувальна (Marena farbuval'na), марена красильна (marena krasyl'na)

LITHUANIAN   Raudė

RUSSIAN Марена красильная (Marena krasil'naja), ализарин (alizarin), зеленица (zelenica), бруск (brusk), крап (krap), красильный корень (krasil'nyj koren'), марина (marina), марзана (marzana)

GERMAN Krapp, Färberkrapp, Echte Färberröte

One of the main criteria we used for choosing a plant for our materia medica was that Mordkhe Schaechter, in his *Plant Names in Yiddish*, identify it with a uniquely Yiddish name. *Rubia tinctorum*, or madder, fell into this category, although it is relatively under-documented in the plant medicinal record. On the other hand, madder was well known for its applications in other diverse folkways of the Pale of Settlement, and, for this reason, we took the opportunity to highlight both *Rubia tinctorum*'s medicinal qualities and its role in the many traditional and often forgotten handicrafts of the shtetlekh and derfer of Eastern Europe.

Rubia tinctorum is a plant with whorls of four or six sharp-edged leaves and axillary, lateral flowers; it is native to western and central Asia, and naturalized in many regions of central and southern Europe, where it mostly prefers hedges, thickets, and waste areas.

Years ago, when I was painting in oils, one of my favorite pigments was the glaze-like rose madder. Mixed with titanium or zinc white, it gave an opaque pink cake-icing texture. At the time, I had only a faint inkling that rose madder was derived from plants.

Rubia tinctorum is not really a component in any contemporary Western herbal remedy, so I was intrigued to note its presence in the medicinal formulations of the Pale of Settlement at the turn of the twentieth century. My curiosity got the better of me, and in my determination to understand the plant's connection with the Jews of Eastern Europe, I followed a trail that led to some very unexpected places.

This is a history of the long-forgotten trades once commonly practiced in the Pale, the lost arts that required a high level of craftmanship, and often a bit of herbal knowledge as well. These "parnosses" (Yiddish for "livelihoods") were handed down in families for centuries. Among the most notable were glassmaking (whence the common Jewish name Glazier or Glazer), rope making (see *Cannabis*, p. 73), iron-mongering, leatherworking, watchmaking, soapmaking (see *Saponaria officinalis*, p. 187), and fabric-related crafts, including linen and wool weaving, sheep shearing, spinning, the manufacture of volikes ("felt or bast boots," see *Tilia europaea*, p. 199), the knitting of socks and other garments, various needlecrafts, and the dyeing of textiles. Also important were cultivation of and trade in medicinal plants such as hops and herbs for making liqueurs and distilled spirits (gentian, wormwood, anise, etc.).

In *A Modern Herbal*, Maude Grieve includes a brief history of *Rubia tinctorum*, reviewing the contributions of this ancient source for pigments on the red spectrum. The plant's roots yield alizarin, the main ingredient in the manufacture of the madder lake pigments that are more familiar to painters as "rose madder" and "alizarin crimson." The term *lake* is derived from the French *lacquer*, a linguistic trace of the pigment's translucent quality. These days, however, the colors once extracted from the plant are more commonly synthesized chemically in industrial quantities, for reasons of economy and greater color stability. Even so, artists can still find a number of paint manufacturers who carry on the age-old tradition of producing plant-based colors such as those from *Rubia tinctorum*.

Of all the forgotten herbal arts necessary to keep communities in the Pale humming along, aside from folk healing, it was the preparation of fabrics that required the most plant knowledge. Fabric dyeing is an ancient art: archaeological evidence from thousands of years ago indicates that woolens and plant-derived textiles were enhanced with plant-based colors.

In the case of wool, it must be stripped of its natural oils before it will accept any tinting. Washing is done according to a process called "fulling" in English, by practitioners known as fullers, or in Yiddish as valkers (think of the door-to-door brush sellers of yore). In ancient times, a combination of the saponin-rich roots of soapwort (see *Saponaria officinalis*, p. 187) along with potash and soda was used in this process. These ingredients are not only important for degreasing wool but are also necessary for manufacturing glass products, such as windows or storage vessels. Both glassmaking and dyeing were skilled trades passed down through generations of Jewish families throughout the diaspora; as is often the case with ancient guilds, manufacturing techniques were generally closely guarded trade secrets. Incidentally, it's interesting to note, as historian Samuel Kurinsky has observed, that if one were curious about the migratory patterns of world Jewry over time, their trail through the diaspora is made visible by consulting the archives for records of soda and potash sales.

A cursory consultation of the yizkor memory books yields nearly two dozen accounts of dyers and dyeing and related fabric crafts. In Białystok, Poland, for example, where Jews made up almost 80 percent of the population at the beginning of the twentieth century, the textile industry was a thriving one, with spinning, weaving, knitting, and dyeing factories throughout the city that employed a large percentage of the population.

Further north, the town of Utena (Yiddish Utian) was home to one of the oldest Jewish communities in eastern Lithuania, dating back to the sixteenth century (in 1897, Jews made up 75 percent of the town's population); their local economy was based on trade in flax, skins, and boar bristles. The Utena yizkor states that all seven dyeing plants in the town, in addition to the wool, flax, knitting, and textile mills, were owned by Jews.

To the west of Utena lies Šeduva, Lithuania (Yiddish Shadeve), famous for its black-headed sheep; for many years the economic life of this town (in 1897, 61 percent Jewish) was dominated by trade, farming, and crafts: many local Jews were farmers who sold their produce to merchants from St. Petersburg and Riga. There were two flour mills, a dye works, and a weaving factory all owned by the Cohen family.

One survivor from Bełchatów (Yiddish Belkhatov), near Łódź, recalled, with some levity, that the lifeblood of the town, its dyeing and tanning factories along the river, gave it "a not so impressive aroma."

The production process for madder would certainly corroborate his memory. The color "turkey red," derived from the root of *Rubia tinctorum* and reputed to be fadeless, was developed in India and spread west from there to Turkey. The ancient process involved more than twenty steps from beginning to finished product; it called for blood, oil, rancid fat, charcoal, cow manure, dog dung, and the liquid contents of the animals' stomachs. Accordingly, many villages where these factories were located housed only the dyers and their families.

The Bełchatów yizkor describes the strength and sophistication of this manufacturing economy, which, given its maintenance of traditional handicrafts, likely continued to rely on natural vegetable dyes even as more "advanced" industrial economies moved toward chemical synthetics like alizarin:

It would be a mistake to picture the Belchatower factories like an industrial unit undertaking, where workers worked at machines in a mechanized pro- duction process. Until the beginning of the twentieth century there were not, in general, any mechanized machinery or factories in Belchatow. The whole production was established by handwork. There were no spinning machines. All of Belchatow and vicinity were working on hand textile machines.

In the literature regarding Jewish dyers throughout the ages, only a handful of dye herbs are disclosed. Perhaps this is because color formulations were, and are, proprietary recipes and hence closely guarded (some traditional dyeing cultures rely on certain dyes to be infused as a protective measure against counterfeiting). The plants most often mentioned in the Jewish plant trade of the medieval era include sumac (Rhus) for red, saffron (*Crocus sativus*) and reseda (*Reseda luteola*) for yellow, and indigo (*Indigofera tinctoria*) for blue.

This last plant was often a source of religious controversy, in the produc- tion of the blue telekhet dye required for making the tzitzit fringes of tallis prayer shawls (various candidates for the "correct" telekhet source include pigments derived from sea snails, cuttlefish, *Isatis tinctoria*, or woad, and indigo, all of which have been proposed by religious and scholarly authorities). It's not difficult to picture a scenario where possible disputes over halakhic fidelity in matters of dyeing might have played out in the shtetl of Dubrowna, near Vitebsk (now Dubroŭna, Belarus). Dubrowna is notable as the site of one of the first and only factories where woolen tallises were produced. The Dubrowna yizkor describes in detail labor struggles at the plant: a culture of cost cutting (both in labor and materials) suggests that the factory owners and managers may well have favored profit over tradition in the dyeing process.

Aside from its commercial exploitation, like that of other vegetable dyes, in the early years of the twentieth century *Rubia tinctorum* was sought out for its healing abilities.

Some applications of the plant may be traced back to ha-Kohen; he identi- fied *Rubia tinctorum* as a medicinal plant, providing its names in Latin, Turk- ish, and Hebrew, פואה (poah).

Mordkhe Schaechter, in *Plant Names in Yiddish*, reports a similar name, khanepoies. Considered together, the names' likeness suggests a very old relationship between Jews and this herb.

The recorded folk medicinal applications of *Rubia tinctorum* in Eastern Europe are concerned primarily with urinary health. This may be a legacy of Dioscorides, who wrote of the plant's affinity for the urinary tract:

> *The root is slender, long, red, and diuretic; it is for this reason that, when drunk with hydromel, it helps the jaundiced, also those suffering from hip ailments and paralytics; it also drives out much thick urine and at times even blood. But the people who drink it must bathe daily. The stem with the leaves, when drunk, helps those bitten by wild animals, and the fruit, when drunk with oxymel reduces the spleen. Applied as a pessary, the root draws the menstrual period and embryos/fetuses and treats dull-white leprosies when anointed with vinegar.*

In twentieth-century official Soviet herbal medicine, according to Nosal' and Nosal', the rhizome and root of madder were valued for their diuretic and antispasmodic properties. They also note that in twentieth-century Soviet folk medicine, madder rhizome decoctions were taken for jaundice, constipation, rheumatic lower back pain, rickets, and as a diuretic. Both Nosal' and Nosal' and Gammerman and Grom report that in Soviet official medicine, madder rhizome and root extracts were clinically tested and approved as treatments for kidney, gall, and urinary stones. In central Asian folk medicine (specific region and tradition not identified), madder rhizomes taken with honey healed jaundice and "memory loss."

In Russian folk medicine, however, according to Deriker, in the mid-nineteenth-century province of Tomsk, *Rubia tinctorum* was used for "cleansing" (treatment unspecified) when menstruation was irregular.

Deriker also provides two regional appellations for *Rubia tinctorum* that we think may shed some light on the secret formulae of the triankas of Eastern Europe (see "Trianke," p. 207): brošč' and brusk. We suspect this might be a clue to one of the mystery ingredients in a complex formulation, the "roots against weakness" offered by Jewish spice merchants in the town of Sobolivka, Ukraine, in the mid-nineteenth century, a recipe that the legendary Russian botanist Annenkov was unable to fully interpret: he left a question mark next to its requirement of twelve "brunški," which, in western Ukraine, may well have been a regional diminutive variation on the Russian brošč' or brusk. Given *Rubia tinctorum*'s role in the folk medicine of the region in matters dealing with the urinary tract and women's health (such as the menstrual treatment mentioned earlier), we think it is a good candidate for the mysterious "brunški" in the complex formulations local folk healers of Ukraine prescribed for postpartum support.

According to Glück, in Bosnia, where we have seen that a similarly interwoven culture of healing among Jewish, Christian (both Catholic and Orthodox), and Muslim healers was well established by the end of the nineteenth century, madder (broć) played a similar role in women's health. Healers relied upon it to treat amenorrhea, and also recommended steam baths of madder leaves to induce labor and hasten the expulsion of the afterbirth (placenta and discharge).

Rubia tinctorum was also credited with magical healing powers. As an apotropaic, madder, along with rue and monkshood, was widely believed to ward off the walking dead. According to Talko-Hryncewicz, in Olchowiec, Poland (a small village with five Jewish families, not far from the town where my grandparents grew up), *Rubia tinctorum* was part of a remedy for dislocations and fractures in young children. If an infant tilted its head to one side, or could not sit up properly, or needed help standing, a sprain or fracture was blamed. One way to cure this was to give the child warm-water baths three times a week in conjunction with "measuring"—pulling the elbows to opposite sides of the child's knees until they met up. This treatment was common among both Polish peasants and local Jews. But in the town of Zwinogródka, children with the same condition were given infusions of the leaves and stems of raspberry or madder root.

SALVIA OFFICINALIS | SAGE

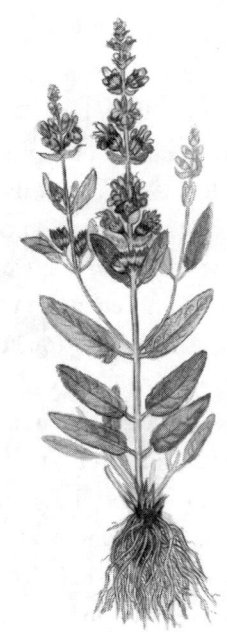

FAMILY   Lamiaceae

YIDDISH   שאַלוויע (shalvie)

POLISH   Szałwia lekarska

UKRAINIAN   Шавлія лікарська (Šavlija likars'ka)

LITHUANIAN   Vaistinis šalavijas

RUSSIAN   Шалфей лекарственный (Šalfej lekarstvennyj)

GERMAN   Echter Salbei, Garten-Salbei, Küchensalbei, Heilsalbei

HEBREW   מרווה רפואית (marvah refuait)

As any herbalist will tell you, deciding which plants to highlight for an audience is a daunting task: you don't want to leave anyone out or feel like you're picking favorites. This was the dilemma that confronted me after I'd written two dozen monographs for this volume and had to commit to the last one. As luck would have it, a good friend had unexpectedly mailed me a surprise package; it arrived just as I was having trouble trying to decide on one more plant ally. Inside the little box I found a treasure trove of fun things like cardamom candies, a notebook, imported watercolors—which would become part of the illustrations for this book—and underneath all this bounty was a small letterpress illustration of a sage plant. As soon as I saw it, I knew the universe had made my decision for me (and unbeknownst to my friend, who told me she didn't even remember putting the card in the package when I called to thank her both for her gifts and for making my decision that much easier).

Like so many of the herbs that were important curatives and spices in the Pale of Settlement, sage is a transplant to Eastern Europe. Possessing a single taproot with many rootlets, and an upright stem branching into twigs with dense and finely notched wrinkled, oblong, and resinous leaves, it's native to the warm Mediterranean climates, but unlike rosemary, another plant in the Salvia genus, sage was able to survive and establish itself in the cooler temperate climes further to the north—and consequently never required drying or powdering to survive the overland voyage. It simply set down roots once it arrived at its destination and was soon adopted by the humans living there as a well-loved and naturalized spice, medicine, and garden habitué.

I wonder about the travails of these migrant plants that travel long distances from their sunny seaside homes to distant lands like Poland or Ukraine or Pennsylvania. How do they survive their long voyages?

My great-grandfather was born in Gomel, Belarus, in the late nineteenth century. Legend has it that as a young boy he was forced to leave home (cruel stepmother) and subsequently joined a caravan. His traveler's life across the length and breadth of the Russian Empire and beyond was peripatetic enough that, according to my father, he spoke Yiddish with a Scottish brogue and could negotiate fluently with the Chinese launderers of South Philadelphia in their native tongue.

To me, this family lore suggests how wide-ranging and well-worn the ancient trade routes must have been. I can picture a procession of dusty conveyances on wooden wheels, bumping along a deeply furrowed track. Inside the wagons, under heavy canvas, a few rows of earthenware pots clink against one another, all protecting tiny sage plants as they trundle along. A young boy like my great-grandfather might have overseen this bounty because sage is an herb that is easily propagated via cuttings in soil, and just as easily transplanted in its new environment given the right seasonal conditions.

Ancient Greeks wrote that, when taken as a drink, sage had properties that could set urination and menstruation in motion, draw down an embryo or fetus, staunch wounds, clean malignant sores, and darken hair; its leaves and branches, decocted in wine, quelled genital itching. In the work of Maimonides, the plant was esteemed for its tonic, astringent, and emmenagogue activities.

By the twelfth century, sage must have been well established in a number of German monastery gardens, because the abbess Hildegard not only wrote a separate chapter for it in her herbal, but also included sage in almost a dozen formulas. She described the plant as warm and dry in nature, noting that it preferred sun to shade, evincing characteristics that almost reveal it as being wistful for its Mediterranean origins. Because of its dry nature, Hildegard found sage useful against noxious humors. She also described a condiment recipe and mouthwash for "stinking breath," or an "overabundance of phlegm," and said that the herb could be cooked in wine to be strained through a piece of cloth and drunk often. For a headache caused by overly moist food, one was advised to anoint the head with a combination of sage, oregano, fennel, and horehound, tossed with either butter or lard, for relief. A similar treatment called for a combination of marshmallow, sage, and olive oil to be applied at night. Sage came well recommended in varied and various preparations for digestion as well. Hildegard also writes that, prior to sleep, watery eyes could be helped by mixing sage, rue, and egg whites, and applying the liquid to the forehead for beneficial results overnight. A recipe that calmed anxious insomnia called for green sage to be sprinkled in wine; this was placed over the heart and around the neck for soothing—and probably aromatic—comfort. It's interesting to note that so many of sage's strengths are best accessed during the nighttime. For a cough, Hildegard recommended that sage be combined in wine with lovage. Paralysis, stitches in the side, gout, and lice were also treated with this powerful plant.

Teller's mid-seventeenth-century Yiddish remedy book recommended sage in four recipes, starting at the head and its potential aches; it first cautioned that care be taken to make certain the patient was not constipated. If suppositories were not sufficient to counter their dry state, herbs were next on the agenda, followed by cephalic vein bloodletting. But for those who were interested in plant remedies, a recipe for a bathing solution for a headache caused by cold, as opposed to heat, called for sage, chamomile flowers, rue, dill, wormwood, lovage, and hyssop to be boiled into a tea with which to wash the scalp. This topical formulation to address headache is similar to Hildegard's but uses a water solution as opposed to one composed of fat or oil. For constipation, sage was also part of a clyster recipe, but if that didn't help, Teller's readers were directed to the apothecary to purchase "Benedicta Laxativa," a well-known electuary that contained purgative plants like scammony and aromatic spices and herbs, plus a sweetener like sugar or honey.

To expel afterbirth, a woman was to smell unpleasant odors such as galbanum, asafoetida, castoreum, or burnt chicken feathers, especially those of the wild fowl. At the same time, she also was to be "fumigated from below" with the smoke of "fragrant things such as cloves, marjoram, civet, ambergris" (from whales, and the description does not sound particularly appetizing), or with specially prepared nutmeg tablets available from the apothecary. Such fumigation seems to have been a common prescription among Jewish healers of this period. According to historian Marek Tuszewicki, a medical pamphlet from the sixteenth century called for a blend of the following herbs and animal substances to be burned at home during an epidemic: juniper, mint, red deer horn, and sage.

In a passage devoted to aches in the midsection, Teller conflates colic and uterine pain (reminiscent of the Polish kolka), without specifically mentioning "the wandering womb," the ancient notion still current in the medical literature of the early modern period. This now-outmoded hypothesis may have influenced the formulation of Teller's recipe for quelling both colic and womb pain that called for "herbs beneficial for the uterus," including sage and rue, which we~e to be boiled in wine and applied warm to the painful abdominal area. Another recipe for stomach (and heart) pain required spearmint, marjoram, oregano, red roses, bayafus (which Teller's translator identifies as sagebrush, bu~ which is probably mugwort), and wormwood, boiled in wine and placed in a small bag to rest on the stomach.

Decades later, in his compendium, Tobias ha-Kohen featured several applications for salvia, and included the herb in a section on laxatives. Per Maude Grieve, the Chinese valued sage for treating digestive weakness in general, preferring it to their own *Camellia sinensis*, which makes me wonder if this plant long ago also wandered eastward from its warm Mediterranean origins along the ancient trade routes.

Ha-Kohen often emphasizes the importance of sweating for treating sickness. To assist the body with this process, he advises submerging specific herbs in warm water, dipping cloths into the resulting tea, and wringing them out a bit before placing the compresses on the back of the neck, under the arms and feet, and finally covering the patient thoroughly to induce a healing sweat. The herbs he specifically recommends for this technique are salvia, rosemary, marjoram, basil, rue, pennyroyal, or chamomile.

Headaches were a complex affair in the Pale. One folk concept surrounding the condition, which may be difficult for contemporary readers to fathom, was known in Yiddish as a kaltine and in Polish as a kołtun, the matted hair that ha-Kohen was the first physician to profile. Ha-Kohen devoted an entire chapter to the Plica Polonica, which was at the time thought to be caused by an evil spirit possessing a person's body, tangling and matting their hair, and consequently creating many painful symptoms, including headaches. Ha-Kohen's advisory begins with very careful and detailed instructions as to how to exorcise the evil spirit without angering it, and concludes with instructions for a topical treatment of the scalp. Sage was one of the capstone herbs in his multistep regimen.

It's curious that ha-Kohen mentions sage and several other plants with warm energetics to treat toothache, specifically in cases caused by cold. This remedy isn't present in Grieve's very thorough section on sage.

For scurvy patients afflicted with painful feet, especially during the night, ha-Kohen again recommended bringing on a good sweat, and he offered sage as one of the plants capable of creating the proper conditions necessary for this healing method.

Podagra, or gout, was another complaint covered by ha-Kohen in a variety of ways. In one striking technique to clear up swelling, which we mentioned earlier, he described taking a piece of iron or ceramic tile to be heated in the fire, whereupon the urine of a young boy would be poured on it and the rising steam could be directed to reach the patient's painful spot. Bathing the area with the same urine was also a possibility for pain relief. Drying up the swollen, gout-ridden area with specific herbs such as sage was prescribed, and above all else, ha-Kohen considered these measures to be easier for young men who were accustomed to physical labor and for those who defecated daily. In all instances, however, he "sagely" recommended that one should go for a walk every day, and eat and drink in moderation.

Lastly, ha-Kohen addressed women's fertility and included a sage preparation that may have been meant to keep the body warm and more receptive to becoming pregnant.

In the late nineteenth century, sage was a much-prized medicinal plant in the Polish lands, as it appears dozens of times in the ethnobotanical studies of the era. In the town of Zwinogródka, for example, sage leaves were applied topically to the breasts of nursing mothers to decrease milk, hastening the weaning of infants. In another application for women's health, sage tea was given to treat vaginal discharges, or leucorrhea.

People of the region at the time generally believed that sore throats were caused by colds, loud talking, or yelling in cold air, especially when it was windy. For this ailment, folk healers turned to many plant remedies, especially rinses and gargles, and sage was a common choice, especially in Lithuanian folk medicine. In Kyiv, Ukraine, for a sore throat, Talko-Hryncewicz reported that the nest of the Eurasian penduline bird was part of a topical cure, but that one had to be careful when buying these from merchants, making certain there was only one hole in the nest, not two, or the remedy would not work.

Coughs were considered serious if they lingered, and folk medicine was dispensed accordingly, requiring stronger herbs for the more dangerous illnesses. Like the sore throat, coughs could be treated with an extremely wide variety of herbs in the folk healer's repertoire, and sage was one of these.

In Ukraine, sage's astringent properties were put to use as an additive in milk to clear up diarrhea.

In the Polish and Ruthenian lands at the turn of the twentieth century, headaches were thought to be caused by bad air, cold, a change in the weather—especially when it rained—and the notorious evil eye. As with other conditions, many plant remedies were at the disposal of the region's folk healers: in the town of Dzianisz, Poland, a sage tea was given to alleviate head pain.

Sweating was reported in the Polish ethnobotanical surveys as an important means of curing cold symptoms such as runny nose, cough, and fever; this method was documented as far more common among Jews and the landed aristocracy than among the lud (Polish, Ruthenian, or Ukrainian peasants), which corroborates the continuity of healing traditions passed down from the age of ha-Kohen (and as reflected in my own family history). While the most popular diaphoretic herbs reported in the late nineteenth century were linden flowers, dried raspberries, marshmallow, and elderflower (which grows everywhere in the region and is readily available to everyone), sage teas were also very common.

Fevers were known by many local names in the Pale, but among Ashkenazi Jews, the most common term was "kaduches." Of dozens of cures reported in Talko-Hryncewicz's surveys, one, noted in the Kharkiv region, offered a sage tea for elevated body temperature. In the town of Żurawka (now Žuravka, Ukraine), near Kaniv, a folk healer, after making certain the patient was covered and warm, applied a formulation that included sage, mixed with vinegar, and dabbed on the pulse of the patient's wrist.

Toothaches were thought to stem from colds as well as eating sweets that might cause painful tooth decay. Dental treatments recorded in late nineteenth-century Poland reflected folk beliefs such as the notion that worms might destroy decaying teeth or that certain phases of the moon were helpful in clearing up dental problems. The new moon was regarded as the best time for folk healers to recite banishing charms that would remove the pain. Many herbs could also be counted upon to relieve toothaches: one of the most commonly reported was an oral rinse of a sage tea, a replica of ha-Kohen's recommendation for quelling tooth pain from two centuries prior.

A superstition held by women in the town of Jurkow for keeping hair healthy required they wash it regularly with an infusion of wormwood, sage, betony, marjoram, and rosemary. This tea must have been meant for brunettes, because at least two of these plants, sage and rosemary, are known to darken tresses.

Sage was also part of a time-honored tea recipe that was enjoyed in Eastern Europe long before black tea, *Camellia sinensis*, became popular. Sbiten, somewhat similar to mead, was made in family samovars, providing an aromatic hot drink for the long, cold winter months. Each person's recipe was unique; ingredients might include honey, berries, and a variety of herbs and spices, such as St. John's wort, valerian, sage, bay leaves, cinnamon, cloves, ginger, and more.

Between the world wars, the Soviet ethnobotanical surveys in Ukraine documented that folk healers in the towns of Berdyansk, Budanovka, Mariupol, Novo-Troitske, Slovyansk, Volnovacha, and Vradiivka applied fresh, dried, or steamed leaves of wooly sage (*Salvia aethiopis*) to fresh or festering wounds. In Starobilsk, the plant's fresh leaves were placed on wounds caused by malignant anthrax, whereas in Volnovacha, the fresh root was placed on an aching tooth. At the time of the surveys, none of these towns had a significant Jewish population, which makes us wonder whether *Salvia aethiopis* and *Salvia officinalis* were in strict complementary distribution geographically in Ukraine, or whether the former is a healing plant whose incorporation into folk materia medica around the Black Sea is correlated with local (e.g., Tatar) or autochthonous traditions.

Among the Karaim, according to Zajączkowski, decoctions of sage roots and wine, or sage leaf tea, were an aphrodisiac; Karaim healers also mixed sage with honey to "cleanse the brain," brighten the eyes, and remove scabies from the skin around the eyes. They also recommended wild, as opposed to cultivated, sage leaves, dried and crushed, and applied with water as a plaster to treat swellings and ulcers. Karaim healers also treated ulcers behind the ears and below the throat with an oxymel mixture of sage seeds or leaves to "completely remove the disease."

In the New World, an Ashkenazi emigré to Argentina wrote that "shalfay" was widespread in Europe and was also known as "Greek tea"; he noted that the virtues of sage leaves lay in easing digestion and as a gargle for oral health.

In the Middle Ages, writes author Sophie Knab, sage was considered a holy plant much revered by the cult of the Blessed Virgin Mary, and that the herb was brought to Poland in the sixteenth century by monks; there it became known in women's reproductive health as an aid to digestion and as an infusion for easing coughs, as well as being valorized in local expressions of Catholic tradition. In the Poznań area, where the earliest Jewish settlements are recorded in the eleventh century, Knab describes a remedy for sore throats to be treated with an infusion of sage with vinegar and honey added, similar to the Karaim oxymel. In other parts of Poland, cooked beets were boiled with sage and given for the same ailment. For a weak stomach, dizziness, or headaches caused by cold conditions, the herb could be mixed with rosemary, marjoram, and thyme in wine and taken for relief.

Russian herbalists today consider sage to be one of their most popular remedies and often make a hot tea gargle to heal a sore throat. Historically, Russian healers relied on the plant to cure female sterility, and it has long been well known in folk medicine for oral and respiratory health, including tonsillitis, laryngitis, and oral cavity infections in general. Official Russian medicine has determined the herb capable of combating many pathogens, and recommends compresses made from infusions of the plant for healing skin wounds and infections. Additionally, sage compresses are found to be helpful in the prevention of hair loss. Other preparations are taken internally to reduce sweating, particularly at night. Like those reported in the nineteenth-century Polish ethnobotanical surveys, babies in today's Russia are still weaned with the assistance of this herb. Although its application in the former Soviet Union extends to teas, both for aiding digestion and urinary system support, folk healers in the region do not recommend its use in pregnancy, or being taken over long periods. (One should never drink more than one cup per day and limit treatment to only fourteen days per month.)

In Lithuania today, Jewish herbalists consider *Salvia officinalis* one of their most helpful plants for improving digestion and as an anti-inflammatory and calmative. To soothe a cough, they boil three to five tablespoons of pine buds for five to ten minutes. After taking the pot from the stove, they either carefully inhale the steam or dilute the tea and drink it. Sage or thyme may be added to this infusion. Sage is also a component in a tea blend for relief of sore throats or inflamed mouth tissues (see *Tilia europaea*, p. 199).

Lithuanian Muslims who were surveyed in a similar study report a greater reliance on sage in folk medicinal practices than their Jewish neighbors. Like

Lithuanian Jews, Lipka Tatar and Azerbaijani healers look to the plant to treat inflammations of the mouth and throat.

I've occasionally added sage to my teas for its strong flavor and also its digestive support, but my main experience with this herb has been much more tactile and sensory than medicinal. Over the years, I've added as many sage species as I can fit onto our tiny plot of land, bewitched by their subtle leaf variations, their small but intensely vibrant flowers, and their cleansing scents—but mostly for their irresistibility to hummingbirds, bees, and the other tiny creatures who frequent our garden.

SALVIA ROSMARINUS | ROSEMARY

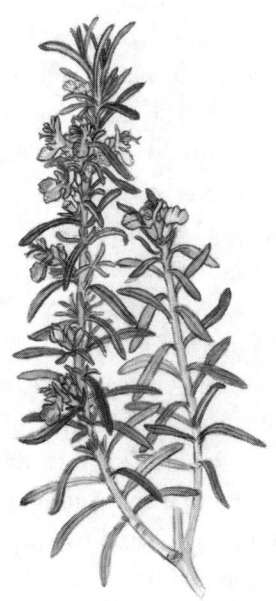

FAMILY Lamiaceae

YIDDISH רפֿואהדיקער ראָזמאַרין (refuahdiker rozmarin)

POLISH Rozmaryn lekarski

UKRAINIAN Розмарин (Rozmaryn), розмарин лікарський (rozmaryn likars'kyj), розмай лікарський (rozmaj likars'kyj), розмарин справжній (rozmaryn spražnij), мария (maryja), розмай-зілля (rozmaj-zillja), розмайран (rozmajran), розмайрин (rozmajryn), розмария (rozmaryja)

LITHUANIAN Kvapusis rozmarinas

RUSSIAN Розмарин лекарственный (Rozmarin lekarstvennyj), розмарин обыкновенный (rozmarin obyknovennyj)

GERMAN   Rosmarin

HEBREW   רוזמרין רפואי (ruzmarin refuai), חילפא דימא (khilpa dima)

In 2017, botanical taxonomists downgraded rosemary's Linnean status from the genus Rosmarinus by folding it into the salvias and conferring the new official designation of *Salvia rosmarinus*, which is synonymous with the now outdated *Rosmarinus officinalis*. The perennial remains in the mint family. Many herbalists were surprised by rosemary's reallocation in the binomial hierarchy, but almost a decade later, this change has become passé.

Just as intriguing as rosemary's nomenclatural switcheroo is the fact that it is one of only five "refue" plants (those with a remedy prefix in Yiddish)—out of hundreds of entries—in Mordkhe Schaechter's *Plant Names in Yiddish*.

On a strictly gut level, for me, the other four refuahdiker herbs (hedge mustard, sanicle, bearberry, and kidney vetch) share a kind of Eastern European flavor, if you will, while rosemary feels a little more exotic, even dramatic, amongst this handful of specially designated entities.

If we explore why that might be so, what immediately comes to mind is this plant's geographic origins. The word *rosemary*, or *rosmarinus*, itself is a clue. It comes from the Latin and translates as "dew from the sea" or "sea dew," signifying the belief that rosemary didn't need to be watered but instead survived solely on moisture from the sea.

When envisioning rosemary, the image that comes up, at least for me, is of an arid landscape with hard-packed soils, under a relentless and blazing sun, none of which conjures visions of Yiddish speakers in the shtetl, conferring about "refuahdiker rozmarin."

Perhaps it's because rosemary is very much at home here on the arid West Coast, and I encounter (and, with frequent inhalations of its sharp scent, smell) this plant nearly everywhere I go.

So how and when did this plant become a refue to Ashkenazim and get to the Pale of Settlement, and why was it considered medicinal? Did it show up dried, and which parts, the leaves, the branches, the roots? The whole plant dried? Does it grow wild in Eastern Europe? Who brought it there at first?

Rosemary's connection with the human world can be traced back thousands of years to the ancient Egyptians, as a plant interred in burials, and later (during the Roman Empire), when Dioscorides included the herb in his *De Materia Medica*. One would think that Dioscorides's entry would have been extensive since rosemary is native to the Mediterranean, but his musings were brief and more prosaic than anticipated, referring mainly to the plant's scent as "oppressive," and its warm properties as a suitable treatment for jaundice or as a component in an analgesic ointment.

In a slightly later historical sighting, medicinal rosemary was discussed in a fourth-century herbal, the Herbarius of Pseudo-Apuleius. It was here that rosemary was promoted as an aid to sufferers of many maladies: as a juice from the plant's root, it relieved toothache; crushed with oil, the herb was rubbed onto fatigued bodies to reinvigorate them; steeped in wine, rosemary served in an anti-itch capacity; boiled in water with either amomum or spikenard, two dates, and some rue, the plant was taken as a drink to treat liver and intestinal pains; to relieve coughs, rosemary was kneaded with pepper and honey into soothing pastilles; for the removal of white spots in the eyes, ash from the plant was rubbed with honey on the affected area; fresh wounds were addressed by applying the herb crushed in a fat; and, mashed in hot water, rosemary was drunk to cool a bout of fever.

Rosemary made its debut in the herbal literature north of the Alps in a decree, credited to Charlemagne in the eighth century, that ordered the cultivation of the herb in monastic gardens and farms, presumably to be protected from the elements, as rosemary does not tolerate severely cold conditions. It appears in England in the mid-fourteenth century, as a gift to the wife of King Edward III. This is the era when European herbalists began documenting rosemary's medicinal strengths as evidenced in the "Rosemary Tractate," which circulated widely in manuscript form. Legends of the time describe the origins of a famous herbal formula whose anonymous inventor cured an unnamed monarchess's headaches with what came to be known as Queen of Hungary Water. Its primary ingredient was none other than rosemary, which was soaked in wine along with a few other well-known resinous and aromatic herbs (such as sage).

In seventeenth-century Prague, rosemary appeared in three of Issachar bar Teller's formulations. To cure a cold, marjoram, rosemary, fennel, false hellebore, and barley, all in dried form, were crushed into a powder that was to be inhaled two or three times a day to provoke the sneezing response and thus expel disease. A second recipe, meant to bring on delayed menstruation, recommended boiling together varying amounts of nutmeg, cloves, saffron, cinnamon, and rosemary. The patient was to drink this brew, warm, several times a day, in bed, thus promoting a curative sweat.

To dispel disease, Teller advises his readers to fumigate a space by simply kindling a fire "because flame consumes the bad air, especially when made with the wood of juniper and the like." If this wood was unavailable, the smoke of burnt juniper berries, hyssop, oregano, mint, rosemary, marjoram, basil, lavender, or the peels of apples or similar plant material would do. And if necessary, premade incense powders and cones were available at the apothecary for those who wished to pay for such things.

During the same period, rosemary was detailed in the Russian *Travnic*, or *Hortus Sanitatis*, a prescriptive materia medica for Russian elites. It was obviously a kitchen or garden plant in Russia at this time, albeit one reserved for the upper classes—by the early nineteenth century, the prescription book for Maria, the Tsarina of Russia, called for rosemary oil to be used in many formulas.

In the early eighteenth century, ha-Kohen praises rosemary in his section on medicinal trees, providing its name in both Ladino (Judezmo) and Turkish and declaring the entire plant as medicinal with hot and dry characteristics. He mentions its affinity for the head and also singles out the plant for its applications for dental health.

Ha-Kohen's plant glossary only provides a handful of names "in the language of Sepharad" for plants: romero, "rosemary," originating as it did in the Mediterranean, has been part of Jewish plant medicinal traditions for many centuries (ha-Kohen also provides a gloss of the plant's Mishnaic appellation: "khilpa ha-dima"). Sephardim have long been familiar with rosemary as a protective agent, carrying it, along with rue, as a shield against the evil eye.

As for the prescriptions themselves, ha-Kohen, in a passage on fevers, calls for rosemary and sage, along with a few other herbs, to be decocted. The resultant tea was to be poured on a cloth that then was applied to the nape of the neck to bring on a healing sweat in feverish cases.

Let's take a short digression to discuss one of ha-Kohen's most remarkable recommendations, in which rosemary plays a part. It's in a very involved regimen he prescribed for curtailing the Plica Polonica, or the Polish plait, the matted, unwashed hair known in Polish as the kołtun and in Yiddish as the kaltine (ha-Kohen himself refers to it "in the language of Ashkenaz" as "ha"r lukir" (cf. German *Haarlocken,* "locks of hair"). Historian Marek Tuszewicki notes that the kaltine was "the most commonplace demonic affliction among East European Jews, and its notorious appellation, Plica Polonica, reflects the fact that it had for centuries been considered endemic to those lands and not documented anywhere else." The disease didn't limit itself, however, to a single group of people in the region. For centuries, Ashkenazim as well as Slavs suffered from the malady. Their common folk belief held that its occurrence signified that a demon had invaded the body and that this foreign entity at times might cause rheumatic pain or other complications and could only find its way out of its host through the mat of tangled hair.

When described this way, it almost seems reasonable that an afflicted person wouldn't dare to anger their tormentor by disturbing the nest it had made on their head. It was this sentiment that dictated the folk healing methods that had to be scrupulously performed before a kaltine and its perpetrator could be safely evicted.

Ha-Kohen might have been one of the first to document the phenomenon of the kaltine, its symptoms, possible causes, and treatment. Aside from his lengthy discussion of the affliction, he also observed in these patients a frequent presence of fever, swelling of the neck, an inability to move comfortably and, as a modern translator interpreted ha-Kohen's words, "[the condition could involve] many more diseases which cannot be enumerated here . . . for the reader would grow tired of reading it."

To relieve a person of the disorder, ha-Kohen suggested a multistep regimen that began with emetic purges to remove toxins from a patient, refortifying their body with chicken soup, and cleansing the blood and the inside of the head, for starters. The eventual removal of the plait was not accomplished by shaving it off, but rather by treating it with herbs such as nigella seeds, tobacco, betony, and verbena, to name a few.

Toward the end of his treatment plan, ha-Kohen contended that it was necessary to extinguish all noxious gases still emanating from the sufferer's head. This was accomplished by softening the scalp with the application of an emollient. Ha-Kohen's offerings of chicken or goose fat luckily were offset by several other more appetizing options including almond oil, rosemary oil, or the fabled Queen of Hungary Water.

By the late nineteenth century, nearly two hundred years later, the kaltine continued to be a familiar affliction throughout the Pale. In an inexplicable twist of reasoning, in the town of Jurkow, if one could not rid themselves of a headache by more conventional means, folk healers cut hair from the patient's head in several places, wrapped it in a cloth, and had them wear it against their heart for two or three days. If the bits clumped together, this determined whether or not they should grow a plait in order to dispel their headaches.

Headaches were believed at the turn of the twentieth century to be caused by a cold, by bad air, or often as the result of having been charmed by an unfriendly person, that is, by the evil eye. Seen in this context, the hair-cutting ritual performed in Jurkow makes more sense: if a demon had invaded this person and caused their headaches, then in order for it to successfully exit the person, it might need the matted hair of a kaltine as a viable exit portal.

In the town of Zbaraż, women burnt their hair to avoid headaches. Married Jewish women in Zwinogródka, Jurkow, and around Zwiahel, who were required to shave their heads and wear the traditional wig (or sheitel in Yiddish), might hide a portion of their shorn locks to prevent headaches. According to historian Marek Tuszewicki, folk healing rituals like this were often performed by Jews to transfer an illness from a patient to an object by taking something such as the person's hair or fingernails and hiding them in a hollow tree, stopped with an aspen peg, in the belief that the ailment would stay in this secret place.

Many plant remedies were also sought to alleviate a headache in Zwinogródka, including a thyme or a juniper-berry tea, or an infusion of rosemary flowers. Another fragrant formula called for tresses to be bathed in a tea in which a handful of wormwood, sage, betony, marjoram, and rosemary had been steeped.

In Latvian folk medicine, one nineteenth-century headache treatment consisted of taking snuff soaked in rosemary oil.

Folk healers in Ruthenia also treated eye conditions with rosemary oil, and sought the plant for dental diseases as well. Bad breath was treated with a variety of strongly flavored herbs, and tooth brushing was also practiced; in the Podolia region, ash obtained from the root of rosemary was used for this purpose, recalling a number of ancient herbal sources, such as Pseudo-Apuleius, Banckes's Herbal, and ha-Kohen.

In the town of Olszana, a formula meant to bring on delayed menstruation shared aspects of Teller's earlier recipe, and required brewing a tea made up of wormwood, juniper, thyme, southern wood, marjoram, rosemary, calamus, centaury, roman chamomile, and bryony that was to be drunk four times a day.

At times, it was necessary to expel a miscarried fetus at the beginning of a pregnancy, and many plants and other means were sought out for this unfortunate situation. Rosemary, documented as such a remedy in the eastern Galcia region, was the least toxic choice in a list of more than a dozen herbs that today are rarely if ever worked with in contemporary Western herbalism.

For women who feared or suspected infertility, there were many options, such as drinking hare fat, which was reportedly a common remedy found in older sources. In the town of Ryżanówka, a cat's placenta was dried and ground into a fine powder and given to both spouses to consume. In Nowa-Uszyca, some women, especially Jewish women, would swallow the blood from a newborn's umbilical cord, but to be effective, they would have to swallow it three times. Another practice in the same town called for an infertile woman to wear the shirt of a woman who had had many children. In Wasylków (Yiddish Vaslkev, in the late nineteenth century 40 percent Jewish; now Vasyl'kiv, Ukraine), swallowing a small fish was recommended. Compared to most of the survey's reported possibilities, the one that seems the least eccentric for us today was recorded in Zwinogródka, where women fumigated themselves with burning rosemary leaves and aloe (this is most likely lign-aloes, or Aquilaria), which they credited to ancient (unnamed) medicinal sources.

If remedies including rosemary were examples of everyday folk medicine in the Pale, how did this herb—which was neither native to the region nor able to grow there because climatic and geographic conditions were too harsh for its survival—travel from the kitchens and covered gardens of the tsars to the towns and villages of the Pale?

If it's a given that rosemary does not grow in colder climates (unless it was cultivated indoors, which precludes anyone without the resources from housing—and pampering—such a plant during the harsh northern winters), it must have been, from its earliest appearance in the Pale, available to the general populace in dried form. This hypothesis is borne out by a late nineteenth-century common folk medicinal formula that was meant to increase fertility in women and girls by mixing a special blend of powdered (signifying dried as opposed to fresh), and mostly imported herbs, including rosemary, in wine and drinking the infusion twice a day. Remarkably, this formulation is very similar to the trianke (see p. 207) in both ingredients and indications.

Considering the plant's natural resinous qualities and the fact that drying its leaves hardly detracts from their potency, it's almost a certainty that "refuahdiker rozmarin" would have been purchased in dried form, from local merchants who specialized in non-native and exotic herbs and spices. Prior to the Second World War and stretching back to the beginnings of the legendary Old World spice routes, it's likely Jewish spice merchants were the conduits for making rosemary and so many other dried herbs and medicinal substances available to local populations of Eastern Europe and beyond.

In those parts of Eastern Europe where rosemary is able to grow wild, specifically multi-confessional, multi-ethnic Bosnia, the plant, according to Glück, had many of the same applications: rosemary brewed in wine countered loss of appetite, while its leaves were employed externally against head dizziness and skin irritations. Among the Roma of southeastern Europe, according to Wlislocki, a magical remedy for toning a postpartum stomach required rosemary, and powdered snails and dung beetles, to be mixed with fresh butter into an ointment that was buried in a new, sealed bowl in horse manure for a week. The wrinkled skin of the stomach was believed to have been caused by an evil spirit, and the application of the ointment, several times a day, was to be accompanied by this charm:

Whoever made this
Let him smell this
So that he may die, so that he may die
Like the worm
In my belly!

In 1940s Argentina, the Ashkenazi Jewish herbalist who had immigrated there prior to the Second World War wrote in Yiddish of "rozmarin blat" (rosemary leaf) as a tea for stimulating the appetite or to calm the nerves.

Author Sophie Knab recounts rosemary's long and circuitous history in Polish plant medicine, starting with King Jan Sobieski III's fragrant plantings in the vast gardens of his summer residence along the Vistula River near Warsaw in the seventeenth century. She also notes the plant's symbolic significance as a component of the bridal wreaths worn during traditional marriage ceremonies, as well as its medicinal role in headache relief, its reputation for soothing coughs and quelling skin conditions, or as part of a formula for repelling moths.

Many of these traditions historically have been shared with various adjacent cultures. For example, according to Nelly Weiss, the Ashkenazi surname Rosmarin suggests the herb's presence in the daily life of the shtetls, derfer, and cities of the Pale as a kitchen seasoning, a medicine, and, "in early times, a flower for brides."

Before we leave rosemary and its healing powers as employed in the Pale, we d like to point out that, for all its importance in treating ailments of the head, rosemary is less associated with memory function in Eastern Europe than it is in the West (we recall Ophelia in Shakespeare's *Hamlet*: "There's rosemary, that's for remembrance"). Perhaps it's because the Jewish diaspora has for many centuries relied upon the Indian marking nut (*Semecarpus anacardium*) for memory retention: one legend around Maimonides, cited in Loew, holds that the sage was never able to retain a single word of the Torah until he defied a warning and ate of the marking nut, whereby he was able to commit all eighteen degrees (of Torah knowledge) to memory.

In my personal acquaintance with rosemary, before I was aware of any of its magical properties, I had two related experiences with this plant revolving around the idea of protection. The first was as a newly minted librarian, substituting at the Claremont branch of Berkeley Public Library. I usually worked in the evenings, and often on cold or rainy nights when more than the usual handful of people would crowd the modest reading room to get out of the weather. It was during these times that an overpowering scent of rosemary dominated the air in that smallish space and made those shifts nearly impossible to endure. The smell at times was repulsive, almost as if someone who had not bathed in a while had made up for this by spending as much time as possible among the branches of an extremely resinous rosemary bush. I never did find out which patron was responsible, but the effect was long-lasting and the result was that I couldn't bring myself to even sniff these plants for many years.

Decades later, having recovered from my fragrant trauma, when we moved to the Central Valley, rosemary was one of the first plants I put along a side fence. A few years later, the neighbor who lived next door and had been relatively friendly retired from her job, and within a few months she unexpectedly became more than a little antagonistic. For some reason, having the rosemary plant between her house and ours felt like a comforting barrier.

These two stories don't explain the mysteries of who brought rosemary to the Pale or in what form it must have been known by those who worked with it as medicine there, but they do explain the more magical side of rosemary as a protector. The library patron who carried with them such a strong force field of scent, and a plant that provided an invisible blockade from hostile forces were both instances of a shielding presence. In my herbal practices today, in winter, I like to infuse rosemary leaves in olive oil and apply this blend to soften dry skin conditions. In a sense, this is also a protective barrier between the body and the weather or whatever harshness one might come into contact with.

SAMBUCUS NIGRA | ELDER

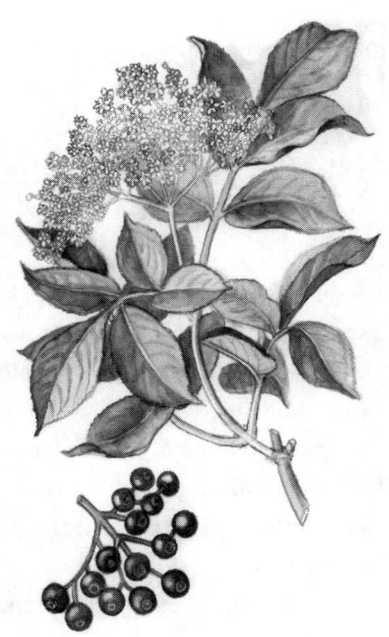

FAMILY Adoxaceae

YIDDISH באָז (boz), בוזינע (buzine); other transliterated names include ruknes-shtekns, sheydim-shtekns, meshugene graypelekh, holder, haldir boim, sambuko-blumen, sambuko bleter

POLISH Bez czarny, bez lekarski, bez pospolity, bzowina, bzina, buzina, hyczka, baźnik, bess, best, bestek, bez apteczny, bez aptekarski, bez biały, bez dziki, bzowina czarna, bzowki, côrny bez, flider, gołębia pokrzywa, hebz, holander, hyćka, kaszka, suk

UKRAINIAN Бузина чорна (Buzyna čorna), бозняк (boznjak), буз (buz), самбук (sambuk), бездерево (bezderevo)

BELARUSIAN   Бузіна чорная (Buzina čornaja), бузіна (buzina), бэз чорны (bez čorny), бэза (beza)

LITHUANIAN   Juoduogis šeivamedis

RUSSIAN   Бузина чёрная (Buzina čërnaja)

GERMAN   Schwarzer Holunder

HEBREW   שנבוג (shenbag), הלונדרא (holundrah), הלדר (holdir), סמבוק (sambuk)

ROMANI   Kast bengeskro

Readers may not be surprised to learn that the elder (both *Sambucus nigra* and *Sambucus ebulus*), like so many of the plants and trees we come into contact with daily, has a long, complex, and uninterrupted relationship with humans.

From its multiple Yiddish names, we can surmise that Ashkenazim and other Jewish communities have long paid close attention to the elder. Maimonides himself identified both of the main species, documenting their distinct appellations in several languages while simultaneously drawing attention to their similar medicinal properties.

Maude Grieve's entry for Sambucus is extensive, and her summary of its associated folk beliefs literally covers a great deal of ground. For instance, she notes that Roma practices have forbidden the use of the tree's kindling: gleaners must carefully sift through firewood lest a stick of elder find its way into their bundles. This custom, posits Grieve, could have come down from the ancient pagan myths of northern Europe (by way of Denmark?), where the magical tree was known to haunt anyone who severed its limbs. In Russia, Grieve writes, it was thought that elder banished evil spirits, while Czechs sought out its power to dissipate a fever. Italians understood its ability to kill snakes and discourage thieves, and in Serbia it brought good luck to weddings. In the British Isles, elder has been associated with many traditions, but today the best known may be the warning to anyone who contemplates dozing beneath its branches. To the uninformed, Grieve counsels:

The whole tree has a narcotic smell, and it is not considered wise to sleep under its shade. Perhaps the visions of fairyland were the result of the drugged sleep! No plant will grow under the shadow of it, being affected by its exhalations.

Yet despite its monitory reputation throughout Europe, elder was an extremely important plant in the folk culture and folk medicine of the Pale of Settlement and beyond. A plant with spreading branches, large compound leaves, white flowers, and dark berries, elder has been sought out for many necessities: its soft pith might be hollowed out from the core to make wood-wind instruments. It could be carved as a basis for toys and for butchers' tools shoemakers' pegs, weaving needles, combs, or fencing. Crushing elder leaves made for an effective insect repellent. The tree entire was also a source for dyes of many colors: from the root, black; from the leaves, green; and the berries yield a whole spectrum of blues. But elder was known most as a healing plant.

This knowledge of elder's healing qualities is shared by many creatures. According to Linnaeus, sheep cure themselves from foot-rot by rooting out and eating the bark and young shoots of the elder. He also observed that elder-berries were salutary for some birds and poisonous to others. It's likely that the first humans to come into contact with elder watched how other animals interacted with it. Could elder be one of our earliest plant teachers?

Elder is long associated with Jewish medicine: known as both sambuk and huldr, and glossed from the Greek of Dioscorides, the tree is found in Rashi, and in the Shulchan Aruch (code of Jewish law).

Certainly, elder has an age-old reputation as a magical plant among Jews. According to Schaechter: "Yiddish ethnobotany has supplied us with terms for the European elder (*Sambucus nigra*)—rúkhes-shtékns, shéydim-shtékns, and meshúgene gráypelekh." It may be this reputation among Jews associating elder with sheydim and madness that informed a broader communal belief common throughout Galicia and Romania in elder's powers as a devil's tree. The source of this belief is sometimes attributed to the Saxon Germans of Transylvania, where it spread among their neighbors. Given the broader demographics of the region until the earlier twentieth century, it's much more likely that this belief was introduced by the Jewish diaspora, although, as we'll see the region's Roma communities share this belief as well.

Regardless, elder has been honored as a healing plant in Europe since the neolithic era: pottery dating from the fourth or fifth millennia BCE found in northern Germany contained plant remains of cleaver, mallow, plantain, poppy, knotweed, vervain, and elder, likely owing to their known healing efficacy.

Teller—whose Yiddish name for the tree, holder, shows how the variety of the language spoken in Prague had close links to southwestern dialects of German—writes of a remedy for headaches in which a well-beaten egg white should be mixed with rose water, one part elder blossom water, wine, vinegar, dill water, and lungwort, to which saffron was to be added and applied as a head compress.

Ha-Kohen recommends sambucus for a number of treatments. Like Maimonides, he distinguished between *Sambucus nigra* and *Sambucus ebulus*, but he focuses on the former in his work. In *Ma'aseh Tuviyah*'s section on scurvy (sharbak, as he identifies it in "the language of Ashkenaz," from German *Scharbock*), sambucus was part of a formula for treating stomach pain that could accompany the disease. This is one of ha-Kohen's simpler recipes: it calls for boiling either chamomile or elder flowers in milk and drinking the infusion for relief.

Ha-Kohen also praises the elder in his separate chapter on the medicinal trees. He identifies it by name in Yiddish as haldir boim (cf. German *Holderbaum*), in Turkish as morbir, and in French as sosian, and echoes the ancient Greeks when he writes of its clean and dry nature that disperses any swelling. Like herbalists of today, ha-Kohen identifies each part of the tree and its associated medicinal actions. He describes the flowers as able to soften and open; if taken internally they are capable of causing perspiration. Externally, they help against colic pain, erysipelas, or burns. He praises the juice of the elderberry: it is good as food as well as medicine and can remove poisons and bad phlegm from the body. The roots and lower bark, he writes, tend to "bad, watery mucus that lies in the outer body." Each of these recommendations follows directly from the teachings of Dioscorides.

In his chapter on children's ailments, ha-Kohen includes elder in several instances, either singly or in formulation. For infants suffering from "cradle cap" (see *Saponaria officinalis*, p. 187), he draws on the Jewish method of encouraging the body to sweat in order to draw toxins from the pores, thus helping free a patient of any pathogenic invaders that might have caused the malady. For such a case in a young child, ha-Kohen calls upon the water of sambukus grass to be imbibed every night by the young patient in order to bring on a healing perspiration.

In an entry on smallpox, which ha-Kohen identifies in Latin as variolae, in "the language of Sepharad" as virgolas, and in "the language of Ashkenaz" as raxen or blatern, based on his understanding of the disease in the era when he studied, practiced, and wrote, he describes the affliction and explains the degrees of severity and the symptoms that a patient might suffer as depending on the level of impurity in the blood. For babies who are still nursing, he advises that the breastfeeding mother take an infusion made with scorzonera (black salsify, *Pseudopospermum hispanicum*) and "karduus sanktus" (blessed thistle, *Centaurea benedicta*). This infusion should be given to an infant several times a day. For children a year or two old, cooked figs with deer horn were recommended to neutralize all sharpness and saltiness of the compromised blood, prevent its overheating, and in addition, cleanse the respiratory tract.

From here, ha-Kohen veers into less charted territory: At one point in his discussion of variolae, he describes the recommendation of the "sage" Itmilirish, who was known for advocating the use of horse manure, strained through liquor or "ashkenaz" (German) beer, to treat smallpox because, according to the original source, it kept the eruption out of the pharynx, reduced the fever, and prevented angina. Ha-Kohen augments the prescription by suggesting several herbs that could be added to the beer concoction, including aquilegia (columbine), raphi (radish), and blessed thistle. But the best infusion, he stresses, is made from the flower of elder, scabiosa, and fennel. If the patient shows signs of epilepsy, he outlines another formula to help them rest, featuring the additional ingredients of white poppy and peony.

Finally, as an afterthought, ha-Kohen offers us a glimpse of the elusive opshprekherin's occult secrets. He reveals, parenthetically, just before invoking alchemy: "In this country, the women are in the habit of putting the seed of the scarlet worm, called in Latin kukus ("coccus"), and in the language of Sepharad pirnigon, but I do not know where they found this, for no author mentions it." This throwaway aside is one more precious glimpse into the secret knowledge of the mysterious Jewish women folk healers, particularly in its reference to coccus: *Kermes ilices,* known in antiquity as *Coccus ilicis,* is one of the oldest known dyes. It was also used in ancient internal medicine for strengthening the heart among other applications. The insect's role in medicine possibly originated due to its vermillion color, which had ritual and supernatural significance. Could its importance for "the women" serve as an echo of long-lost remnants of a prehistoric legacy that were later co-opted by patriarchal physicians?

In the German lands, prior to the nineteenth century, elder had several distinct medicinal applications in Jewish health and healing. According to historian Herman Pollack, "During the rite of circumcision, the mohel would dip an elderberry in the wine to deepen its color and make it more appetizing." As part of a formula, elder helped bring on menses, and the plant was a key ingredient in the eponymous hollerkuchel, an elderberry cookie for relieving toothache.

Incidentally, when we consider syncretic care in the Pale, we should mention that circumcision was practiced by both Muslim Lipka Tatars and their Jewish neighbors. Because Tatar communities were small and scattered, they relied on the mohel for this observance.

By the late nineteenth century, it was common across villages and towns throughout Poland and Ruthenia for folk healers to administer infusions of elder flowers as a remedy for uterine disorders. This remedy may be a variation on Dioscorides's method in which he writes of "root boiled with water and used in a sitz bath to soften and open the uterus and correct conditions associated with it."

In the Pale, hemorrhoids were associated with the landed gentry and Jews, and several folk treatments were common among the region's Jewish communities. One such curative attested in Talnianki, near Uman (now Tal'janky, Ukraine), required crushed elder leaves in unsalted butter to make an ointment for opening infected hemorrhoids.

In Odessa during the same period, edema was treated with the fresh bark of the tree: The green peel would be scraped from the inner side of the bark and to it would be added a half-pint of fresh melted animal fat or unsalted butter, to be fried at low heat until the peel turned yellow, whereupon the ointment was applied to the swollen areas of the body several times a day. This remedy also recalls both Dioscorides's and ha-Kohen's writings on elder's medicinal capabilities.

According to the Polish ethnobotanical surveys, it was noted that gout was treated by folk healers as a symptom of rheumatism, and for this complaint, "rubbing the body with the fats of various animals and birds was widely employed across Ruthenia, not only among the common people [lud], but also among the Jews, a legacy of ancient medicine." Dioscorides specifically mentions elder leaves plastered on suet or goat fat to "help the gout."

The Polish surveys state categorically that diaphoretics were generally "more widely used among slightly more civilized classes, the landed gentry and the Jews, than among the common people." According to the surveys, diaphoretics addressed ailments with symptoms including a runny nose, fevers, shortness of breath, and the like. All the remedies employed by folk healers for this condition were plants. First and foremost among these was elder flower, the most popular of medicines because it grew close to every household and was employed internally for many maladies.

Externally, the flower and leaves were also helpful for erysipelas, a skin condition believed by many, including the region's Jewish communities, to be caused by the evil eye. Even as late as the mid-twentieth century, erysipelas would be treated with an application of plants, minerals, or animal products, or with the aid of magic ritual. Or a combination of all of these. One of the most remarkable folk remedies for the treatment of erysipelas commonly reported in towns surveyed by Talko-Hryncewicz was a prescription for elder to be employed in several ways. After first being sprinkled with chalk or rye flour, softened wood was placed over infected skin, or elder bark and flowers were boiled in lye and then applied to the skin. In some cases, the berries were also spread onto the affected area. What is extraordinary about this herbal remedy is its direct lineage from ha-Kohen, who mentions erysipelas exactly once in his *Ma'aseh Tuviyah*, and the sole topical curative he prescribes for the disease is sambucus.

According to Wlislocki, the Roma of nineteenth-century Eastern Europe also relied upon elder (which they, similarly to the Ashkenazim, called "devil's wood": kast bengeskro) to treat erysipelas: they would mix bullfinch blood in a new pot with scraped elder bark, put the ointment on a cloth, and bandage the affected area overnight. This application, which had to take place after sunset, was accompanied by an incantation:

I have two eyes
I have two feet
Pain from my (eyes)
Goes into my feet
Goes out of my feet
Down into the earth
Climb out of the earth
Into death!

The following morning, the bandage was to be thrown into the nearest river, to ensure that the erysipelas would not return.

The yizkor book of Shidlovtse (Szydłowiec, Poland) also attests to elder's prominence in the home medicine cabinet, observing that linden, raspberry, and elderberry cordials were specifics for inducing perspiration, in order to draw disease from the body.

Immediately after the Second World War, in the diaspora Jewish communities of Argentina, the healing powers of elder's flowers and leaves were part of communal plant medicine. Known as sambuko-blumen and sambuko bleter, "elder flowers" and "elder leaves," and in Spanish as sauco, this tree was praised for its ability to bring on perspiration to ameliorate colds, soothe rheumatism, and serve in a compress to hasten the eruption of ulcers, an application that recalls the late nineteenth-century Polish Jewish remedy for hemorrhoids.

According to Veckenstedt, traditional Sorbian folk medicine, in Lusatia, southeast of Berlin and bordering Poland, called upon elder teas to treat malaise. In traditional Romanian pediatric folk medicine, bathing in elder leaves helped underweight children; taken internally as tea, elder leaves treated cramps and intestinal parasites.

Traditional Lithuanian folk medicine, according to Henneberg and Stasuliewicz, has relied upon elder as an emetic, anti-inflammatory, antitussive, diaphoretic, diuretic, emmenagogue, and laxative, and as a treatment for erysipelas, headaches, hemorrhoids, catarrhs, dropsy, stomach and duodenal ulcers, colds, and rashes.

In modern Russian folk medicine, a tea of elder flowers has been a traditional way of treating several conditions, including rheumatism, gout (reminding us of ha-Kohen and Dioscorides, as well as the nineteenth-century Polish surveys), and kidney issues, as well as allergies of the respiratory system. A tea made from the flowers is also known as an antiseptic skin wash that's rubbed on infected areas. A combination of the flowers of elder and chamomile is steeped in boiling water and used as a compress to reduce swelling around joints and muscles. For chronic constipation, an infusion of early leaves with berries ripened in the fall is combined with honey. The same extract is recommended for kidney complaints accompanied by swelling. Also applied for kidney and bladder complaints is elder bark. Russian folk medicine also calls upon elder to treat colds and promote sweating, and the leaves of young shoots may serve as a laxative.

In the last few years, we planted an elder on the edge of our garden. It's grown so quickly that the local jays have already built two nests in its branches, and there have been so many flowers and berries that even when I give most of them away to friends and family for making their own recipes, there are still plenty for the birds and squirrels who come to visit every day.

My medicinal experience with elder has revolved around boosting immunity curing "the cold and flu season." A simple elderberry syrup can be modified with warming herbs like cinnamon, cardamom, and ginger, or cough-soothing herbs like wild cherry bark. The ratios are one part decocted dried elderberries to one part brandy and three parts honey. It's helpful to warm the honey before adding in the berry infusion, to make sure these two liquids are thoroughly combined. It's best to allow this mixture to cool to room temperature before adding the brandy. Don't forget to label your container with all the ingredients and the date you made it. The syrup can be stored for up to a year in the refrigerator. A tablespoon can be taken three times a day for supporting immunity if you feel under the weather or when you have a cold or flu.

SANICULA EUROPAEA | SANICLE

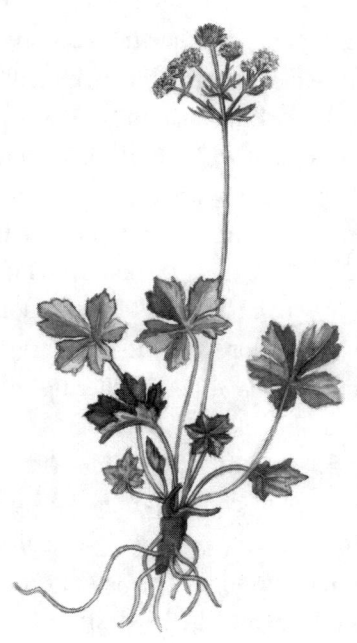

FAMILY   Apiaceae

YIDDISH   רפֿואַהכל (refuahkhl)

POLISH   Żankiel zwyczajny

UKRAINIAN   Підлісник європейський (Pidlisnyk evropejs'kyj)

BELARUSIAN   Падлеснік еўрапейскі (Padlesnik eŭrapejski)

LITHUANIAN   Girūnė

RUSSIAN   Подлесник европейский (Podlesnik evropejskij)

GERMAN   Wald-Sanikel, Waldsanikel, Sanikel, Wundsanikel, Waldklette

Sanicle is one of only five plants—out of hundreds—in Mordkhe Schaechter's *Plant Names in Yiddish* that has the word "remedy" (refue) in its name. When I first noticed the handful of Yiddish refue plants, I found myself at a total loss as to why these were singled out when so many other plants in his work clearly warrant medicinal appellations than this seemingly random assortment.

In sanicle's case, Schaechter identifies it as refuahkhl, which very loosely translates as "little cure-all" or "little heal-all" in English. I couldn't find much information about sanicle, a plant with a dark shallow root, upright stem, palmate leaves, and small flowers, as a panacea in contemporary Western herbalism, although Maude Grieve's entry on the herb sheds a bit of light on why this might be the case. She writes that "wood sanicle has locally often been known as self-heal, a name which belongs rightly to another quite distinct herb, *Prunella vulgaris*, of the Labiate order." With this insight in mind, I wondered if Schaechter's informant may have been adhering to this convention when they identified sanicle as a refuahkhl?

Nevertheless, and regardless of its possible Yiddish misnomer, sanicle, which has fallen out of favor in contemporary Western herbalism, was historically a well-respected medicinal plant with a history of incorporation into healing modalities that continues today in Eastern Europe.

Grieve also notes that the plant's genus designation comes from the Latin word *sano*, "I heal/cure," which is a direct testament to the herb's medicinal virtues.

Hildegard, who practiced in Germany nearly a millennium ago, found the plant's juice to be good for a sick stomach and for infected wounds. She sweetened its medicine with honey and licorice to make a more palatable remedy for patients suffering from either of these conditions.

In medieval Europe, sanicle's reputation as both an internal and external vulnerary was legendary.

Ha-Kohen formulated a drink for lacerations that featured sanicle, the well-known wound-healing comfrey, and the possible addition of boneset (*Eupatorium perfoliatum*) and chickweed (Stellaria). This herbal combination was to be sweetened with sugar before consuming. Ha-Kohen also recommends an external salve that calls for the skin of the anguilla fish (an eel) and some egg white mixed together and applied topically for external traumas.

By the late nineteenth century, ethnographers Hovorka and Kronfeld reported that feldshers in Bavaria prepared an ointment with the green juice of the sanicle root that was to be stirred with good lard. These paramedics would make sure they carried a bit of root with them in a vest pocket at all times. When it was necessary to heal a wound without causing scarring, they moistened the root and brushed it on the cut. The "melted" leaves of the plant were also drunk as a tea with milk to help against congestion.

Grieve describes sanicle's flavor as very bitter at first, astringent in the mouth, and this, she explains, is mostly due to its membership in the Umbelliferae family. Aside from its astringency, she reports that in early twentieth-century western Europe, sanicle was a highly esteemed alterative to be taken in combination with other herbs to improve the blood. Sanicle was also well regarded for a variety of respiratory complaints and was beneficial as a gargle for sore throat, inflamed tonsils, and other oral concerns whenever an astringent was needed.

For children's rashes, Grieve writes that sanicle was also a popular topical choice. In France and Germany a century ago, the plant was a specific to staunch bleeding from the lungs, bowels, and other internal organs. Teaspoon doses of the fresh juice were also given to relieve symptoms of dysentery.

Sanicle's adoption in Eastern Europe is likely conditioned by geography. A common medicinal plant elsewhere in Europe (especially central Europe: Germany, Bohemia, etc.), it has less of a presence to the east. For instance, while sanicle is known and prescribed in contemporary Lithuanian folk medicine, it is not a common wild plant there.

In mid-twentieth-century Polish herbal medicine, sanicle was prized for its diuretic, diaphoretic, strengthening, and astringent properties. Leaves, flowers, and roots were all incorporated into infusions or decoctions to strengthen the urinary and respiratory tracts and to assist in digestion. Similarly, in the Subcarpathian hill country of western Ukraine, sanicle is considered an excellent treatment for lung bleeds. Folk healers prescribe leaf infusions for coughs, and crushed leaves are applied to heal nasal passages; in powdered form, sanicle is applied to furuncles. A decoction is also good for stomach and intestinal catarrhs. In modern Ukrainian folk medicine, according to Grodzins'kyj, sanicle serves as a hemostatic, anti-inflammatory, anti-bacterial, and analgesic aid.

Herb infusions or rhizome decoctions, taken internally, treat bleeding in the lungs, stomach, intestines, and kidneys, as well as gastrointestinal ailments and coughs; externally, they are vulneraries. Root tinctures are thought to enhance male potency.

Considering its illustrious past as a reliable and versatile curative in western Europe, one wonders why sanicle disappeared from the materia medica of mainstream contemporary herbalism. As far as Ashkenazim are concerned, it's probable that Yiddish-speaking folk healers who considered the plant a cure-all did continue to rely on sanicle prior to the Second World War, but its application must have vanished along with the traditional healers of the Pale in the early decades of the twentieth century. It's likely that Ashkenazi Jews became acquainted with the plant in medieval Germany and took this knowledge (and sanicle's magical reputation as a protective plant) with them during their eastward migrations.

SAPONARIA OFFICINALIS |
SOAPWORT

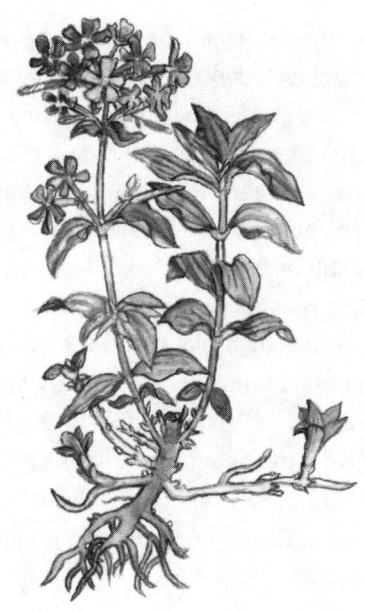

FAMILY Caryophyllaceae

YIDDISH זײַפֿגראָז (zayfgroz), זײַפֿן–װאָרצל (zayfn-vortsl)

POLISH Mydlnica lekarska

UKRAINIAN Собаче мило лікарське (Sobače mylo likars'ke), мильнянка лікарська (myl'njanka likars'ka), дике мило (dyke mylo), зірки білі (zirky bili), мило псяче (mylo psjače), мильний корінь (myl'nyj korin'), стягач (stjahač), сороканедужник (sorokanedužnyk)

LITHUANIAN Putoklis, vaistinis putoklis

RUSSIAN Мыльнянка лекарственная (Myl'njanka lekarstvennaja)

GERMAN Gewöhnliches Seifenkraut, Echtes Seifenkraut, Seifenwurz, Waschwurz

HEBREW בורית (borit)

What was everyday life like in the shtetls and villages of the Pale of Settlement? Some aspects are well recorded, preserved, and remembered: the religious observances, the mitzvot, the cheder, the latkes, and the kugel. But what about the material factors like the shape and construction of cottage roofs? What was clothing made from? What were the most popular methods of washing clothes? Or hair? So many of these minutiae have been (nearly) lost to history, but with a little excavation, we can still reconstruct some of our not-so-distant past.

Unsurprisingly, plants have played a large role in our daily lives, often in obscurity. Soapwort is one such plant, and it's been known, variously, in English as soapwort, soaproot, bouncing bet, latherwort, fuller's herb, bruise-wort, crow soap, sweet Betty, and sweet William. In the monograph on *Rubia tinctorum* (see p. 145), we write about the valkers or fullers of the Pale, and, judging from the plant's English moniker "fuller's herb," one can imagine the village spinners sitting at their wheels, having relied upon this herb for its attributes, which are so specific for degreasing freshly shorn wool.

The stout saponaria plant is a perennial that commonly grows in the Mediterranean basin and is renowned for its sudsing roots and leaves; it sports five-petalled flowers ranging in color from pink to lilac, as well as lanceolate waxy smooth leaves that arise from a narrow stalk-like base. It has a bitter and slightly sweet taste that causes a numbing sensation in the mouth. I'm not personally familiar with this herb, but it must be visually interesting, as Maude Grieve mentions it specifically as part of her garden's array of herbs.

In the early eighteenth century, ha-Kohen referred to the plant in two ways. In his alphabetical medicinal index, he lists saponariah (from the Latin *sapo*, "soap") as an external remedy. In the body of the text he calls upon it as בורית (borit), as an ingredient for formulas to be taken internally.

For a young child's rash on the face or head, ha-Kohen identifies a skin condition by names in several languages that seem indecipherable today. In what he identifies as French, he calls the condition krosta latika, which can be translated as "milk crust"; in "the language of Sepharad" he glosses the disease with the mysterious names krusmin and mastihini. In "the language of Ashkenaz," an even more curious name, דער לאזי ברנה (der lazi burnah), is invoked. All things considered, ha-Kohen may have been referring to what today we know as "cradle cap," a childhood malady that even now is not well understood by modern Western medicine and that can be misdiagnosed.

Ha-Kohen approached this affliction as a toxin that needed to be sweated from the body. Encouraging perspiration to cure an illness is a particularly Jewish remedy; my mother would tell me how sweating was a common method to combat sickness in her parents' community back in the old country. For this particular situation, ha-Kohen recommends that the juice of sambucus be given to an infant to drink at night so as to promote a healing sweat. Cleaning the affected skin was also important, and in this case, he suggested an external wash of chelidonium, fumaria, or saponaria, together or separately, as purifying herbs. Intriguingly, while ha-Kohen does not relate saponaria to his description of the kaltine (Plica Polonica or Polish kołtun) or how to treat it, physicians a century after him recognized soapwort's utility in relieving this affliction, recommending that the patient submit to decoctions of "soapy" plants, according to H. Rosenberg in his 1839 study of the Polish plait, *Der Weichselzopf* (The Vistula Plait).

In *Ashkenazi Herbalism*, we wrote about *Chelidonium majus,* a significant herb in many Jewish communities of the Pale, one often applied for cleansing the scalp in the shtetls of Polona (now Polonne) and Tchan (now Teofipol). In Romen (now Romny), Luben (now Lubny), Kyiv, Anopol (now Hannopil), Bohslov (now Bohuslav), Balte (now Balta), and Monasterishtche (now Monastyryšče), shvalbn milekh, "swallow's milk"—as chelidonium was called in Yiddish—was helpful when rubbed on locally or in a bath to heal skin disorders such as itching, eczema, and rash. Over two hundred years after ha-Kohen, Maude Grieve writes of a decoction of fumitory (another plant in ha-Kohen's remedy) that made a curative lotion for "milk crust" on the scalp of an infant. Her modern recipe reminds us that the ancients' medicinal knowledge was, and continues to be, an enduring gift to the healing arts.

Ha-Kohen was also concerned with children's regularity. For those with constipation that lasted more than two or three days, he recommends chicory with rhubarb or apple syrup. Also, the abdomen could be softened with an enema or suppository of borit, "soap," depending on the size or nature of the child. This aperient promoted by ha-Kohen could still be found in the practices of those living in the Polish lands two centuries later; it was described by Talko-Hryncewicz as "a common suppository made of gray soap that was especially common among the Jews," which reminds us again that one of the distinctive features of Jewish folk medicine in Eastern Europe was its attention to digestive health.

Talko-Hryncewicz described jaundice as a "disease caused by the spillage of bile throughout the body, or by shock or impact to the kidneys, causing the skin of those affected to become discolored." To heal this condition, home remedies as well as magical treatments were sought out throughout the Pale. One recommendation from Zwinogródka included having the patient hold a live pike in each hand and stare at the fish until they died, thus passing the disease from the human to the fish. A similar remedy relied upon young, defeathered pigeons, and yet another called for the sick person's urine to be boiled with a chicken egg and thrown to dogs to eat, thereby transferring the disease away from the patient.

In persistent cases of jaundice, *Saponaria officinalis* was considered quite effective in the Polish lands of the late 1800s, a remedy corroborated by Maude Grieve some decades later. In Czerkasy, it was found to be helpful to ingest pieces of soapwort to break up bladder stones. In the town of Nowa-Uszyca, the herb, dissolved in water, was taken to stimulate delayed menstruation.

In mid-twentieth-century Polish plant medicine, saponaria was recommended for its actions on the mucous membranes of the respiratory tract, on digestion, and for its metabolism-stimulating qualities; it was also recommended as a blood cleanser and anti-rheumatic. It is a very powerful plant: per Bieganski, official Polish herbal medicine recommended it be limited to one-twelfth of compound formulas treating chest ailments, rheumatism, and for cleansing the blood.

During the same period, in Ukrainian and Russian folk medicine, according to both Nosal' and Nosal' and Müller-Dietz, decoctions of saponaria have long been relied upon for gastrointestinal, kidney, liver, rheumatic, and spleen ailments, as well as diseases related to metabolic disorders leading to skin inflammations such as eczema, furuncles, boils, or abscesses; folk healers in mid-nineteenth-century Russia relied upon decoctions of saponaria root mixed with charcoal powder to be applied to scabies. Soapwort is also part of the modern Russian folk medical kit as a laxative, diuretic, and cholagogue.

Contemporary Ukrainian folk medicine, particularly in the Subcarpathians, still adheres to these traditional applications (decoctions, infusions, and compresses) as a diuretic and expectorant, as a metabolic stimulant, and for skin diseases (eczema, psoriasis, furuncles, etc.).

In twentieth-century Lithuanian official herbal medicine, according to Gudelytė, infusions of soapwort flower are applied for conditions of the menstrual cycle, coughing, or skin diseases, and also to treat rheumatism and stimulate the secretion of bile and the excretion of urine, as well as for diaphoresis.

Polish folk medicine reveals a very intriguing parallel to saponaria remedies on both sides of the Atlantic Ocean. Yiddish-speaking Jews who settled in South America were advised to apply the bark of the Chilean soap bark tree (*Quillaja saponaria*) for both laundry and the scalp. Polish plant medicine of the same period, according to Biegański, specifically recommends saponaria as a substitute for Quillay, as a soap, as a compress for bruises, and as an expectorant.

According to author Sophie Knab, pharmacies in early nineteenth-century Poland that adhered to the directives of the *Pharmacopoeia Regni Poloniae* were making six different varieties of soap, some of which were regarded as internal medicines for treating illnesses such as venereal disease, gallbladder stones, and, by the administration of small doses of saponaria on thin wafers to be ingested, to relieve constipation. This remedy was very similar to those described earlier by ha-Kohen in his children's laxative, and the Polish surveys reported the same treatments as common among Jews in the late nineteenth century.

For anyone who has wondered about hair care in the towns and villages of the Pale, Knab sparks our imagination when she describes how women in Poland grew the beautiful saponaria plant in their kitchen gardens to have it on hand for shampooing hair or washing delicate fabrics. Because commercially made soap products were often too expensive (or less available) for the average villager, and concocting one's own cosmetics could be extremely labor-intensive, "for personal use and laundry, sometimes it was easier to use the stems, leaves, and roots of the soapwort plant, which lathers when mixed with water." In fact, in the village of Zwinogródka, *Saponaria officinalis* was the plant of choice for washing one's hair, especially among girls and women. Soapwort could also be combined with burdock root and nettle leaves for imparting one's tresses with more softness and luster.

Nowadays, we can still find saponaria's sudsing virtues in unexpected places, such as making consistent the distinctive texture of halva, as a stabilizer in the commercial production of tahini, and as a component in enhancing the foaming quality of American beer.

SISYMBRIUM OFFICINALE |
HEDGE MUSTARD

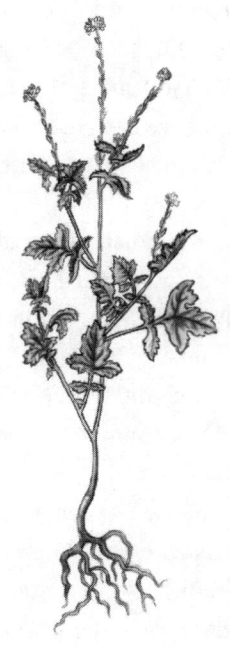

FAMILY Brassicaceae

YIDDISH רפֿואה–טודרע (refuah-tudre)

POLISH Stulisz lekarski

UKRAINIAN Сухоребрик лікарський (Suxorebryk likars'kyj)

BELARUSIAN Гуляўнік лекавы (Huljaŭnik lekavy), кудзер лекавы (kudzer lekavy)

LITHUANIAN Pikulė

RUSSIAN   Гулявник лекарственный (Guljavnik lekarstvennyj)

GERMAN   Weg-Rauke, Echte Rauke, Gewöhnliche Rauke

HEBREW   תודרה (tudrah)

Sisymbrium officinale, or hedge mustard, is one of the five plants in Mordkhe Schaechter's *Plant Names in Yiddish* that include the mysterious designation *refuahdiker,* "remedy," in their Yiddish name. There's very little written about hedge mustard in the West or otherwise. Historically, however, hedge mustard was quite the popular remedy in the Pale of Settlement, even as late as the turn of the last century.

The herb's other mysterious Yiddish name, tudre, can be explored in Fred Rosner's *Moses Maimonides' Glossary of Drug Names.* Rosner's translation informs us that *Sisymbrium officinale*'s Yiddish name comes from Persian tudari and that Maimonides himself mentioned "tudari asfar" in his medical works. When considered as a whole, the appellation *refuah-tudre* suggests that hedge mustard must have been known as a healing plant by Jews for quite some time, perhaps millennia.

Sisymbrium officinale, formerly *Erysimum officinale,* is in the Brassicaceae, or mustard, family, and is native to Europe and North Africa and is naturalized throughout the world. It has a long stem, serrate-pinnate leaves, and small crowning flowers. Issachar bar Teller warned against the consumption of mustard, and other plants classified as warming, whenever the patient suffered from "redness of the face." Ha-Kohen later wrote of khardal, the Arabic word for mustard, but he didn't specify which mustard family herb he was referring to in his remedy for scurvy or as part of a dietary caution against the consumption of plants he considered hard on the body.

In the West, Maude Grieve and other herbalists refer to hedge mustard as an herb known since antiquity to soothe a singer's irritated vocal tract. In fact, one of the plant's French names is herbe aux chantres, "singer's plant."

In the late nineteenth-century Pale of Settlement, *Sisymbrium officinale* was a plant known for its many medicinal applications. For children and adults, "mustard plasters" were effective for soothing coughs, reminiscent of Nicholas Culpeper's treatment of the plant. Mustard seed was also useful as a laxative.

In eastern Galicia, snuff tobacco mixed with mustard powder cured a runny nose caused by a cold.

In the town of Hussakowa, to dispel stomach pain, distention, wind, and nausea, folk healers gave a teaspoon of hedge mustard to be drunk with water.

Headache relief treatments could be surprisingly harsh. For instance, lubricating the head with fried squirrel brains was reported in Płoskirow, and it was common practice throughout the region to inhale grated horseradish or snuff. Even the common practice of kneading mustard into dough and placing it behind the ears or back of the neck seems extreme, but no more so than attaching leeches to the skin behind the ears to remove excess blood, or pulling the hair of a person suffering from a headache so as to distract them from the original source of pain, both of which were popular remedies of the Pale.

Perhaps the most curious of the sympathetic medicinal remedies for a headache reported by informants in the Pale in the late nineteenth century was the belief that not combing one's hair would cure headaches. This prophylaxis could sometimes be achieved by growing out the matted, unwashed hair known to Poles as the kołtun. It's curious that in the Polish lands, the kołtun, or ka_tine (as it was called in Yiddish), might be either the affliction or the cure.

Should a person suffer from sudden paralysis or fainting, many folk remedies were available in the Pale in the late nineteenth century. Physical methods included blowing into a patient's face and eyes (possibly borrowed from Tatar siufkaczes), giving them powdered black pepper or hellebore as a sneezing agent, giving them an emetic, opening their mouth and tickling the back of their throat with a goose feather dipped in olive oil, making them sniff a strong spirit or ammonia, moving them into fresh air and loosening their clothing, or squeezing their little finger or entire hand. For paralysis, a hedge mustard tea was given to drink, or if someone was suffering from a numb patch on their body, a mustard plaster or grated horseradish was applied to the numb area.

Plasters for painful hips and other sores were commonly derived from plants other than mustard. According to Zajączkowski, Karaim healers, in particular, relied upon mosses (species not specified), an approach their Turkic ancestors may have brought with them from distant Siberia: one Karaim remedy book recommends that for pain in the hips, one should collect moss from stones, boil in water, and drink at night. Similarly, a Karaim treatment for ulcers called for brewing moss taken from an old thatched straw roof and applying topically.

Fevers were one of the most common illnesses in late nineteenth-century Eastern Europe. In parts of Ukraine, a widely held belief was there were ninety-nine kinds of fevers. Throughout the Pale, almost every region had its own local name for the condition: in Ukraine, it was called propastnycija, trastija, trepetuxa, or potepuxa; in Volhynia, xvebra and trjasuxa; in Podolia, gnietuxa and lyxomanka; and around Chełm, znobycia and titka. Ashkenazim referred to it as kaduches.

At that time, there were many superstitious beliefs throughout the Pale regarding the cause of fevers, among them the evil eye. Folk healers of various regions considered many herbs beneficial for ridding the body of fever, including strong teas of sage (brewed in the Kharkiv district), either a strong brew of madder or young willow branches (in Podolia), or a tea of forest garlic or dried wild strawberry leaves and flowers (in Zwinogródka). Among the most common herbal remedies reported were those of hedge mustard, bogbean, rowan berries, or garlic. Most of these plants are considered to be energetically warming in the body, thus causing a person to sweat.

Besides plant material for treating fever, healers turned to other substances such as crayfish eyes, dried and powdered frogs, breast milk, the dung of various animals, spiderwebs, tar, or clay, any of which could be prepared in a multitude of combinations. Sympathetic magical remedies were also prevalent. One such treatment required fumigating a patient with burning parchment on which were written charms. This treatment, which seems to have originated in the Jewish community, and which was universally associated with Tatar healers, became widespread throughout Podolia. In general, wearing specially prepared amulets was also found to be effective for the relief of fever and other ailments.

In the popular imagination of the time, many diseases were believed to be caused by poisoning via magical means. This malevolent practice was a complex one and called for the use of powdered animal material, which allegedly revivified in an unsuspecting victim's digestive tract. One Polish story mentions a Jewish man who claimed to have been the victim of such a poisoner and as a result vomited up thirty-five frogs, which conjures up an image of the Perrault fairy tale "Diamonds and Toads."

In my family lore, it's said that one of my ancestors (from Tarnogród, Poland) died from poisoning (see *Armoracia rusticana*, p. 51). No other details were passed down to me, but reading about a decoction that was recorded as an antidote for poison in Zwinogródka made me wonder if the power of hedge mustard could have saved my great-grandfather's life. The belief that the herb was a cure for all poisons and venoms may have its origins with the ancients, or at least as far back as the age of Nicholas Culpeper, author of *The English Physitian* (1652), also known as *Culpeper's Complete Herbal*, the greatest authority on healing plants of the early modern era.

Another health concern, multivarious in both cause and location, was hemorrhage. For this, plants were very helpful when staunching was needed, including compresses of mustard or horseradish. Many other styptic remedies were popular in the towns and villages of the late nineteenth-century Pale, such as applying clean spiderwebs or the soft center of a loaf of bread.

And of course magical means were called upon to staunch the flow of blood from a wound. One of many such examples was recorded in Zwinogródka, where an eighty-three-year-old Jewish woman, whose name is only given as (Mrs.) Panarowska, recited an incantation to help stop a hemorrhage. An approximate translation of her charm, which was repeated three times, runs as follows: "By God's will, there are three horns. One with water, one with honey, one with blood. I pour out the honey, I drink the water, I order the blood so that it does not flow."

As if all of this weren't enough, hedge mustard had at least one more documented power in the Pale before the Second World War. Eye complaints were sufficiently common enough in the region to warrant a plethora of ready remedies. Although the conditions varied, their causes, according to Talko-Hryncewicz, were often attributed to "spoiled blood," "heat effects" among those who brought in the harvest, or overzealous attention to kitchen duties around the hot oven (known in Yiddish as the pechka or petzerke) by the women of the house (gospodyni).

Some remedies against eye complaints were prophylactic: in Zwinogródka, coral beads were worn around the neck; throughout the region, children, particularly young girls, would wear earrings. Taking snuff was also thought to prevent future eye problems. It's interesting to note that these are highly gendered remedies, as is the association of eye complaints with overzealous housewives. As for plant medicine, here again we find hedge mustard pounded into dough and applied behind the ears or on the nape of the neck to relieve eye pain. For epidemic eye diseases, in the towns of Zbaraż and Załuże, healers used more sympathetic cures, such as fumigating victims with the smoke from a fried frog.

Most fascinating of all, however, was the summoning of a medicine man in the town of Ryżanówka to heal an eye affliction by licking it. Today, this seems very strange, and possibly dangerous, but in the Pale it was an extremely common remedy that is attested in many yizkor books, such as those of Slutsk, Gorodets, and Mlave.

Twentieth-century Russian folk medicine, according to Müller-Dietz, has relied upon hedge mustard seeds and leaves to treat asthma, diarrhea, and parasites. Externally, it has served as a remedy for ulcers or abscesses. In Romanian pediatric folk medicine, the aerial parts were to be taken internally (unspecified) as a treatment for epilepsy.

So many of these Old World remedies that survived well into the mid-twentieth century, while incongruous with our contemporary understanding of medicine, can remind us that we're just a small part of the animal kingdom, of the world, and of the cosmos in general. Not very long ago, our ancestors had to learn how to take care of themselves and each other by closely observing everything around them. Although some of their methods appear worrisome or merely ineffectual to us today, those who came before us survived well enough and long enough using their ancient ways to bring us to the present moment.

TILIA EUROPAEA | LINDEN

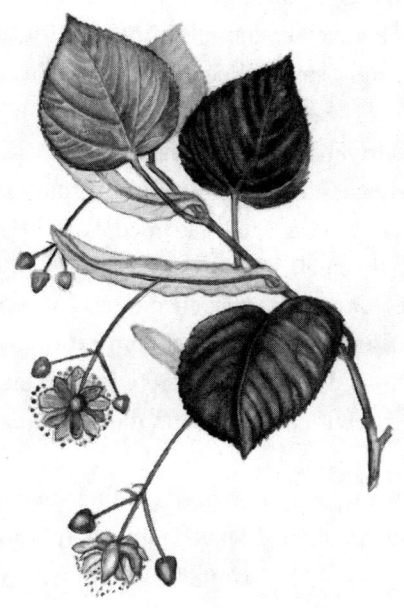

FAMILY Malvaceae

YIDDISH ליפע (lipe), לינדנבוים (lindnboym)

POLISH Lipa

UKRAINIAN Липа (Lypa)

BELARUSIAN Липа (Lipa)

LITHUANIAN Liepa

RUSSIAN Липа европейская (Lipa evropejskaja), липа обыкновенная (lipa obyknovennaja)

GERMAN Linden

Years ago, before I studied herbalism formally, I would often encounter a subtle fragrance in the spring air that was familiar yet unidentifiable. I came to think of it as the "candy smell," and for a long time its source remained a mystery. Fast-forward some years later to a late-spring afternoon meandering the cobbled streets of an ancient central European city, and I caught an unexpected whiff of the candy smell. Needless to say, I was determined to find its source and eventually wandered into a tiny wedge-like park. In one of the sharp angles of the courtyard, where the back walls of the old stone apartment buildings met, a lonely café patiently awaited customers under the canopy of an enormous tree in full bloom. This, I learned, was the European linden, and from it wafted the candy smell.

In the years since that momentous encounter, I've come to rely on linden in my daily tea blend, and it's been a real comfort in many ways. In modern Western herbal traditions, linden is considered a nervine and a cardiac tonic, but the tree's connection with humans is far more complicated and, unsurprisingly, ancient.

In Eastern European communities, including those of the Ashkenazim, linden (which bears heart-shaped leaves with sharply toothed margins, dark green above and pale below, and whitish flowers with yellowish bracts) has been a well-known and well-loved tree. Prior to the Second World War, it was known in Yiddish as di lindnboym (cf. German *Lindenbaum*) or lipe (cf. Polish *lipa*). Linden's importance to European onomastics is obvious, as one can tell from the sheer number of places, particularly in Eastern Europe, whose names are derived from linden: Berlin's Unter den Linden boulevard, Leipzig in Germany, Liepava in Lithuania, and Russian Lipetsk, where my aunt was born just before the Nazi invasion of the USSR.

And yet—despite such deep and obvious roots and their long entanglement with the many peoples of the region—our relationship with this sacred tree remains shrouded in mystery, especially for Ashkenazim. Most puzzling to me was one of ha-Kohen's several names for linden, "asherah tree." When I first encountered this name in ha-Kohen's plant glossary, I was unclear about the association he was making between the ancient Near Eastern deity Asherah and the medicinal tree. Fortunately, it was his habit to provide multiple names for plants in the pre-Linnean age: ha-Kohen also records the name of the tree in "the language of Ashkenaz" as lindinboim, in French as tillet (cf. modern French tilleul), and in Turkish as flamur (from Greek φλαμουριά, Tilia tomentosa, leaving no doubt that linden is his asherah tree.

As someone who identifies as "ethnically" Jewish but who has never been religious, I wasn't acquainted with this ancient goddess, so I was surprised to learn Asherah was a significant Semitic nature deity, the female counterpart to Yahweh himself. Asherah is mentioned at least thirty times in the Tanakh, mostly positively. But from a very early date, the honoring of Asherah was strongly discouraged, and finally prohibited. This scenario is borne out from conversations I've since had with observant friends who know of Asherah as a sacred figure, but not in Judaism.

Francesca Stavrakopoulou, a contemporary historian of Judaism, has spoken of Asherah's biblical association with ancient midwives, lamenters, bonesetters, and women who interceded with the dead on behalf of the living. Readers may recall these as the professions of bobes and opshprekherins. Is it presumptuous to posit that these women folk healers may well have been practicing a distaff tradition so ancient it can be traced back to the pre-Judaic Semitic world?

That a Semitic goddess so closely linked to the natural world has been maligned and neglected in Judaism is, to say the least, disappointing. But if ha-Kohen or contemporary biblical reinterpretations of the ancient texts are any indication, Asherah's deliberate erasure as a Judaic deity seems irrelevant, especially to someone like me who has little or no connection to religious teachings. When I consider my own experiences with linden, it feels as though the entity ha-Kohen named as the tree of Asherah has been patiently calling to me over the years, waiting until I was finally able to recognize her significance.

But regardless of its association with contested belief systems in the ancient Near East, linden has long been a revered healing tree for the many peoples of the Pale.

Teller writes that linden helps with a headache, but only if constipation is not present. His recipe is a tea "for a cold flow from the head" that requires a few handfuls each of the flowers of chamomile, rue, sage, dill, wormwood, linden, lovage, and hyssop, all to be boiled in water and used as a headwash for pain relief.

Teller also offers a concoction to bring on menstruation, by soaking laurel leaves, pimpernel root, and the blossom of nutmeg, then crushing and mixing these components with linden water. He advises drinking the infusion warm in the evening when in bed.

Ha-Kohen also advises linden for many conditions, including as a general tonic for health. More specifically, he writes of the herb as a treatment for oral lesions. As a poultice, he calls for the flowers to be mixed with vinegar for skin conditions, especially for swelling in the legs. While these ancient remedies may seem at odds with what we understand of linden's nervine and cardiac attributes, they are reflected in contemporary Russian herbal formulas that rely on linden for soothing mouth lesions or as a topical application for skin conditions, or even for headache relief.

In a complicated section on spasms in children, ha-Kohen surmised that "the forced disease" (epilepsy, or "the falling sickness"), so called because it had an external origin (possibly malignant spirits), could be brought on by a variety of causes, including prolonged nursing, undigested milk, intestinal worms, fevers, toothache, or even sudden fear. One of his formulas includes peony root, followed by the water of linden flowers as part of a more complex regimen. Another one of his multifaceted formulations for spasms requires pulverized emerald or crystal dust.

Two centuries later, childhood epilepsy, known as czarna słabość ("black weakness") in Poland, was considered a disease of the nervous system, and many believed it was caused by fear in a pregnant woman that in turn affected her unborn child. The illness was treated with special linden flower distillations made in the old Polish apothecaries. Another belief held that seizures were contagious: watching someone having a seizure would cause enough fright in the onlooker to bring one on as well. In such cases, it was a common practice to cover an epileptic with a black cloth. Ashkenazim would use a tallis for such purposes as well. Linden was also part of a formula for seizures in Kyiv (see *Valeriana officinalis*, p. 213).

In the Polish lands in the late nineteenth century, people believed that linden offered protection against lightning and evil, and healers found many applications for the tree's medicinal properties as well. Some of these Polish prescriptions closely parallel both Teller's and ha-Kohen's remedies, especially for the relief of headaches, where the linden leaves were applied to the head or given as a tea made from the tree's flowers.

For children's breathing difficulties, linden was a common remedy in the Pale during this period. A linden flower tea was recommended for general coughing and also for the coughing associated with tuberculosis. In Podolia, fresh linden leaves were advised. For consumptives in Nowa-Uszyca, healers offered linden wood charcoal with camphor. Remedies in the town of Zwinogródka also recall ha-Kohen's recommendation for edema in the legs by covering swollen areas with linden bark, boiled and applied warm, or just applying the leaves.

Looking back once more to ha-Kohen's writings on treating damaged skin, in Zwinogródka folk healers more than a century ago applied dry compresses of linden leaves to soothe burns.

As I've said, my mother told me that sweating was an important component for restoring health among our ancestors in southeastern Poland. And in fact, diaphoretics were a common remedy among both Jews and the landed gentry in the Polish lands of the late nineteenth century. One of the most common curatives to produce sweat in a feverish patient was a tea made with linden blossoms.

As we wrote in *Ashkenazi Herbalism*, in the Pale, a common condition among children was fear (Yiddish shrek, Polish przestrach), and it was generally treated with herbs and magic. Because many of the healers who removed this affliction were women—bobes and opshprekherins—their methods were infrequently recorded. Treatments, including diagnosis through divination (wax or lead pouring, for instance) and relief via plants and charms, were similar, if not identical, among the region's various communities.

In the late nineteenth-century Polish lands, children's bedwetting was a condition believed to be caused by fear, and it was treated by opshprekherins and other women folk healers by means of rituals such as wax or lead divination in order to discern the source of the child's unease. In Eastern Europe, this could be further addressed with remedies made from animal ingredients—for example, burnt hedgehog skin, or ash from burnt goat, or sheep dung mixed with vinegar and water, a recipe Talko-Hryncewicz documented in the town of Zwinogródka. But the most effective method noted was a magical one that required hollowing out a linden log and having the afflicted child hop over it several times a day for nine days. This was a common treatment in Volhynia, Podolia, and Bessarabia. The number nine is associated with magical rituals among the peoples of the region, including Ashkenazim.

A distinctly related treatment described by Isaac Lévy and Rosemary Lévy Zumwalt in their *Ritual Medical Lore of Sephardic Women*, known as sara-dura or ensaradura among Sephardim in Rhodes, Greece, specifically requires linden combined with marjoram as a nurturing tea for working with anxiety, fear, or depression.

Herbalist and author Naomi Spector writes that in her Sephardi tradition, linden was part of a tea given to help alleviate cold symptoms. In *The Jewish Book of Flowers*, she offers a recipe inspired by a traditional cold remedy known by the Separdi community of Rhodes. Two parts dried linden leaf and flower is combined with one part cinnamon bark chips and simmered in boiling water for a few minutes, allowing the flavors to extract. After straining, you can add a spoonful (or more, depending on your preference) of freshly squeezed lemon juice and then drink the tea while still hot.

In the yizkor memory books, linden trees have a strong presence, both medicinally and in other surprising ways. For instance, one yizkor book, from Ostrolena (Ostrołęka, Poland), memorializes the trusting and positive relationship the town's Jews had with their neighbors the Kurpies, a Polish community who lived close to the land, practiced apiculture, and made sandals from the bast of the linden tree. Kurpies called their neighbors "starozakonni" (Old Testament) and engaged in a lively trade in both honey and bast shoes with them.

Linden bast was an important product in other parts of the Pale as well. In mid-nineteenth-century Zawiercie, Poland, several Ashkenazi entrepreneurs founded a large "linden wool" factory and exported bast as a substitute for shearling.

A century later, linden was still enjoyed in the shtetls for its healing scent, as described in the memory book of Sanok.

Time-tested folk healing traditions prevailed in Poland in the early twentieth century, where infusions of elder and linden flowers, along with dried raspberry or raspberry cordial, were the medicines of choice for inducing perspiration to draw disease from the body.

Folk healers in the shtetl of Antopol also looked to "popular grasses such as chamomile, linden, nettles, and the like" for soothing illnesses such as fever or stomach pain.

Linden was also known for its specifically magical properties: in Nowa-Uszyca, one belief held that boiling linden bast in water and pouring the mixture out before the threshold of one's home would cause one's enemy, if they passed by, to be transformed into a wolf. In the yizkor book for Bobruisk (now Babrujsk, Belarus, near Mogilev), a heart-wrenching scene was described by a survivor from that town: "On a hill near the railroad depot, they will show you a spot circled by linden trees, and they will tell you that it was once a Jewish cemetery."

But not all of linden's healing stories among the Ashkenazim have been tragic or even melancholy. In postwar Argentina, survivors continued to look to the tree for its healing qualities. In Buenos Aires, "di lindn" was referred to by one Ashkenazi herbalist as a true panacea; he recommended linden tea to quell nervous disorders, to aid difficult digestion, and to drive away insomnia.

A different application for linden was observed among the Roma of Serbia in the late nineteenth century: For eye infections, they would carefully remove the outer bark of fresh linden and juniper branches and scrape off the white inner bark. On this they would pour river water, beating it with a clean stick until it produced a mucilage, which was then applied to a linen cloth to wipe and bandage the afflicted eye.

Among contemporary Lithuanian Jewish healers (mostly women), linden and chamomile are the most highly regarded plant remedies. These healers collect the blossoms shortly after opening, and make a tea from the flowers to treat upper respiratory conditions, improve expectoration, promote sweating, and cleanse the oral cavity of any potential infection. They also take equal parts linden blossoms and diced raspberries and steep them in boiled water for ten to twenty minutes, recommending drinking this tea three to four times a day to promote sweating, especially in the presence of a low-grade fever.

For a sore throat, these Lithuanian Jewish folk healers mix two parts three-lobed beggartick, four parts chamomile flowers, two parts linden flowers, and two parts sage leaves. Once this dried plant matter is assembled, they take two to three teaspoons of the mixture and simmer in one glass of boiling water for fifteen minutes. They advise rinsing the mouth and gargling with the cooled liquid several times a day as needed.

Every contemporary Lithuanian healer from the formerly majority-Jewish region of Kaišiadorys surveyed relies on linden: in a tea for colds, for flu symptoms, fevers, coughs, and to promote sweating. One healer recommends inhaling the scent of linden flowers as a treatment for respiratory diseases, and chewing linden buds to address stomach acidity.

Lithuanian Muslim herbalists have a similar understanding of linden: they offer this herb to those with colds or inflammations of the mouth and throat.

According to Müller-Dietz, in his survey of the medicinal plants of the former Soviet Union, linden is much less employed there than it is in the west, which makes the treatments of Ashkenazi Jewish healers and their neighbors something of an outlier. In other parts of the former Russian Empire and Soviet Union, however, the powdered seeds of linden serve as a styptic for nosebleeds and wounds; the powdered leaf buds are used externally to treat abscesses and burns. Powdered linden wood has been relied upon to treat meteorism and diarrhea; as a disinfectant for clothing and other household objects, known as "tsar's water," it has treated infectious diseases.

THE TRIANKE

While researching *Ashkenazi Herbalism*, we happened upon something more significant than we could have known at the time. This was a story within a story, a brief interlude in Pauline Wengeroff's *Memoirs of a Grandmother*. She recollected the career of her grandmother-in-law, Beile, a folk healer and midwife who attended the author's pregnancy, childbirth, and postpartum recovery in Konotip (present-day Konotop, Ukraine) in the nineteenth century. What we found remarkable was the passage that described an herbal formula Beile administered to a mother-to-be—the ingredients were so casually itemized it seemed as if di gantse megillah (Yiddish for "the whole thing") was common knowledge. Beile's recipe calls for several specific plants, describes in detail how they are to be prepared, and identifies the formula merely as "the trianka," a title that suggests, inevitably, the number three.*

During this early stage of our research, to find any mention at all of plants as applied by a Jewish woman folk healer in the Pale of Settlement was revelatory. Beile's recipe was the first of its kind that we had encountered, and its significance was in no way lost on us.

Ashkenazi women folk healers in particular are scarcely mentioned in the literature of the Pale. We have called the resulting lack of information one of the many "erasures" that obscure the world of healing in the Pale, which has made finding out more about the lives of the healers very challenging. One significant erasure was established by the healers themselves, by simply never setting their methods on paper but rather passing down their wisdom from one generation to the next through word of mouth or direct instruction.

At that stage of our research, just to locate and situate this formula and its significance seemed sufficient. Aside from the documentation of the recipe itself, we noted that most of the ingredients (galangal, anise, nutmeg, cinnamon, clove, figs, and carob bean) were not native to the Pale. This realization led us to include a monograph devoted to nutmeg (*Myristica fragrans*). We traced that herb's distant origins in Oceania, trying to understand how such

---

* While this formula has many spellings, our preference is for its Yiddish name, trianke.

an exotic spice came to be a common ingredient in a specialized remedy for postpartum healing administered by an unknown folk midwife from an obscure shtetl in a forgotten corner of Eastern Europe.

Several years after the publication of *Ashkenazi Herbalism*, while reading through Talko-Hryncewicz's nineteenth-century ethnobotanical surveys, we again stumbled upon a recipe with an undeniable resemblance to Beile's. This "famous Russian recipe," as attested in the town of Sobolivka (in the late nineteenth century 20 percent Jewish; now Sobolivka, Ukraine), was known not as trianka but as korni ot slabosti, "roots against weakness." This formula appears in Talko-Hryncewicz's section on childbirth; he emphasizes that this preparation was always recommended for women who needed to regain their strength after childbirth. The ingredients are nutmeg (*Myristica fragrans*), yellow ginger (*Zingiber montanum*), white ginger (*Zingiber officinale*), galangal (*Alpinia officinarum*), star anise (*Illicium verum*), "brunški" (likely *Rubia tinctorum*), cloves (*Syzygium aromaticum*), "English pepper" (allspice, the fruit of the New World tree *Pimenta dioica*), senna (likely *Senna alexandrina*), cinnamon bark (*Cinnamomum verum*), chicory (*Cichoria intybus*), "staroduba" (likely *Adonis vernalis*), carob (*Ceratonia siliqua*), and camphor (*Camphorum officinarum*).

This new encounter with the world of healing in the nineteenth-century Pale made us take a closer look at Beile's story, beyond merely observing that exotic spices were commonly available in the shtetls of Eastern Europe. It became clear that Beile's Konotip trianke (or the "roots against weakness" of Sobolivka) was a widely known remedy, the basis for which was invariably non-native (i.e., imported) plants. But even more remarkably, we learned that the main source for these exotic spices and plants in the towns and villages of the Pale was the mostly Jewish spice traders and merchants of the region.

Our discovery is fascinating: it underscores just how entwined the peoples daily lives were in the Pale of Settlement and beyond. From our close reading of the nineteenth-century Polish ethnobotanical surveys, we now can say with certainty that these recipes were in use in the mid-nineteenth century in highly mixed communities more than three hundred miles distant from one another, and that the recipes consisted of exotic herbs and spices acquired from Jewish vendors. This (along with other evidence we've uncovered) testifies to the centrality of this complex formulation for supporting postpartum recovery, and that it is perhaps the defining remedy of women healers of all faiths and ethnicities throughout the Pale.

The rediscovery of the trianke offers a rare opportunity to more closely examine the contents of Beile's secret black bag that she carried with her when called into action for a laboring woman, a feverish child, or any other ailing community member who knew and trusted her healing abilities. Prior to discovering the Polish surveys, we only had very tiny, keyhole glimpses into the lives of these women—in this instance, a midwife's half-remembered trianke recipe as administered nearly two centuries ago and recalled almost fifty years later. But with the Polish surveys, a panoramic view of the region's rich and tightly woven herbal embroidery comes into much clearer focus than the passing glances we'd uncovered earlier. The tantalizing statement by Abraham Rekhtman from the An-sky expeditions that "these women knew hundreds of ways to cure a patient" could now be expanded upon.

In a general sense, the "roots against weakness" formula exemplifies just how prevalent herbalism was in the shtetls of Eastern Europe up until the Second World War. Moreover, it's remarkable to find that towns with comparatively small Ashkenazi populations, such as Sobolivka (20 percent), had a thriving Jewish herbal tradition and practice.

Returning to the spice merchant's role in this story, we must point out that the majority of the plants in the two recipes would not have been possible to cultivate in the climate or geographic conditions of Eastern Europe. Therefore they would have been imported, and it's probable they traveled along the age-old spice routes. It's only natural to surmise that the spice trader in Sobolivka would have had "connections" from whom he secured his wares wholesale. These wholesalers would have had their own sources, and so on, suggesting a complicated chain of wheeling and dealing. Jewish merchants of the Pale have a long and colorful history of taking part in wide-ranging, complex commercial navigations that required arduous travel, linguistic acrobatics, and elaborate negotiations that spanned borders, jurisdictions, and eras. Imagining this lattice of trade, whether by sea (to the Baltic ports of Gdańsk or Hamburg, or the Black Sea port of Odessa) or by land (across central Asia and Siberia, or up the Volga and across the Caucasus), begs the question: Over how many centuries had this system developed, and what were the methods for transporting the plants from their distant origins in the Far East (and the New World) to the obscure shtetls of the Pale of Settlement? Some historians think this trade was established by those legendary Jewish traders known as the Radanites (or Radhanites), whose routes, according to Arab historians of the Middle Ages, spanned the known world.

It may come as a surprise to readers (it did to us) to learn that the trianke even made its way to the New World, complete with its mysterious moniker. A 1907 issue of *The Druggist's Circular* (p. 211) provided the responses from several pharmacists to a query about the ingredients of the "trojanka." A. Weinstein, A. Kaufman, J. A. Klein (a "Russian pharmacist"), and L. Hirshon, all practicing in Northeastern cities in the United States, responded to the journal's query by writing in to describe the plants their personal trianke formulas required. Every one of these American pharmacists included the herbs in both Beile's remedy and the Sobolivka recipe. Were these American transplants recalling their bobes' remedies?

Almost a century and a quarter later, in contemporary Lithuania, the trianke continues to heal those who seek its medicine. At least two proprietary commercial formulations under the names Trianka and Trojanka are advertised as effective for boosting immunity and maintaining strength.

Here's a linguistic puzzle we think we may have solved. The name trianke (or *trianka* or *trojanka*) in Eastern Europe invariably reminds us of the number three. But the trianke not infrequently has a dozen ingredients. In Lithuania, the remedy is also known as "the three nines" (trejos devynerios), which is also the brand name of one of the local commercial formulations (vodka-infused bitters). Like Goldilocks and the three bears, we would seem to have not enough and too many ingredients—why none that are just right?

We believe that *trianke* (or *trianka* or *trojanka*) is likely a (peasant) corruption of *theriac*, the fabulous antidote for all poisons, for two reasons: one pharmaceutical and one phonological. The trianke recipes of the Pale (and the Jewish diaspora) are generally similar if not identical to many theriac formulations once found in European apothecaries.

One distinctive characteristic of Polish is its nasal vowels (similar to French). The phenomenon of hypercorrection by analogy—wherein "majority rules"

A. Kaufman, also of this city, sends the following formula:

Orange peel	1	ounce.
Cut gentian	1	ounce.
Cardamom	½	ounce.
Galangal	½	ounce.
Star anise	½	ounce.
Caraway seed	½	ounce.
Centaury	1	ounce.
Red clover blossoms	½	ounce.
Blood root	½	ounce.
Cinchona	1	ounce.
Cinnamon	1	ounce.
Cloves	½	ounce.
Senna pods	½	ounce.
Orange flowers	½	ounce.
Nutmeg	1	only.

J. A. Klein, "a Russian pharmacist" doing business in this city, says that for trojanka he always dispenses—

Gentian	50	grammes.
Galangal	50	grammes.
Sarsaparilla	50	grammes.
Red clover blossoms	50	grammes.
Centaury	50	grammes.
Orange peel	15	grammes.
Star anise	8	grammes.
Cinnamon	8	grammes.
Nutmeg	4	grammes.
Nux vomica	2	grammes.

These, he says, he directs to be made into a tea.

Still another formula is supplied by L. Hirshon, of Boston. It is—

Valerian	1	ounce.
Calamus	1	ounce.
Gentian	1	ounce.
Sarsaparilla	1	ounce.
Cinchona	1	ounce.
Star anise	1	ounce.
Juniper berries	1	ounce.
Purging cassia	1	ounce.
Fennel	1	ounce.
Cardamom	½	ounce.
Nutmeg	½	ounce.

Bruise all and mix.

Three recipes for trianke from the 1907 issue of *The Druggist's Circular*.

become universalized—is not uncommon in cases of language contact. Think of how in English many people say "habañero" pepper rather than the correct Spanish "habanero," modeling their pronunciation on the "jalapeño" pepper. We suspect that illiterate Polish peasants, used to nasal vowels (specifically *ą*) in stressed positions, "regularized" the unfamiliar foreign word *theriaka* as *theriąka*, and ultimately to the familiar *trianka* (later *trojanka*).

And because it has many ingredients and magical qualities, the trianke, in Lithuania, was (sensibly) renamed to associate the number of its ingredients (much higher than three) with an appropriate magical number, the three nines, a number so powerful that Lithuanian Roma call their regional idiom in Lithuanian "trins devineres kalbas" ("three nines language"). Roma throughout Eastern Europe regard the number nine as a magical one: one cure for headaches, which are known to be caused by the nagaza, or evil eye, is found among the Roma of Serbia and calls for taking water from nine different places into which glowing embers of charcoal have been thrown.

On a personal note, for decades one of my favorite teas has been the traditional Indian chai, made with variations on the powdered dried spices found in the trianke. Might the chai be the original source for the much-loved and well-traveled trianke?

VALERIANA OFFICINALIS | VALERIAN

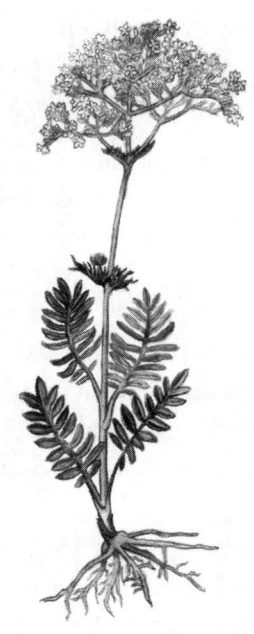

FAMILY Caprifoliaceae

YIDDISH וואַלעריאַן (valerian)

POLISH Kozłek lekarski

UKRAINIAN Валер'яна лікарська (Valer'jana likars'ka), маун (maun), кадило (kadylo), горобинка (gorobynka)

BELARUSIAN Валяр'ян лекавы (Valjar'jan lekavy), аўрыян (aŭryjan), валерыана (valeryana), валяр'ян (valjar'jan), дуброўка (dubroŭka), валяр'яна (valjar'jana), капроўнік (kaproŭnik), капроўнік лесавы (kaproŭnik lesavy), валяр'янка (valjar'janka), рута (ruta), грудоўка (hrudoŭka)

LITHUANIAN Vaistinis valerijonas, baldrijolas, budrijonas, karštžolė, velnio barzda

RUSSIAN Валериана лекарственная (Valeriana lekarstvennaja), кошачья трава (košač'ja trava), балдриян (baldrijan), маун (maun), земляной ладан (zemljanoj ladan), глухой серпый (gluxoj serpyj), аверьян (aver'jan), мариян (marijan), стоян (stojan), лихорадочная (lixoradočnaja), дигол (digol), трясовичное коренье (trjasovičnoe koren'e), очной корень (očnoj koren'), кошкина трава (koškina trava), козлек (kozlek)

GERMAN Echter Baldrian, Arzneibaldrian, Großer Baldrian, Katzenkraut, Stinkwurz, Hexenkraut, Augenwurzel, Augenwurz, Mondwurz, Bullerjan, Tolljan, Katzenwargel, Theriakswurz, Denmark, Dennenmark

HEBREW ולריאן רפואי (ualerian refuai)

Many years ago, when I was having trouble sleeping, I tried a few different herbal remedies from my first herbal medicine book, *The Family Herbal* by Barbara and Peter Theiss. At that time, I didn't realize that different factors contribute to insomnia, and all that interested me was the idea (and the activity—or inactivity) of sleeping.

In their chapter on the nervous system, the Theisses recommend valerian as a calming herb, ever helpful throughout the day, but especially for getting a good night's rest. However, I don't think it was understood at the time that some people are agitated rather than calmed by valerian. I was one of this small number of humans, but because I wasn't aware of this possibility, over the course of a few weeks I gave up working with valerian, coming to the conclusion that it wasn't the herb's fault, but rather it just didn't have the desired effect on me.

Even though my initial contact with valerian didn't help with my insomnia, I've had much more luck with this dreamy perennial in our garden, where it loves to relax beneath the shade of the walnut tree, close to the elecampane and the mugwort, generously sharing its striking scent and little pale pink flower bouquets with visiting insects and birds, and, occasionally, me.

Dioscorides, writing of its root, described the scent of marsh valerian (*Valeriana phu*) that grew in the Pontic region (along the Black Sea coast of modern

Turkey) as a "somewhat foul-smelling oppressiveness," and that when drunk it warmed and activated micturation (urination), was good for pains in the side, and drew down the menses.

It's true that valerian root does have a distinctive scent that some liken to sweaty socks. One of valerian's names in German is Katzenkraut, "cat's herb," because even a tiny whiff of the root's sharp smell can mesmerize felines the same way catnip does.

Valerian does not play a large role in the older works of Jewish medicine. Maimonides hardly mentions it. Teller does not include valerian in his medical text at all. Ha-Kohen's index entry echoes Dioscorides and Galen, naming both Valerian and Phu without actually citing any valerian remedies in the main text of his materia medica. In one curious index entry, however, he identifies a plant called both baldrian and tsikotah. Baldrian is the German word for valerian. Tsikotah suggests the Yiddish *tsig* (cf. German *Ziege*), "goat." In Polish, valerian is called kozia bródka, "goat's beard." This may seem like an herbal game of what we called whisper-down-the-lane in Philadelphia (telephone, elsewhere), but these kinds of tracings sometimes lead to unexpected discoveries. Ha-Kohen's account of tsikotah associates this herb with helping with digestive issues, recommending a stomach plaster made from the plant.

At times it can be helpful to look to Hildegard as a baseline for early recorded herbal applications in Europe, and her reference to valerian is associated with remedies for pleurisy and gout, both of which deviate from the earlier Greek recommendations.

In the Pale of Settlement, in late nineteenth-century Olszana, goat's beard root was drunk in a decoction to stop heavy menstrual bleeding. If someone suffered from "hysterical attacks," it was common to offer a valerian plant infusion or root decoction to calm the patient.

Another condition folk healers in the Pale associated with the nervous system was epilepsy. There were various commonsense folkways for ameliorating this malady. For instance, many people believed it was unwise to move a person while they were having a seizure. Jews covered someone having convulsions with a tallis (prayer shawl), while other communities of the region covered the person with a black cloth, until their spasms subsided. In the towns of Szczepanów and Zabełcze, in Poland, another belief held that anyone who saw the first mole cricket of spring should squash the insect lest they become afflicted with epilepsy. One remedy for epilepsy that folk healers in Zwinogródka administered was powdered root of valerian to be taken morning and evening. In Kyiv, a very specific mixture of valerian, dug up in the autumn, combined with peony, nutmeg, horse hooves, and dried mole hearts, all grated together, was taken in coffee and drunk at the full moon; at the new moon the same blend was to be taken in a linden blossom tea. It's unnerving to contemplate how some of these highly specific ingredients, particularly the animal components, were so readily at hand for on-the-spot care.

To cool fever, valerian was one of the remedies commonly offered in the town of Zwinogródka (according to Deriker, also a popular treatment among the Bashkirs of Siberia, a Turkic people closely related to Tatars). In Kyiv, wounds were washed with a brew of valerian.

The act of poisoning seems to have been fairly widespread in the Pale. In the late nineteenth century, poisonings were attributed to the activities of "wizards" ("czarodzieje"), znachors, or "unfriendly people." Many of the reputed poisons were the dried and powdered essences of small animals or other substances considered unclean. They were put in food or drink to be given to the unsuspecting victim. Most people believed that when someone was poisoned in this way, the snake, or frog, or other small creature was revivified once ingested to roam around inside the victim's body, wreaking havoc. Invaders had to be purged from the victim as quickly as possible, first by sticking a finger down their throat, then tightening and untightening the belt, and administering emetic plants. In the town of Zwinogródka, a brew of valerian was found to be an effective antidote for poisons.

The yizkor books compiled by survivors after the war mention many instances of valerian prescriptions. One of these is a recipe for the popular Russian tea called sbiten that was brewed and kept warm all day in the family samovar, if they were prosperous enough to own one. As we've noted, sbiten is similar to mead and other honey-based drinks. Its main ingredients are water, honey, and berries, but everyone in the Pale would have their own unique herbal combination. The more exotic herbs would have been purchased dried for easy storage, and later ground by the woman of the house with her trusty mortar and pestle. This suggests these non-native herbs had been procured from a spice vendor, having traveled long distances before arriving in the Pale to add their unique flavors and aromas to the meals, beverages, and even incenses known in the shtetls and villages.

"The Rebbetzin," a short story by the Yiddish writer Chaim Grade, tells of the Rebbetzin Perele, who suffered from a litany of ailments and was given to fits of moodiness. She self-medicated by sucking on valerian-soaked sugar cubes to wash down her many other homemade remedies.

In the town of Wasylków, at the beginning of the Yom Kippur fast, "some men would use a pinch of strong tobacco to sniff for relief [from hunger], or ammonia and valerian."

In the shtetls of Zhetl (now Dzjatlava, Belarus), Stashov (now Staszów, Poland), and Smorgon (in the late nineteenth century 76 percent Jewish; now Smarhon, Belarus), yizkor authors describe how just a few drops of valerian and cold water could revive a person who had fainted, a condition which may have been the result of over-enthusiastic fasting on Yom Kippur.

Herschel the scribe had a sideline as a feldsher in the town of Amdura (now Indura, Belarus), where he relied heavily upon valerian in his healing repertoire.

In Suwałki before the Second World War, Moshe Punsker, the beloved feldsher, was never without his medic's bag when visiting patients. Inside could be found many of the tools of his trade: bankes for cupping, a jar of leeches, thermometers, an enema, castor oil, bandages, and valerian.

Another story, from the Jewish community Łódź, Poland, recounts a young girl's task in attending to a dying man one cold night by counting out twenty-five valerian drops to soothe him.

The Jewish midwife from Borshtshiv (in the late nineteenth century 42 percent Jewish; now Boršćiv, Ukraine) carried all her professional tools in her bag, which included valerian tincture to calm a woman having a difficult labor, in addition to various plasters for treating boils and abscesses.

In Romania, up until the 1970s, valerian was a folk remedy for children's health, including digestive considerations such as dysentery, which was treated by placing a valerian compress on the abdomen—this very reminiscent of ha-Kohen's prescription—or by drinking one teaspoon of the plant decocted in an earthen pot. Valerian was also given as a bath for children with insomnia.

In the 1920s and 1930s, Soviet officials were interested in further exploring valerian's various health benefits; the ethnobotanical surveys undertaken in Ukraine during this period found that folk healers in the towns of Bohslov, Kresilev, Ritzev (now Hrytsiv), Slovita (now Slavuta), Anopol, Polona, and Olt-Kosntin relied on valerian in combination with other herbs for digestive health such as pain in the pit of the stomach. As with the midwife of Borshtshiv, the plant was also sought after to calm overly anxious women in labor. A healer from Bohslov reported the importance of valerian for relief from rheumatic pains and colds.

Valerian has also been valorized in the Jewish diaspora: the Polish herbalist who emigrated to Argentina before the Second World War describes the plant's root as helpful in cases of insomnia and for calming the nerves in general.

In present-day Lithuania, Jewish folk healers continue to rely on valerian to quell anxiety and help with sleep. For depression, these folk healers put one tablespoon of dried, hardened valerian root and chopped aloe leaves into boiling water and then simmer for an hour before drinking small portions of the decoction twice a day. To decrease stomach acidity, they assemble a premixed tea blend of equal parts dried peppermint, St. John's wort, calendula, chamomile, cumin, and valerian. From this blend, they put one tablespoon in boiling water, then simmer for ten minutes, recommending that a tablespoon of this decoction be drunk three times a day before meals.

Folk healers of the local Azerbaijani community of Lithuania look to the root, taken as an infusion, to relieve migraines. Lipka Tatars rely on valerian root tea to help with cardiac arrythmias and as a sedative. Overall, Muslim folk healers in Lithuania report a somewhat greater reliance on valerian than do Jewish folk healers. Folk medicine among ethnic Lithuanians emphasizes valerian infusions as a calmative (nerves, heart, throat, stomach, and bronchial spasms) and for reducing abdominal swelling.

Maude Grieve reminds us that valerian has a remarkable influence on the cerebrospinal system, which is why it is such an effective herb for nervous disorders and is especially apt for those suffering from stress. As an added benefit, valerian produces none of the aftereffects other sedative herbs may cause.

According to Zevin, contemporary Russian herbalists also look to valerian for working with a variety of maladies such as digestive disorders, insomnia, anxiety, migraines, hysteria, epileptic seizures, and menstrual cramps. But like Grieve, they recommend caution when employing valerian because "if taken in excessive doses it may create intestinal problems and cause drowsiness and lack of alertness." Even though "symptoms disappear rapidly after taking the herb is discontinued, it's advised to limit courses of treatment to no more than once or twice a day for a period of up to three weeks, and to limiting a course of treatment to two months per year."

Many herbal advisories describe valerian as a potent medicine that, like all healing plants, should always be employed with proper care and knowledge.

Although valerian isn't quite right for me, at one point a family member was having trouble sleeping. I offered them some valerian, still not realizing that its effects could vary, and they reported that almost immediately after taking a few drops in a little bit of water, they were quickly out for the night. This makes me wonder whether the plant's interactions are more random, and not based upon genetics.

VERBASCUM THAPSUS | MULLEIN

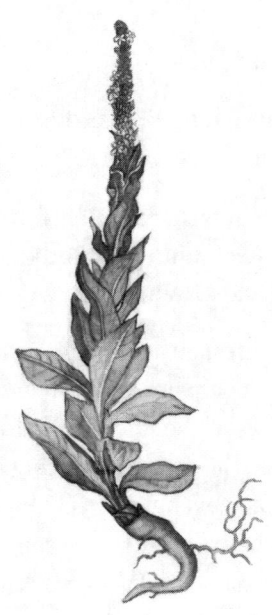

FAMILY Scrophulariaceae

YIDDISH קבֿרים–מנורות (kvorim-menoyres)

POLISH Dziewanna drobnokwiatowa, gorzykrot, knotnica, dziwizna, szabla, królewska świeca

UKRAINIAN Дивина ведмеже вухо (Dyvyna vedmeže vuxo), довган дикий (dovhan dykyj), дообідниця (doobidnycja), дрябчак (drjabčak), жовтяки (žovtjaky), коров'як (korov'jak), лопушанка (lopušanka), царські свічі (cars'ki sviči), воловий хвіст (volovyj xvist)

BELARUSIAN Дзіванна звычайная (Dzivanna zvyčajnaja), дзяванна (dzjavanna), каўтунічнік (kaŭtuničnik), панна-дзяванна (panna-dzjavanna), дзевана (dzevana), дзівана (dzivana), дзівана белая (dzivana be_aja), дзівана касматая (dzivana kasmataja), касмак (kasmak), лісяк (lisjak), трава касматая (trava kasmataja), шальнік (šal'nik), дзівена (dzivena), мядзведжае вуха (mjadzvedžae vuxa)

LITHUANIAN Smulkiažiedė tūbė

RUSSIAN Коровяк обыкновенный (Korovjak obyknovennyj), медвежье ухо (medvež'e uxo)

GERMAN Kleinblütige Königskerze, Echte Königskerze, Marienkerze, Frauenkerze, Wollblume, Kleinblütiges Wollkraut, Himmelsbrand, Fackelkraut, Wetterkerze, Feldkerze, Brennkraut

Mullein begins its two-year lifespan as a fuzzy, light-green rosette that closely hugs the ground, often in the company of family members in various stages of development. In its second year, the plant's basal leaves send up a stalk that can reach well over eight feet. Like steps ascending either side of a tower, more downy leaves cling to this stalk, eventually reaching the densely packed flower spikes. These bloom over the course of a season, only a few at a time, like kernels of popcorn, for the remainder of the plant's life. I've seen both katydids and praying mantises hidden in the felted foliage, along with many bees and other insects. Once flowers have finished blooming, the dried stalk becomes a brittle husk and home to thousands, if not millions, of tiny black seeds that make a barely audible rattling sound when the stalk is shaken.

According to Wisconsin's cooperative extension service, mullein prefers "disturbed" areas, which probably means broken or turned soils like those along roadsides where you can often find the herb towering above other "invasive weeds." But "disturbed" can also describe places that are troubled or traumatized, such as those subjected to wildfires. Mullein thrives in these zones, almost inviting us to work with its healing qualities when we might need them most.

In the Western herbal canon, mullein has many medicinal virtues. The flowers, infused in olive oil, are known to help with earaches; the demulcent wooly leaves, tinctured in alcohol, have an outstanding reputation for respiratory relief from coughs and asthma; and tinctures of the stalk and root, although less widely employed, are sought for relief from chronic spinal pain.

Most of these medicines are straightforward to make, although if one attempts to macerate the root, it's best to slice it into pieces when first unearthed, as it can be very woody and difficult to break up once it's dried.

These are the well-known Western herbal Verbascum remedies I was taught, most of which I've tried myself, so discovering mullein's more obscure history in the eastern lands where my ancestors once lived has been no less than utterly fascinating.

British herbalist and author Maude Grieve tells us that *Verbascum thapsus* has more than thirty common English names and that "all the various species of Mullein found in Britain possess similar medicinal properties, but *Verbascum thapsus*, the species of most common occurrence, is the one most employed." For the purposes of this monograph, we will focus on the genus Verbascum since several species are included in our research, and as Grieve points out, they all possess similar medicinal qualities.

At least three of Grieve's thirty-plus English common names refer to candles. This recalls the plant's Yiddish name as attested in Schaechter's plant dictionary, קבֿרים–מנורות (kvo'rim/kvu'rem-menoyres), which translates to "cemetery candelabrum" in English. This Yiddish appellation is particularly interesting because it alludes to a nuanced story of the plant within the Ashkenazi communities of the Pale, one we have not found elsewhere in Europe. Although mullein plants have served as tapers in many places, the Ashkenazi association of the plant with funeral rites is distinctive. The closest analogue is found in southern Germany and Austria (Carinthia): Heinrich Marzell, in the *Handwörterbuch des deutschen Aberglaubens,* records this tradition: If mullein blooms in the yard or on the grave of the recently deceased, it is a sign that the soul of the departed is in purgatory, and a pilgrimage must be made on their behalf.

The Ashkenazi "cemetery candelabrum" mullein may be a faint echo of an ancient Roman tradition, found in Parkinson's 1640 *Theatrum botanicum,* which tells us how mullein was known among the "Latines" as "Candela regia and Candelaria, becaufe the elder age ufed the ftalkes dipped in Suet to burne, whether at Funeralls or otherwise."

In ancient times, before more sophisticated methods of illumination were introduced, the long stalks of second-year mullein were dried and dipped in fatty substances such as tallow, then lit and carried as torches, hence Grieve's colorful mullein glossary. But the additional Yiddish designation as a grave or cemetery plant suggests mullein's more tender disposition, like that of a trusted companion, lighting the way not only in darkness but also while accompanying mourners in places of great sorrow. Mullein's Yiddish name also conjures the long-lost image of klogerins and zogerins, the women lamenters who wailed and sang soulful and ancient melodies at burials or called upon those in the other world, the departed, beseeching them to intercede on behalf of the living.

Mullein's role as a medicinal as well as mourning plant is well established in Jewish medicine of the modern era. Hemorrhoids, a frequent affliction documented as early as the ancient Egyptians, are mentioned several times in the Torah. By the twelfth century CE, Maimonides had devoted an entire treatise to this ailment, which even today is still praised by contemporary researchers for its forward-thinking treatment plan that emphasizes dietary changes and exercise as prophylactics before other interventions for this painful condition. In his treatise on hemorrhoids, Maimonides offers many herbal remedies, one of which is the regular application of lubricating oils and a fumigation with the smoke of burning rue seeds.

However, we first see mullein recommended for hemorrhoids in the seventeenth century: Teller addresses this complaint via a delicate euphemism for those suffering from an "urgency" and "for someone whose bowel comes out." He offers the following recipe to address the ailment:

> Soak lady's mantle, spurry, mullein, and oak leaves. Place these moistened herbs into two little bags and boil in water. Place one after the other on the lower back of the patient. For urgency, take the crust of rye bread, bake it on coals, rub it well with nutmeg, and pour brandy over it. Then place it warm on the navel.

Decades later, ha-Kohen modernized some of these formulations with an alchemical twist by prescribing crushed rue leaves with an iron rinse and the juice of ווירבאסקום ("virbaskum"), none of which sounds as soothing as Teller's earlier Yiddish-language remedies. Incidentally, Maude Grieve in her time mentions mullein's moistening qualities as providing an excellent remedy for hemorrhoids in both a decoction to be taken internally and also as a serviceable fomentation or poultice, both of which sound quite reasonable, provided the plant's tiny hairs are strained out before applying to sensitive tissues.

Another ethnobotanist who explored folk medicine in Poland in the late nineteenth century noted that mullein was regarded as very helpful against illnesses of the chest, and that mullein and green pine cones, when collected in the spring, were also effective for treating coughs (method unspecified).

Throughout Poland from the nineteenth century up to the Second World War, mullein was most widely recommended for respiratory diseases. Around Zamość and elsewhere in Poland, according to Fischer, mullein baths were often taken to give strength, particularly for newborn, sickly, or consumptive children. For such baths, the mullein root was immersed facing upward. If the patient themselves were to cut their own mullein (three plants were required), the angle of the cut was always applied upward, never downward.

In the early twentieth century, in the Ukrainian town of Bohuslav, Verbascum phlomoides was mixed with plantain to make an infusion for grippe, also known as the flu.

By the late nineteenth century, Talko-Hryncewicz's ethnobotanical surveys also covered hemorrhoids but pronounced them to be unfamiliar among "the people" (lud), the Slavic peasants of the region, be they Polish, Ukrainian, Rusyn, Beskid, or others; for the two other primary demographics, the region's Jews and the landed gentry, they were, unfortunately, rather common.

The nineteenth-century Polish surveys reveal that informants were following Maimonides's ancient recommendation that hemorrhoid sufferers avoid acidic, spicy, or burning food and drink. This advice was assiduously observed in the Podolia region, often accompanied by compresses made of the liquid squeezed from horse dung for extra protection.

Talko-Hryncewicz states that the hemorrhoid remedies cited in his surveys were taken from those healers regarded as most familiar with treating the ailment, viz, Jewish folk healers. Several plants are listed as common treatments for the malady, including mistletoe, a plant understood in the region by many local cultures to be a powerful curative, including for warding off evil. Demitsch, another chronicler of plant medicine in nineteenth-century Russia, notes that Russian folk healers employed mullein flower extract for hemorrhoids and diarrhea.

In the town of Zwinogródka, the folk healers interviewed looked to many plants for the relief of hemorrhoids, including leaves from the ash tree, powdered yarrow, warm baked onion compresses, a decoction of cabbage cobs and clay used to steam the affected area, and poultices made of mullein leaves and flowers. Contemporary Polish author Sophie Knab corroborates this last cure and offers the additional option of bathing in an infusion of the herb.

According to Fischer, therapeutic remedies used by the Polish nobility in Volhynia around 1830 recommended pouring a decoction of mullein, mugwort, and lemon balm over a hot stone and infusing painful areas with this formulation to treat broken bones. Around Stryj (Yiddish Stri, in the late nineteenth century 42 percent Jewish; now Stryj, Ukraine), *Verbascum phlomoides L.*, known in English as orange mullein or wooly mullein, was taken for rheumatism by soaking the affected arm or leg in a decoction of the mullein root, to which a little salt was added, for half an hour a day for a whole month. In the early twentieth century, around Jędrzejów, Poland (Yiddish Yendzhev, at the time almost 40 percent Jewish), applying *Verbascum thapsus* leaves or roots to painful eyes brought relief. For stomach pain combined with cramps, patients in Kielce province and around Oszmiania were given a mullein decoctior to drink. Around Kraków, mullein was used to fumigate maternity wards, and it was, like many other plants, a popular medicine for gynecological ailments among the Polish landed gentry of Volhynia in the early nineteenth century.

Many cures have been associated with mullein in the Polish lands. The sixteenth-century Polish herbalist Szymon Syreniusz claimed that mullein could remove wrinkles and its flowers were good for dyeing hair; such beauty treatments persisted in some parts of Poland until the twentieth century: around Bóbrka, washing oneself daily in an infusion of dried mullein flowers was deemed effective.

Mullein was also reported as helpful for other skin-related conditions. In Jurkow, the flower, fried in butter, was applied to edemas, or to dress cuts, both fresh and unhealed. Also in Jurkow and around the local region, it was common to apply a cataplasm of mullein flowers and leaves to accelerate the accumulation of pus in a boil (to draw it out).

In eastern Galicia (contemporary western Ukraine), juice squeezed from the mullein was applied to older, infected wounds.

In Zwinogródka, to relieve pain, the pulp from leaves and flowers of the plant, boiled in water or milk, was applied warm to soothe burns. Aside from the well-known specific celandine, it was common in Vinnytsja and around Zwinogródka to rub the juice of the mullein leaf or flower on the skin to get rid of warts.

In the Polish ethnobotanical surveys of the late nineteenth century, we find that mullein was helpful for relief of rheumatic pain, especially (again) in Zwinogródka, where the afflicted were washed in a decoction of the plant.

In the Pale, as in the West, folk healers trusted mullein for soothing many ailments including respiratory conditions. With its moisturizing properties and its affinity for the lungs, mullein possesses a perfect combination of attributes to ease a dry cough. These herbal actions were much loved in the small towns and villages of the region, especially for children's health. Talko-Hryncewicz reports that in the late nineteenth-century Pale, for all types of coughs, children were commonly given internal decoctions of mallow roots. A tea of mullein or linden flowers was also often offered to ease a child's cough.

It's very interesting to learn that Russian folk medicine—in common with folk traditions from various parts of the world, including the Mediterranean and the Near East—relied on mullein to stun fish in order to catch them (the Spanish word for stunning fish is *embarbascár* < *Verbascum*). According to Demitsch, Russian folk healers have also prescribed mullein for the same range of ailments as in the Pale: decoctions for postpartum complaints (documented in Perm, Russia), powdered leaves to heal wounds, flower and leaf infusions for shortness of breath and coughing (Moscow), and flower and leaf infusion for pains in the urethra (Saratov, Russia).

In nineteenth-century Latvia, according to Alksnis, peasants relied on mullein to treat a constellation of ailments relating to overextending oneself or overwork: symptoms included abdominal and back pains, headaches, vomiting, internal tissue ruptures or stresses, and "wandering" kidneys, hernias, abdominal separation associated with pregnancy, intestinal tearing, and the like. Treatments for such overextension would include mullein or arnica (*Arnica montana),* or the juice of *Veronica beccabunga* or peppermint teas. Intriguingly, one very important prescription was to take the truhkuma akmins, or "stone of tearing," a mysterious brown stone that was grated for its brown powder to be taken with brandy. According to Aronson, another Latvian ethno-botanist of the period, the main remedies for all internal illnesses were chamomile tea, St. John's wort in a brandy infusion, wormwood, rowan tea, and a mullein decoction.

To the north, in Estonia, Krebel tells us that folk healers would boil mullein flowers with cow's milk as an ointment for rashes, and, kneaded in butter, as a cough suppressant (calendula was relied upon as well). Ointments of mullein mixtures (with, variously, coltsfoot, comfrey, or linden) and fat (butter, lard, goose fat, etc.) were common remedies for many skin afflictions, from cuts and wounds to rashes, impetigo, and edema.

In nineteenth-century Hungary, which included what is now Slovakia, Temesváry tells us mullein was part of a recipe against postpartum urinary retention. While doctors and midwives recommended catheterization, people in rural communities esteemed their age-old remedies, which included taking internally a number of herbs, including juniper berries, brandy spiced with pepper and paprika, southern wood (*Artemisia abrotanum*), celery, oat straw, cooked mullein, red or yellow turnips, Jew cherry (Judenkirsche, or *Physalis alkekengi*), corn husk, and watermelon seeds; also employed were teas of white mallow or lilac root.

In Russian folk medicine, according to Müller-Dietz, mullein is relied upon for catarrhs of the stomach and respiratory tract, and as a diuretic and antirheumatic. Wounds and swelling are treated with leaf infusions, and the roots can be employed as an insecticide.

In my own herbal practice, the plant grows happily in clay soil beneath the unrelenting summer sun in our garden. Every year I offer mullein seeds to anyone interested in growing this amazing, majestic herb, and I gather the leaves and flowers to make the alcohol and oil extracts, respectively. I find the tincture not only helpful for dry coughs, but also very relaxing for tense nerves and muscles, especially in the neck and shoulders, and I sometimes take just a few drops before bed to help me sleep.

VERBENA OFFICINALIS | VERVAIN

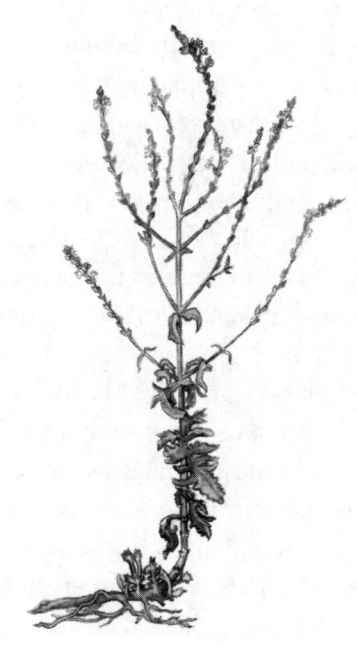

FAMILY Verbenaceae

YIDDISH ווערבענע (verbene); also recorded as ayznkroyt

POLISH Werbena pospolita, ostudnyk, zeliźniak, ostudnik

UKRAINIAN Вербена лікарська (Verbena likars'ka)

BELARUSIAN Вербена лекавая (Verbena lekavaja)

LITHUANIAN Vaistinė verbena

RUSSIAN Вербена лекарственная (Verbena lekarstvennaja)

GERMAN Echtes Eisenkraut, Verbene

HEBREW וירבינה (virbinah)

Like most medicinal plants, vervain's entanglement with humans has a long, intricate history.

The English name *vervain* comes from the Celtic, meaning "to drive away a stone," because the plant, at one time, was known to disrupt accumulated calculus in the bladder. Other linguistic theories regarding the origins of the plant's name are, according to British herbalist Maude Grieve, based on speculation around its possible historic place on Roman altars (the ancients, according to Pliny, knew the plant they called verbenaca as a hierabotane or "holy herb"). For their part, druids employed vervain in their lustral or sacred water purification rituals. Magicians, sorcerers, amulet makers, and those who performed rites and incantations all honored this plant. Vervain also provided protection against headaches and snakebites and was found to bring good luck in general.

In many European languages (including Slovak, Finnish, and others), the herb's name is associated with the element iron: it's known as Echtes Eisenkraut, "true iron herb," in German, and in Danish as læge-jemurt, "medicinal iron herb." Iron is a magical element that occupies a place of honor in many of the world's folk medicinal traditions. It is a guardian: An iron blade under the bed will protect both mother and baby during childbirth (in the shtetl of Zawiercie, mother and child were protected against witchcraft by putting a knife and a cleaver underneath the pillow). It is honored in charms asking for strength. Among Ashkenazim, according to scholar Marek Tuszewicki, iron's magical powers would heal the trauma of the bris, strengthen children's teeth, and when placed in a dwelling, protect its occupants against evil spirits.

In Yiddish, *Verbena officinalis* was known as both verbene and ayznkroyt, and in the Pale of Settlement, it had a variety of applications.

By the time I discovered the ways recent Ashkenazi ancestors worked with the plant, I had already become acquainted with its healing qualities. During a class session, one of our herbal program's more illustrious instructors vaguely hinted at the plant's existence, almost with a subtle wink, and suggested that vervain's place in the Western herbal tradition had faded somewhat, despite its uncanny affinity for quelling the agitated energy so common in society these days. Of course, my curiosity was immediately piqued, and that night I brought home a small vial from the school's apothecary.

When I got home, I put one droplet on the back of my hand and took a hesitant taste. Vervain, I quickly discovered, is exceptionally bitter, almost like unsweetened dark chocolate, and when tinctured, elicits a similar rich dark-brown color. Within seconds of sampling it, I had a strong sensation of being rooted down by the earth's gravity. After my long drive home, this was a very noticeable feeling. I can only describe it as feeling grounded. Instead of the frazzled buzz I often feel after driving in the dark or on a crowded freeway for over an hour, I felt calm—and, more than that, the swirling thoughts that sometimes overwhelm me seemed to dissipate, leaving me with a feeling of relief and an ability to focus on what I was doing in that moment. Just before getting into bed, I tried a second droplet. This had the effect of releasing whatever tension I still held in my muscles and nerves. I slept very well that night.

Vervain's ability to calm a racing mind is well known, especially among those who work with flower essences. Strangely enough, I've held on to the same vial of Bach's Vervain for almost thirty years. I cannot remember why I bought the flower essence of the plant so many years ago, but I must have intuited its influence even back then. Patricia Kaminsky, doyenne of flower essences, writes that "vervain soul types naturally possess strong forces of passionate idealism," and that vervain helps with finding "the middle way," a Taoist concept to which I've long aspired.

Like many people, I have a tendency to spend a lot of time thinking, or stuck in my head, as opposed to being more aware of my body. In the folk medicine of the American South, according to herbalist Phyllis Light, this is characteristic of an "air" personality that can cause anxiety or possibly even insomnia. So when racing thoughts present these kinds of difficulties, one or two droplets of vervain are very beneficial to me. This subtle remedy has helped people I know who have difficulty falling or staying asleep because of an overactive mind.

In recent years, I've grown *Verbena officinalis* in our garden. The plant has a delicate branching form, and its unscented flowers are small but luminous and, to me, give an impression of strings of tiny lights or floating lightning bugs. I find the herb's presence in the garden very comforting, and vervain seems so content growing nearby a magenta sage and a shock of fleabane.

The ancestors had their own unique relationship to this herb. The historian Herman Pollack tells us that in the German lands, Jewish women had many folk medicines to help them get pregnant. Taking "Karlsbadwasser" (mineral water sourced in Karlovy Vary, Czechia, for centuries a very popular spa for "taking the cure") or a drink made with vervain were among their remedies.

For a woman who could not achieve ritual purity, according to Teller, vervain boiled in white wine was prescribed to drink on an empty stomach for three or four mornings while still in bed. The herb was also recommended to clear the sight and cool the eyes. For this purpose, equal amounts of vervain, fennel leaves, celandine leaf and root, and "good roses" were chopped up together and then distilled, and a few drops of the resulting liquid were to be dropped into irritated eyes morning and evening.

In a related condition, Tobias ha-Kohen, in his section on diseases of the head, echoes Maude Grieve's summary of the plant's medicinal qualities by advising a patient to wear an amulet containing plantain around the neck while drinking vervain water to relieve a headache.

Ha-Kohen recommends the iron herb for two other conditions affecting the head. One is a salve for a rash-like affliction, and the other addresses the infamous Plica Polonica, the kaltine or kołtun. Until the twentieth century, many communities of the Pale believed that supernatural influences caused this ailment, which might affect various body systems, but its worst effect was most noticeable as severely matted hair. Because of the kaltine's association with malignant forces, simply removing the plait was believed to cause even more difficulties for the person suffering from the disease. One of ha-Kohen's remedies was an elaborate method of softening the affected skin so that contaminated vapors could pass through the pores as sweat, thus eliminating the cause of the mat. Vervain was one of several herbs required for this procedure (for more on matting, see *Salvia rosmarinus*, p. 163).

In the Polish lands of the late nineteenth century, folk midwives in Lwów (now Lviv, Ukraine) gave laboring women a tea with vervain to speed childbirth.

During this era, it was thought that touching a swallow or even removing its nest could lead the bird to take revenge by giving the transgressor freckles (an angry swallow could do so by changing one's blood from red to white). Most people treated this skin condition with facial washes and sometimes by mystical means. In Podolia folk healers recommended washing the face with a decoction of vervain to get rid of freckles, also an effective remedy against harmful magic.

Russian folk medicine, according to Müller-Dietz, has also relied upon fresh vervain juice to treat anemia (including menopausal anemia), general debility, headaches, colic, liver ailments, jaundice, enlarged spleen, venereal ulcers, fevers, and rheumatic pains; leaf infusions are part of the Russian folk medicinal arsenal against tumors, bruises, and rashes. In Romanian pediatric folk medicine, the plant's aerial parts have been called upon in children's health to treat digestive issues and aid weak or underweight children. Vervain baths soothe teething discomfort, as well as skin conditions such as wounds or scabies.

Vervain accompanied Jews in the diaspora to South America. In Argentina, the plant was known to Yiddish speakers as ayznkroyt ofitsineler and helped induce sleepiness. The herb was also recommended for liver pain or stomach support, reminding us that its strong bitter taste has the ability to aid the digestive process, while its overall effect relaxes the body as a whole.

In her novel *Beyond the Pale*, Elana Dykewomon brought to life the character Gutke Gurvich, an Ashkenazi midwife and folk healer who offered her patients vervain "particularly during the waning moon," for relaxation to bring on sleep.

The half-remembered tales of our plants are so complex. When I think of vervain as the Yiddish ayznkroyt, "iron herb," I'm reminded of the iron objects that were placed under the bed of a woman in labor. Could it be that the iron herb is a substitute for these objects, protecting someone at their most vulnerable, especially during sleep?

Plant names can reveal so many long-forgotten parts of our ancient intimacies with these beings, and reimagining our shared roots is a powerful way to reweave the tapestry of our larger collective healing past.

THE KITCHEN TABLE OF THE PALE: A GATHERING OF HERBS AND SPICES

A simple list of every plant known to and employed by Jews and their neighbors in Eastern Europe would be a lengthy book in its own right. To accompany the preceding monographs, we present a sprinkling of the Eastern European herbal kitchen: those healing plants that have long had a place on the table, whether on a plate or in a bowl, cup, pitcher, or glass. In some cases, we've included plants not commonly employed in cuisines, such as gentian, but which are often (secret) ingredients in the digestive bitters that accompany meals.

ALLIUM CEPA | ONION

FAMILY   Amaryllidaceae

YIDDISH   ציבל (tsibl)

POLISH   Cebula zwyczajna

UKRAINIAN   Цибуля городня (Cybulja horodnja)

BELARUSIAN   Цыбуля рэпчатая (Cybulja repčataja)

LITHUANIAN   Valgomasis svogūnas

RUSSIAN   Лук репчатый (Luk repčatyj)

GERMAN   Zwiebel

We could have written a hundred books on onion. A staple of our own kitchen, onion serves as a general prophylactic and friend to all dishes—while we were finishing this book, a chance encounter in the bulk aisle led us to quinoa latkes (heavy on the onion). We prefer sweet to yellow or purple, and shallots are part of our chicken soup recipe. In many Jewish communities of the Pale, vegetable-dyed eggs were a colorful component of the Lag B'Omer holiday: boiling the eggs in onion skins lent them a reddish hue.

The world of Ashkenazi Jewish plant healing is consumed by onions: the yizkor memory books provide us with many old-country remedies. In Antopol, wounds, blisters, and bleeding were treated with cobwebs, little balls of dough mixed with honey, grated potatoes, milk bread, and roasted onions. In Mlɛve, nursing mothers would eat onions to soothe colicky babies. In Lipowiec, nursing mothers whose babies were weaning would smear their breasts with the juice of crushed onions, followed by cold compresses, several times a day, to stop the production of milk.

In the shtetl of Voronovo, mothers would attach an onion with salt to children's underwear to ward off the evil eye.

Yiddish literature honors the humble onion in this excerpt from Rɛyzl Zikhlinsky's charming "Di alte lid" (The Old Song):

די ברייטע ציבעלע זיצט אין בלומען-טאָפּ
און שמעקט
– אירע בלעטער זענען גוט צו אַ געשוויר
זאָגט אײן באָבע

Di brayte tsibule zitst in blumen-top
un shmekt
ire bleter zenen gut tsu a geshvir
zogt ayn bobe

The hefty onion sits in a flower pot
Smells great
Its leaves are good for an abscess
Says a bobe

ALLIUM SATIVUM | GARLIC

FAMILY Amaryllidaceae

YIDDISH קנאבל (knobl)

POLISH Czosnek pospolity

UKRAINIAN Часник городній (Časnyk horodnij)

BELARUSIAN Часнок (Časnok)

LITHUANIAN Valgomasis česnakas

RUSSIAN Чеснок (Česnok)

GERMAN Knoblauch

ROMANI Siv, sir

We could have written two hundred books on garlic. It is an essential plant among Ashkenazim and other diaspora Jews for cooking and protection (to be worn inside one's clothing). Just a shmek ("taste") of the vast literature on garlic as a traditional healer of the Pale: among the Karaim, one vermifuge recipe calls for boiling garlic (along with burned and powdered elk horn) in goat's milk and drinking the mixture. And for Gagauz healers of Moldova, garlic is one of the most powerful apotropaic plants against evil spirits and the evil eye, and is a well-known antibacterial, particularly for treating diarrhea.

It's also one of our most beloved staples—there's always a couple of heads on our kitchen counter. When I feel I might be exposed to an airborne infection, it's often helpful to swallow one clove of minced garlic with a little juice or tea. I always take some before traveling. The volatile oils from the herb are said to leave the body via the lungs, effectively incapacitating any possible infections that may have compromised the respiratory tract. Garlic is known to affect the blood's viscosity, so consult with a health care provider before trying this prophylactic remedy.

ALPINIA GALANGA | GALANGAL

FAMILY Zingiberaceae

YIDDISH גאַלגאַן (galgan); galganvortsl

POLISH Galangal, galanga

UKRAINIAN Калган (Kalhan)

LITHUANIAN   Alpinija

RUSSIAN   Калган (Kalgan)

GERMAN   Galgant

Galangal, a valued medicinal plant in the Zingiberaceae family (along with ginger and zedoary), likely originated in the Far East. An important component in the trianke, it has been a standard materia medica plant for Jews throughout the world for many centuries. From the Cairo Genizah, we know that galangal was sold by Jewish pharmacists in medieval Cairo; in Egyptian traditional medicine, galangal root is an aphrodisiac, aromatic, and carminative. Interestingly, Maimonides notes that galangal root was sold in Cairo "in cylindrical pieces as big as a finger" as an aphrodisiac. In the traditional medicine of the Jews of Yemen, galangal aided digestive function as well as abdominal organs themselves. Iraqi Jews relied on galangal for eye diseases and as an aphrodisiac. Moric Levi tells us that in Bosnia, where during the Ottoman era Sephardim were the community healers, galangal root (havlendžan) was part of their materia medica.

ANETHUM GRAVEOLENS | DILL

FAMILY   Apiaceae

YIDDISH   קאָפּער (koper), קריפ (krip)

POLISH   Koper ogrodowy

UKRAINIAN   Кріп запашний (Krip zapašnyj), кріп пахучий (krip paxučyj)

BELARUSIAN   Кроп (Krop)

LITHUANIAN   Krapas

RUSSIAN   Укроп пахучий (Ukrop paxučij), укроп огородный (ukrop ogorodnyj)

GERMAN   Dillkraut, Gurkenkraut, Dillfenchel

The leading role dill plays in chicken soup (and pickles) testifies to its importance in plant healing among Ashkenazi Jews and their neighbors. This kitchen plant is a well-known carminative and digestive.

ARACHIS HYPOGAEA | PEANUT

FAMILY Fabaceae

YIDDISH סטאַשקע (stashke), רעבי־ניסל (rebi-nisl); Schaechter also lists the following transliterated terms: erets-yisroel-niselekh, rebe-nislekh, moyse-rabeyne-nislekh, ertsisrol-nislekh, amerikaner nislekh, marokaner nislekh, kitayske nislekh, shtroyene nislekh, fistashkes

POLISH Orzacha podziemna, orzech ziemny, fistaszki

UKRAINIAN Арахіс підземний (Araxis pidzemnyj), арахіс культурний (araxis kul'turnyj), земляний горіх (zemljanyj horix)

LITHUANIAN Valgomasis arachis, žemės riešutu, arachis

RUSSIAN Арахис культурний (Araxis kul'turnyj), арахис подземный (araxis podzemnyj), земляной орех (zemljanoj orex)

GERMAN Erdnuss

HEBREW אגרוי אדמה (agrui adomah)

We mostly encounter the peanut in Eastern Europe as a rare and imported treat for children of the shtetls. Earlier generations of Jews living in the Muslim world knew it by its Arabic names, which point to its African roots, and its likely route up the Nile to Egypt: fūl dar-fūrī (Darfur bean), fūl kordofānī (Kordofani bean), fūl sudānī (Sudani bean).

Peanuts are grown in the Caucasus. For heartburn, one rural Russian feldsher of the late nineteenth century whose notes were preserved in *Zapiski russkogo feldšera* (Notes of a Russian Feldsher) recommended taking a teaspoon of peeled, roasted, and crushed peanuts three times a day, an hour before meals. This feldsher also recommended peanuts as a children's remedy and held that peanut butter (or ointments of boiled peanuts) would soothe fistulas and hemorrhoids and serve as a mild laxative.

ARTEMISIA ABSINTHIUM | WORMWOOD

FAMILY   Asteraceae

YIDDISH   ווערעמקרויט (veremkroyt), ביטערער פּאָלין (biterer polin)

POLISH   Bylica piołun, psia ruta, absynt, wermut, bielica piołun, bilica piołun

UKRAINIAN   Полин гіркий (Polyn hirkyj)

BELARUSIAN   Палын горкі (Palyn horki)

LITHUANIAN   Pelynas, kartusis kietis, pelūnas, metėlis, kartėlis

RUSSIAN   Полынь горькая (Polyn' gor'kaja)

GERMAN   Wermut, Wermutkraut, Bitterer Beifuß

We devoted a great deal of attention to wormwood in *Ashkenazi Herbalism.* For Jews and their neighbors in the Pale of Settlement, it has always been a respected plant. Ha-Kohen includes wormwood in many of his formula-tions, and it is a component in no less than nine of Teller's remedies. Most contemporary Lithuanian Jewish folk healers rely on wormwood (gathered around the time of its blossoming) as a bitter to improve digestion and curb diarrhea. Its psychoactive qualities have been much valued in the Pale: Zalman Schachter-Shalomi, a contemporary scholar of Hasidism, in his book *A Heart Afire: Stories and Teachings of the Early Hasidic Masters,* recalls:

> *My papa, Reb Shlomo Schachter, of blessed memory, was a Belzer Hasid, and once I remember he told me a secret he had learned in Belz. In Poland, before the Holocaust, they used to make a green-tinted schnapps called pyel-lum bronfen. It was made with bitter herbs (hence its greenish tint) and was supposed to be good for the stomach. But Papa told me he had learned in his time among the Belzer Hasidim that "you should never buy pyellum bronfen from a Hasid." "Why?" I asked. "Because a Hasid doesn't let it steep long enough . . . he drinks a lot faster than the ordinary person!"*

Two other species in the Artemisia genus have been highly revered plants in the communal cultures of the Pale. *Artemisia vulgaris*, or mugwort, generally known in Yiddish as געוויינטלעך ביטערגראָז (geveyntlekh bitergroz; in Teller, it is probably the plant he identifies as bayafus), is widely esteemed for its affinity for women's health, digestive support, and its ancient applications in flavoring fermented beverages, as well as its magical properties, especially with regard to sleeping and dreaming. It's an extremely important women folk healers' plant, known to Poles as bylica pospolita and Ukrainians as полин звичайний (polyn zvyčajnyj) or чорнобиль (čornobil'). Like so many other healing herbs, mugwort deserves its own book.

Artemisia abrotanum (European sage or southern wood: Mishnaic Hebrew קסים) is not a kitchen plant, but it is called "God's tree" by Poles (bylica Boże drzewko) and Ukrainians (полин Боже дерево). Ha-Kohen mentions it a number of times, as part of a formula to promote hair growth and as a dewormer in children. Along with calendula, women healers in mid-nineteenth-century Borysów (now Barysaŭ, Belarus) relied on southern wood as a prophylactic against miscarriage. Sicinskij reports that midwives in Belarus would also rely on a mixture of *Clinopodium vulgare* (wild basil), *Artemisia abrotanum*, and *Sedum acre* to fumigate a woman suffering from eclampsia. In the late nineteenth-century Pale, cutting southern wood directionally was a magical remedy for menstruation (cutting the bark upward to induce, cutting downward to arrest).

AVENA SATIVA | OAT

FAMILY Poaceae

YIDDISH האבער (haber)

PCLISH Owies zwyczajny

UKRAINIAN Овес посівний (Oves posivnyj), овес звичайний (oves zvyčajnyj)

BELARUSIAN Авес пасяўны (Aves pasjaŭny), гавес (haves), шавіль (šavil')

LITHUANIAN   Sėjamoji aviža

RUSSIAN   Овес посевной (Oves posevnoj), овес кормовой (oves kor-movoj), овес обыкновенный (oves obyknovennyj)

GERMAN   Hafer, Saat-Hafer

HEBREW   שיבולת-שועל (shibulot-shuel)

TATAR   Игуле солы (Igule soly)

Oats, according to Pauline Wengeroff, are part of a midwife's formula to strengthen a woman after childbirth. In the late nineteenth-century Pale of Settlement, oat decoctions were taken internally against catarrhs. In eastern Galicia, an oat divination was consulted to gauge whether the patient's con-sumption was curable ("worldly") or fatal, wherein the healer would pour some oats in water: if they sank to the bottom with hairy parts on top, the patient might recover. If not, the disease was considered incurable.

BETA VULGARIS | BEET

FAMILY   Amaranthaceae

YIDDISH   בוריק (burik)

POLISH   Burak zwyczajny

UKRAINIAN   Буряк звичайний (Burjak zvyčajnyj), бурак (burak), бурак звичайний (burak zvyčajnyj), борак (borak), буряк (burjak), буряк столовий (burjak stolovyj), бут (but), румпля (rumplja), рункля (runklja), рунтля (runtlja), свекла (svekla), свекловиця (sveklovycja), свікла (svikla)

BELARUSIAN   Буракі звычайныя (Buraki zvyčajnyja)

LITHUANIAN   Paprastasis runkelis

RUSSIAN   Свёкла обыкновенная (Svëkla obykvnovennaja), буряк (burjak), бурак (burak)

GERMAN   Rüte, Zuckerrübe

HEBREW   ביטה רוברה (bita rubrah), תרדין (tardin)

Along with potatoes and cabbage, the humble beet is one of the most important staple crops of the Pale of Settlement and its varied cuisines (so many of which claim borscht as their own). Along with chicken soup and garlic, the beet is an Ashkenazi prophylactic: Adam's father, a lifelong runner, would drink a bottle of Manischewitz borscht to improve his overall fitness when he was in training. Ha-Kohen recommends beets as part of an aperient formula to cleanse the stomach and intestines.

In Lithuania, Lipka Tatars and Karaim Jews were renowned for their skill at gardening and raising vegetables. According to Stanisław Kryczyński, the chronicler of Lipka Tatars, it was observed that "[a] Tatar devotes the greatest part of his time and effort to his garden. Every clod of earth is dug up meticulously and fertilized abundantly. Tatars plant beets, radishes, carrots, turnips, cabbage, cucumbers, watermelons, etc.; thanks to his perfect care of the garden, it provides the Tatar an abundant harvest. Tatars sell their garden products in the markets of the nearest cities or towns at very low prices." Kryczyński goes on,

> Only the Karaites of Troki, whose cucumbers have enjoyed a deserved fame at the Vilnius market for centuries, can compete with them. Here again, we are dealing with a traditional profession common to both Turkish groups in the Polish lands. The gardening culture characteristic of warmer regions (cucumbers, onions, watermelons) was adopted by both the Tatars and the Karaites in the mild climate of the southern coastlines of the Crimea, where, as all travelers have emphasized [. . .] the gardens and vineyards were perfectly maintained.

BORAGO OFFICINALIS | BORAGE

FAMILY   Boraginaceae

YIDDISH   בוריטש (buritsh)

POLISH   Ogórecznik lekarski

UKRAINIAN   Огірочник лікарський (Ohiročnyk likars'kyj)

BELARUSIAN   Агурочнік лекавы (Ahuročnik lekavy), Бурачнік (buračnik), агурочная трава (ahuročnaja trava), агурэчнік (ahurečnik), Масляная капля (masljanaj kaplja)

LITHUANIAN   Vaistinė agurklė

RUSSIAN   Бурачник лекарственный (Buračnik lekarstvennyj), огуречная трава (ogurečnaja trava), огуречная трава лекарственная (ogurečnaja trava lekarstvennaja), бурачник (buračnik), огуречница (ogurečnica), борач (borač)

GERMAN   Borretsch, Boretsch, Gurkenkraut, Kukumerkraut

TATAR   Кыяр үлэн (Kyjar ùlän)

In his *Ma'aseh Tuviyah*, ha-Kohen cites several formulations containing borage for heart, digestive, and women's health.

Boswellia | Frankincense

FAMILY   Burseraceae

YIDDISH   וויַרעכניק (vayrekhnik)

POLISH   Kadzidla, kadzidłowiec, ładon

LITHUANIAN   Ladanas

UKRAINIAN   Ладан (Ladan)

BELARUSIAN   Ладан (Ladan)

RUSSIAN   Ладан (Ladan)

GERMAN   Weihrauch

This plant has a fumigant reputation that dates back to the Song of Songs (4:72–75):

Thy shoots are a park of pomegranates, with precious fruits
Henna with spikenard plants
Spikenard and saffron, calamus and cinnamon
With all trees of frankincense; myrrh and aloes, with all the chief spices
Thou art a fountain of gardens, a well of living waters
And flowing streams from Lebanon

Ha-Kohen counts it as an ingredient in a number of incense-based remedies (along with the rotem tree, juniper, and aloe). Throughout late nineteenth-century Ukraine, ear pain or tinnitus were treated with frankincense. In Łysianka, yarn dipped in spiritus and sprinkled with frankincense was applied to the abdomen as a treatment for uterine disease (unspecified).

BRASSICA OLERACEA | CABBAGE

FAMILY Brassicaceae

YIDDISH קרויט (kroyt)

POLISH Kapusta warzyna

UKRAINIAN Капуста городня (Kapusta horodnja)

BELARUSIAN Капуста агародная (Kapusta aharodnaja), капуста звьчайная (kapusta zvyčajnaja), капуста (kapusta), качанне (kačanne), качаны (kačany)

LITHUANIAN Kopūstas

RUSSIAN Капуста огородная (Kapusta ogorodnaja)

GERMAN Gemüsekohl

HEBREW כרוב (kheruv)

TATAR Бакча кәбестәсе (Bakča käbestäse)

Along with the native beet and the imported potato, without this brassica, Eastern European cuisine is unimaginable. Much loved (soups, sauerkrauts, wrapping for stuffed foods), it is very nutritious and rich in vitamin C; unsurprisingly, ha-Kohen advises it as an antiscorbutic. He also recommends it, along with chicken soup, as a postpartum stimulant for both digestion and blood flow. In late nineteenth-century Uszyca, an elaborately prepared cabbage sitz bath healed hemorrhoids by drawing out the blood:

> In autumn, preferably during the new moon, they take out the cabbage cobs left over after the harvest, and, after cleaning, washing, and cutting them, throw them in a cauldron and boil the mixture, covering it tightly for three hours. They then pour this water into a vessel, put white clay without sand in it, and boil again, before pouring it into a basin for the patient to sit in for a half an hour until the hemorrhoids start to bleed.

Similarly, contemporary Lithuanian Jewish folk healers apply cooked cabbage leaves to the skin to reduce swelling, pain, inflammation, and bruising.

CAMELLIA SINENSIS | TEA

FAMILY Theaceae

YIDDISH טשײַ (tshay)

POLISH Herbata chińska

UKRAINIAN Чай (Čaj), чайний кущ (čajnyj kušč), чай китайський (čaj kytajs'kyj)

LITHUANIAN Kininis arbatmedis

RUSSIAN Чай (Čaj), чайный куст (čajnyj kust), камелия китайская (kamelija kitajskaja)

GERMAN Tee

HEBREW צמח התה (tsemah ha-teh), קָמֶלְיָה סִינִית (kamiliyah sīnīt)

Herbalists and folk healers rely on any number of infusions for their remedies, but the most popular leaf infusion in the Pale of Settlement must be tea, usually black, taken with sugar. The Chinese loanword for *Camellia sinensis* ("ča") first appeared in Russian in 1567; the plant was likely "introduced" to the court of the Russian tsars in the early seventeenth century by Chinese diplomats via the Tatar khanates of central Asia. The Tatars had been drinking tea for a long time before it reached the Pale: "After tea, in your soul a summer" runs one Tatar proverb.

Beginning in the eighteenth century, *Camellia sinensis* largely supplanted or augmented local Russian hot or cold infusions such as uzvar (dried fruits and berries) and sbiten (honey and herbs such as ginger, sage, St. John's wort, cinnamon, and nutmeg). In almost every home, the samovar (whether brewing sbiten or tea) occupied pride of place. And, of course, tea was relied upon as medicine throughout the Pale, particularly for children. According to one yizkor memory book recalling a folk healer in Tishevits (Tyszowce, Poland): Aunt Gitl was beloved by her young patients because "she always prescribed the same remedy: a teaspoon of raspberry juice and lots of tea."

In the Pale, tea was often sold at Jewish-owned stores known as kolonyal gesheftn (cf. Polish *sklepy kolonialne*), the "colonial stores," so called because they mostly sold exotic commodities imported from abroad. Today, we honor the importance of tea in the Old Country whenever we say "האַק מיר נישט קיין טשײַניק" (hak mir nisht kayn tshaynik), literally, "Don't knock the tea kettle at me," meaning "Quit bothering me."

CARUM CARVI | CARAWAY

FAMILY   Apiaceae

YIDDISH   קימל (kiml)

POLISH   Kminek zwyczajny

UKRAINIAN   Кмин звичайний (Kmyn zvyčajnyj), дикий аніс (dykyj anis), польовий аніс (pol'ovyj anis), ганус (hanus)

BELARUSIAN Кмен звычайны (Kmen zvyčajny), кмiн (kmin), кмен (kmen), тмень (tmen'), цьмен (c'men), каралёк (karalёk)

LITHUANIAN Paprastasis kmynas

RUSSIAN Тмин обыкновенный (Tmin obyknovennyj), кмин посевной (kmin posevnoj), индийская зира (indijskaja zira)

GERMAN Echter Kümmel, Wiesen-Kümmel, Gemeiner Kümmel

GAGAUZ Çor otu

In Lithuanian folk medicine, caraway tea or ground caraway (taken by the teaspoonful three times a day) is useful as an appetite and lactation stimulant, an expectorant, and remedy for constipation. Most contemporary Ashkenazi Jewish healers of Lithuania rely on caraway for digestion and to promote lactation. These traditional healers have found that the herb reduces bloating and soothes spasms of the bile duct and urinary tract.

Caraway is an important magical plant for Turkic healers of Eastern Europe. Contemporary Lipka Tatars and Azerbaijanis of Lithuania promote caraway as a preferred remedy for treating diseases of the digestive and respiratory systems. According to Kvilinkova, Gagauz healers of Moldova rely on caraway for its apotropaic qualities: a protective plant, it serves in the production of amulets (muská).

CERATONIA SILIQUA | CAROB

FAMILY Fabaceae

YIDDISH באָקסערבוים (bokser)

POLISH Szarańczyn strąkowy, drzewo karobowe, karob, ceratonia

UKRAINIAN Ріжкове дерево (Rižkove derevo), цареградський стручок (carehrads'kyj stručok), солодкий ріжок (solodkyj rižok)

BELARUSIAN Ражковае дрэва (Ražkovae dreva), цэратонія струкавая (ceratonija strukavaja)

LITHUANIAN Saldžioji ceratonija

RUSSIAN Рожковое дерево (Rožkovoe derevo), цератония стручковая (ceratonija stručkovaja), цареградские рожки (caregradskie rožki)

GERMAN Johannisbrotbaum, Bockshörndlbaum, Karubenbaum, Karobbaum

Carob, a tree in the legume family, is native to the Mediterranean region and the Near East. Carob was an extremely well-known plant in the Pale of Settlement and was sold by spice merchants in every town and village. Many yizkors attest to the fruit being eaten on Tu B'shvat as part of the holiday celebrations. One of its Yiddish names, khamishosser, refers to its significance on this commemorative day ("fruits of the fifteenth"). Children in the shtetls played games with the dried pods. Carob was also an integral component of both the trianke and the "roots against weakness" formulas offered to women after childbirth.

CICER ARIETINUM | CHICKPEA

FAMILY Fabaceae

YIDDISH נאהיט (nahit)

POLISH Ciecierzyca pospolita, groch włoski, barani groch

UKRAINIAN Нут звичайний (Nut zvyčajnyj), турецький горох (turec'kyj horox)

BELARUSIAN Нут культурны (Nut kul'turny), нут пасяўны (nut pas-jaŭny), бараноў гарох (baranoŭ harox)

LITHUANIAN Sėjamasis avinžirnis

RUSSIAN Бараний нут (Baranij nut), турецкий горох (tureckij gorox), культурный нут (kul'turnyj nut), бараний горох (baranij gorox), воложский горох (voložskij gorox), грецкий горох (greckij gorox), нохут (noxut)

GERMAN Kichererbse, Echte Kicher, Römische Kicher, Venuskicher, Felderbse

HEBREW חומוס (humus), אפון (afun), אפונים (afunim)

TATAR Бәрән ногыты (Bärän nogyty), төрек борчагы (terek borčaɣy), нут (nut), шиш борчагы (šiš borčagy), пузырник (puzyrnik), нахат (nahat)

Chickpeas are an ancient staple of the Jewish diaspora and have retained their status throughout the Jewish world, whether in hummus or in the Sabbath cholents. The Ashkenazi Jews of Lite relied upon the beans to give them strength, according to one yizkor book.

It turns out that chickpeas, for such a humble legume, are mentioned fairly often in the Mishnah; their Hebrew name, afun, "little nose," is derived from the resemblance of the bean's sprout to a little nose. Many yizkor books attest to the chickpea's role as a special treat for children attending a bris circumcision ceremony.

According to Asaph ha-Rofe (and derived from Galen), a chickpea decoction is good for treating kidney pain and breaking up stones; a warming herb, it also encourages mucus secretion and is beneficial for bile and jaundice. Drinking a mixture of ground chickpea, honey, cinnamon, and pepper is sound prophylaxis against illness.

In nineteenth-century Russia, according to Rudolph Krebel, chickpeas were sold as medicaments in the Persian apothecaries of Astrakhan, the erstwhile capital of the Tatar khanate in southern Russia on the Volga River, alongside such plants as poppy, crocus, calamus, licorice root, orchid tuber flour, turpeth (*Operculina turpethum*), myrobalan (*Phyllanthus emblica*), beleric (*Terminalia bellirica*), pomegranate, asafoetida, galbanum, ammoniacum, caraway seeds, anise, oak galls, and so on. This indicates once more that within the Russian Empire, including the Pale, traders and vendors could source even the most exotic herbs, spices, and medicaments and carry them to every corner of the realm.

CINNAMOMUM VERUM | CINNAMON

FAMILY   Lauraceae

YIDDISH   צימערינג (tsimering)

POLISH   Cynamon

UKRAINIAN   Кориця (Korycja), цинамон (cynamon)

BELARUSIAN   Карыца (Karyca), цынамон (cynamon)

LITHUANIAN   Cinamonas

RUSSIAN   Корица (Korica)

GERMAN   Zimt

An exotic import sold by spice merchants in the Pale, this aromatic bark has various beneficial qualities that make it an ideal ingredient in many formulations. According to the *Oxford English Dictionary*, the English word *cinnamon* derives from the ancient Greek *kinnámōmon*, which in turn was borrowed from a Phoenician word related to the ancient Hebrew name for the tree, *qinnamon*.

In the Pale, cinnamon had many culinary and medicinal applications, including its role in both the trianke and the "roots against weakness" recipes. In my own herbal practices, I add cinnamon to teas for its warming qualities, its balancing and harmonizing abilities, and also its sweet demulcent properties.

COFFEA ARABICA | COFFEE

FAMILY   Rubiaceae

YIDDISH   קאווע (kave)

POLISH   Kawa

UKRAINIAN   Кофе (Kofe)

LITHUANIAN   Kava

RUSSIAN Кофе (Kofe)

GERMAN Kaffee

HEBREW קפה (kafah)

Coffee, commonly held to originate in Ethiopia, is alleged to have been introduced to the Polish lands by the Ottoman Turks, who left this fragrant and stimulating bean behind during their unsuccessful siege of Vienna in 1683. The same trading networks via which Ashkenazi Jews, Greeks, Armenians, and other diasporic communities brought spices and other imported foodstuffs to the Pale seem to have added coffee to their manifests during the eighteenth century.

The yizkor books tell of the beans being ground in the household mortar and pestle, and many lekach (or honey cake) recipes call for coffee—to lend the pastry a little bitterness, perhaps?

FAGOPYRUM TATARICUM | TATAR BUCKWHEAT

FAMILY Polygonaceae

YIDDISH טאַטערקע (taterke)

POLISH Gryka tatarka

UKRAINIAN Гречка татарська (Hrečka tatars'ka)

LITHUANIAN Totorinis grikis

RUSSIAN Гречиха татарская (Grečixa tatarskaja)

GERMAN Tatarischer Buchweizen, Falscher Buchweizen

In the Polygonaceae family, this cereal (its name derived from its introduction by the Tatars in the late Middle Ages) may have been one of the ingredients in the beloved "kasha and bowties" dish popular in Eastern Europe and a familiar staple in the New World as well. Tatar buckwheat has been widely employed in the folk medicine of the Pale of Settlement. According to Adam Fischer, around Pińczów, a Tatar buckwheat latke (ground, mixed with egg, and fried) or infusion, eaten or drunk, respectively, would cure diarrhea. Around Lublin it was applied to treat all manner of childhood illnesses. Buckwheat flour would dry wounds (method unspecified); and ointments of buckwheat flour were a treatment for smallpox. In early twentieth-century Polish folk medicine, Fischer tells us that cataracts would be fumigated with Tatar buckwheat.

FERULA ASAFOETIDA | ASAFOETIDA

FAMILY Apiaceae

YIDDISH טייבֿלס קוט (tayvls kut)

POLISH Asafetyda, smrodliwa

UKRAINIAN Асафетида (Asafetyda)

RUSSIAN Асафетида (Asafetida), вонючка (vonjučka), вонючая смола (vonjučaja smola), чортово говно (čortovo govno), гной чертов (gnoj čertov), дрек (drek), чертов кал (čertov kal)

GERMAN Asant, Stinkasant, Teufelsdreck, Teufelskot, Stinkendes Steckkraut

Asafoetida is the key ingredient in the long popular and frankly repulsive materia medica known in German as the Dreckapotheke ("feculent pharmacy"). The Dreckapotheke was part of both official and folk medicine throughout much of Europe for centuries (it can be traced back to Babylonian medicine, three millennia ago; moreover, there are strong Dreckapotheke traditions in Chinese, Indian, and Islamicate medicine). The term stems from a book by Christian Franz Paullini published in Germany around the time ha-Kohen was writing *Ma'aseh Tuviyah,* and in good early modern fashion, the full title (of the third and final edition, published in Frankfurt am Main in 1699) summarizes the entire work: *Die Neu Vermehrte / Heylsame Dreck-Apotheke, - Wie nämlich mit Kot und Urin Fast alle / ja auch die schwerste gifftigste Krankheiten, und bezauberte Schäden vom Haupt biß zun Füssen, inn- und äusserlich glücklich curiret worden* (The Newly Expanded / Beneficial Dreck-Apotheke: How Almost Every Disease and Magical Affliction, Even the Most Poisonous, May Be Happily Cured, Head to Toe, Inside and Out, with Excrement and Urine). Paullini's motto was "Im Kot und Urin liegt Gott und die Natur" (God and nature may be found in excrement and urine), and his work provides many recipes for treating all manner of disease with all manner of excrement and urine (human, dog, chicken, sparrow, cow, sheep, and so on) as well as semen, spit, blood, earwax, scabs, spiderwebs, ad nauseam. My mother once told me that my grandparents and their neighbors in Józefów relied on fresh dung (cow or horse) to apply to wounds, which I've subsequently learned was a common practice in the Pale.

I've since wondered if this remedy was based on the idea that these vegetarian animals somehow processed plant material through their digestion, thus creating a ready-to-use medicinal substance. However, my supposition may be undermined by Tatar remedies of the region: Talko-Hryncewicz reports that people from Ruthenia who had been displaced to Crimea, where they lived among Tatars, learned from their new neighbors that the most common and effective remedy for rheumatism was the application of warm dung, especially dog dung (which was most likely not plant derived).

This Turkic note in the Dreckapotheke of the Pale turns up again among the Karaim (karamekk, they called their magical medicine): for diseases of the uterus ("kolki," possibly derived from "colics"), folk healers recommended a decoction of dried foal's excrement (or similar "black" ointment) be taken to relieve acute pains. In the Pale, the Dreckapotheke was thought to be indicated for uterine disorders, in order to "repulse" or "disgust" the uterus into rejecting the affliction.

Back to asafoetida: It is the dried resin of the root of a few species of plants in the Ferula genus, which belongs to the Apiaceae (or Umbelliferae) family; they are native to Iran, Afghanistan, and central Asia. Asafoetida is both a cooking and a healing spice, with a very long tradition not only in India (where it is known as Kandaharee Hing), Iran, and Afghanistan but in ancient Rome as well. In modern Eastern Europe, it is making something of a comeback in regional cuisines, as households rediscover formerly common but now exotic spices, along with cardamom, tamarind, and the like.

According to ha-Kohen, its strong and fetid odor was employed by Jewish women healers to make incense that would protect a newborn from the evil eye. Jews of the Pale—both Ashkenazim and Karaim—would wear it around their necks as an amulet to affect the same purpose (according to Zajączkowski,

Karaim healers would also protect children from the effects of k'oźukm'ak, "casting the evil eye," by having them wear their clothes inside out). Teller also advises its use:

> *Give the patient distilled Aqua Coquet* [boiled water] *for the delivery of the placenta. This woman should be given unpleasant things to smell such as the Gummi Galbanum* [Ferula gummosa] *plant, Asafoetida, castoreum, or chicken feathers, especially the feathers of a wild chicken. Burn them and hold them to the nose. But from below, one should fumigate her with fragrant things such as cloves, marjoram, civet, ambergris, and with the tablets from the apothecary which are made from nutmeg.*

Could this represent two contrasting approaches to childbirth, the masculine above, and the feminine below? This may be related to the widespread magical practice of opening all enclosures, including every door, window, and cabinet in the house, and undoing all knots and fasteners, in order to ease childbirth, a process that was further assisted by the widespread practices of encouraging childbirth through vomiting or sneezing.

FICUS CARICA | FIG

FAMILY Moraceae

YIDDISH פֿײג (fayg)

POLISH Figowiec pospolity

UKRAINIAN Інжир (Inžyr), фігове дерево (fihove derevo), фіга (fiha), смоківниця (smokivnycja), смоква (smokva)

BELARUSIAN Інжыр (Inžyr), вінная ягада (vinnaja jahada), смакоўніца (smakoŭnica), фігавае дрэва (fihavae dreva)

LITHUANIAN Skiautėtalapis fikusas

RUSSIAN Инжир (Inžir), фига (figa), фиговое дерево (figovoe derevo), смоковница обыкновенная (smokovnica obyknovennaja), смоква (smokva)

GERMAN Echte Feige, Feigenbaum, Feige

Another surprise staple in the pantries of the Pale of Settlement, figs, native to the Mediterranean region, were easily dried and transported, playing a prominent part of the spice merchants' imported offerings throughout Eastern Europe. Along with carob, dates, and raisins, the sweet fruit was eaten on Tu B'Shvat as part of the holiday festivities to remind revelers of the Holy Land. Figs were also considered medicinal and were included in the formulas of Teller and ha-Kohen for digestion and other bodily support.

Nor were figs, although not native to the region, unknown to the folk medicine of the Pale: In Poland, according to Fischer, boiled barley and figs were good for stomach aches. Crushed figs were applied to scrofulas and swollen glands. A boiled fig milk rinse was held to alleviate toothache.

FOENICULUM VULGARE | FENNEL

FAMILY   Apiaceae

YIDDISH   קימלגראָז (kimlgroz), קעפּערעק (keperek), פֿענכל (fenkhl)

POLISH   Fenkuł włoski

UKRAINIAN   Фенхель звичайний (Fenxel' zvyčajnyj), фенхель (fenxel'), копрій (koprij)

BELARUSIAN   Фенхель звычайны (Fenxel' zvyčajny)

LITHUANIAN   Paprastasis pankolis

RUSSIAN   Фенхель обыкновенный (Fenxel' obyknovennyj), укроп аптечный (ukrop aptečnyj), укроп волошский (ukrop vološskij)

GERMAN   Fenchel

A member of the Apiaceae (or Umbelliferae) family and native to the Mediterranean, fennel is a frequent ingredient in many of Teller's and ha-Kohen's formulas. Even though it doesn't appear in any of Fania Lewando's recipes in her *Vilna Vegetarian Cookbook*, one of the book's beautiful illustrations is identified in both Yiddish and English as fennel, alluding to the herb's presence in the Ashkenazi culinary repertoire at the turn of twentieth century.

GENTIANA LUTEA | GENTIAN

FAMILY   Gentianaceae

YIDDISH   געָנצ'אַנע (gentsiane)

POLISH   Gorzyczka żółta

UKRAINIAN   Тирлич жовтий (Tyrlyč žovtyj), джинджура (džyndžura)

LITHUANIAN   Geltonasis gencijonas

RUSSIAN   Горечавка жёлтая (Gorečavka žëltaja)

GERMAN   Gelber Enzian

Gentian was a component in both the trianke and the renowned liqueur Riga Black Balsam, a remedy invented in Riga by the apothecary Abraham Kunze, who created the formula to save the life of Catherine the Great. In the shtetl of Felshtin (now Hvardijs'ke, Ukraine), gentian was given as part of a tea formula for children to stimulate their appetite and improve digestion. Contemporary Lithuanian Jewish folk healers also find bitter gentian helpful for digestive support.

Gentian was one of the more important healing plants among the Karaim (along with hazelnut leaves): according to Zajączkowski, its root would be rubbed until it softened to heal open wounds caused by venomous bites.

Here's a personal story that I can't help but associate with gentian, which flourishes across the mountains and valleys of central and Eastern Europe.

In the summer of 1947, hundreds if not thousands of refugees crossed the Austrian Alps on foot in the hope of reaching Italy for the possibility of safety after surviving years of flight and displacement. My mother was part of this wave of humanity.

I didn't hear the story of their sojourn until I was well into my forties, and the specifics are hazy. What I do know for certain is that summer my grandmother was nearly nine months pregnant and so was somehow ferried to Rome, where my aunt was born, leaving my mother and her older sister (just five and six at the time) in the care of my grandfather, to continue their trek from a Displaced Persons camp outside Salzburg over the mountains into Italy. Somewhere along the way, my grandfather gave his daughters a small tool chest to carry, maybe to amuse them, but more likely because he didn't want the box or its contents to attract any attention—a child's toy might be less of a target for bandits. But I really don't know what motivated his decision. The important part of the story, my mother told me many years later, was that the chest contained a hammer, and hidden in its hollowed-out handle was a small cache of gold coins.

Because they were children, I'm certain my mother and my aunt had no idea what they were carrying. And like all children, they must have been trying to eke out some pleasure from their situation and find some distraction from all the heaviness—not only the weight of this small box, but the fear, illness, hunger, and dread they had carried with them from birth as they sought refuge across the breadth of Europe.

Two little girls crossing the Alps on foot, carrying a heavy box, in search of a haven: this is where my imagination wends its way into the tableau, and I see them, dressed in the ragged clothes my grandfather the tailor stitched together from various castoffs. They're exhausted, hungry and thirsty, and probably more than a little cranky, but they're still playful so they set the chest down and begin to quarrel over who gets to sit on it and rest. Because my aunt is the elder, she gets to sit down on the chest first, with a sigh of satisfaction and relief.

I see my mother making a half-hearted protest, but then looking around for something to make her sister jealous . . . and seeing all the wild flowers dotting the slopes and declines they've been traversing, across the Hohe Tauern of the Austrian Alps: bright white stars of edelweiss, sprays of the more delicate pink-tinged bladder campions, a few arnica dotting a nearby meadow. But right there, growing next to the rocky path, a little group of bright blue gentians, impossible to resist. My mother making a show of gathering up the flowers, so enticing that her sister abandons her seat, and after each has made a bouquet, they set off carrying flowers instead of a chest and run off to catch up with the procession.

This story doesn't have a terrible ending. Yes, they forgot the chest alongside the trail, but it was recovered. I'm guessing no one else was tempted to carry a box full of tools across the Alps. But in my imagination, I'm wondering whether gentian offered these little girls a respite and provided a signpost to the place where they had set their burden down, making it easy to find again. My mother and her family spent more than a dozen years in Italy, eventually emigrating to the United States, to Philadelphia, where I was born.

HELIANTHUS ANNUUS | SUNFLOWER

FAMILY Asteraceae

YIDDISH זונרויז (zunroyz); Schaechter also provides royz, reyz, zunreyz, zinroyz, zinreyz, zunblum, levone-kveyt, levone-tshatshke, levone-soneshnik, soneshnik, shontshenik, tshondzhenik, aylbit, shaynperl, zumerglants, eyerblumen, ayerblimen, tabikblimen

POLISH Słonecznik zwyczajny

UKRAINIAN Соняшник звичайний (Sonjašnyk zvyčajnyj), соняшник однорічний (sonjašnyk odnoričnyj)

BELARUSIAN Сланечнік аднагадовы (Slanečnik adnahadovy), сонечнік звычайны (sonečnik zvyčajny)

LITHUANIAN Paprastoji saulėgrąža

RUSSIAN Подсолнечник однолетний (Podsolnečnik odnoletnij), подсолнечник масличный (podsolnečnik masličnyj), подсолнух (podsolnux)

GERMAN Sonnenblume, Gewöhnliche Sonnenblume

HEBREW חמנית מצויה (chamonim matsuih)

In the Pale of Settlement, sunflowers grew in abundance. The seeds, roasted, were a popular shtetl snack. Raw, they also yielded an oil that was often part of the culinary and medicinal recipes of the late nineteenth-century Pale, such as salves, balms, cough suppressants, aperients, anti-diarrheals, fever reducers, or even as part of a magical formula along with an incantation to counter gastritis. The shtetl of Belz (now Bălți, Moldova) was one of the great commercial centers of sunflower oil production in the late nineteenth century. According to the Yiddish plant guide published in Buenos Aires after the Second World War, the seeds calmed a fever brought on by a cold with their ability to encourage perspiration. In twentieth-century Russian folk medicine, according to Müller-Dietz, the leaves and flowers are understood to be anti-malarial and the oil important for folk veterinary medicine as a mild laxative.

HERACLEUM SPHONDYLIUM | COW PARSNIP

FAMILY   Apiaceae

YIDDISH   באָרשטש (borshtsh)

POLISH   Barszcz

UKRAINIAN   Борщівник (Borščivnyk), цвиндух (cvyndux)

BELARUSIAN   Баршчэўнік (Barščeŭnik), баршаўка (baršaŭka), бядрыца (bjadryca), баршч (baršč), баршчэўнік звычайны (barščeŭnik zvyčajny)

LITHUANIAN   Barštis

RUSSIAN   Борщевик (Borščevik), болячечная трава (boljačečnaja trava), борщь (boršč'), роженец (roženec), опаль (opal'), вонючка (vonjučka), пучька (puč'ka), бадран (badran), акант (akant)

GERMAN   Bärenklau, Bärentatze, Heilkraut, Unechte Bärenklau, Bartsch, Kuhpastinak

TATAR   Балтырган (Baltyrgan)

The Slavic name for this plant in the Apiaceae (or Umbelliferae) family derives from an ancient sour soup that originated in Eastern Europe and was made with a pickled herb in the Heracleum genus (a caution for foragers: many plants in this family that are similar in appearance are toxic or even deadly). Just as over time *Camellia sinensis* took over the samovar from the traditional sbiten, so did other vegetables, especially beets and cabbage, eventually replace the cow parsnip as borscht. Ashkenazi immigrants to North America popularized the dish in the New World and contributed the Yiddish word *borscht* to the English language. Today, there are many Eastern European variations of this renowned soup. In my own family, my grandmother made both red (with beets) and green (with shchav, or *Rumex acetosa*, sorrel).

At the turn of the twentieth century, the broth made from the herb was also given by traditional healers to relieve headache pain in the town of Nowa-Uszyca. Around Kamieniec, a combination of horseradish and cow parsnip was given to quell toothaches. According to Deriker, in the late nineteenth-century Voronezh region of Russia, a pinch of crushed cow parsnip seeds was a "wonderful" treatment for dysentery.

HIPPOPHAE RHAMNOIDES | SEA BUCKTHORN

FAMILY   Elaeagnaceae

YIDDISH   זילבערקוסט (zilberkust)

POLISH   Rokitnik zwyczajny

UKRAINIAN   Обліпиха звичайна (Oblipyxa zvyčajna), щець звичайний (šček' zvyčajnyj)

BELARUSIAN   Абляпіха крушынападобная (Abljapixa krušynapadobnaja)

LITHUANIAN   Dygliuotasis šaltalankis

RUSSIAN   Облепиха крушиновидная (Oblepixa krušinovidnaja), облепиха крушиновая (oblepixa krušinovaja)

GERMAN   Sanddorn, Fasanenbeere, Haftdorn, Seedorn

In Russian folk medicine, per Müller-Dietz, sea buckthorn oil is a painkiller and also treats stomach ailments, scurvy, and rheumatism. In contemporary Lithuania, Jewish folk healers look to sea buckthorn for its oil, which they know to reduce inflammation, improve wound healing, and treat stomach ulcers. Here in the United States, grocery import stores sell the juice, which is unlike any fruit juice I've ever had. It's tart and refreshing. Hydrating skin care products containing oil from the fruits and seeds of sea buckthorn, also exported from Europe, can sometimes be found in American stores.

HORDEUM VULGARE | BARLEY

FAMILY   Poaceae

YIDDISH   גערשט (gersht)

POLISH   Jeczmień zwyczajny

UKRAINIAN   Ячмінь звичайний (Jačmin' zvyčajnyj)

BELARUSIAN   Ячмень звычайны (Jačmen' zvyčajny), ячмень шматрадковы (jačmen' šmatradkovy)

LITHUANIAN   Paprastasis miežis

RUSSIAN   Ячмень обыкновенный (Jačmen' obyknovennyj)

GERMAN   Gerste

HEBREW   שעורה תרבותית (sheurah tarvutit)

TATAR   Арпа (Arpa)

For anyone who's ever had mushroom barley soup, this grain is one of the dish's main ingredients. It could also be the "groats" so often found in the literature of Isaac Bashevis Singer. I make mushroom barley soup with fresh shiitakes, but I've often wondered which mushrooms were part of the ancestral recipe. So many yizkors tell of the berry and mushroom gathering that was so popular in the forests of the Pale of Settlement, but it's very difficult to decipher which fungi were being sought out. Both mushrooms and barley are found in the folk medicinal literature of the region. Ha-Kohen and Teller have numerous barley recommendations in their medical works. In the Pale at the turn of the twentieth century, barley continued to be an important medicinal plant and was one of the more nutritional remedies given to children with "wasting diseases." Barley's popularity is understandable owing to its abundance, relative inexpensiveness, good flavor, and nutritional and demulcent qualities; it seems a natural, enduring choice for the kitchen and medicine cabinet.

HUMULUS LUPULUS | HOPS

FAMILY   Cannabaceae

YIDDISH   הָאָפֿן (hopn)

POLISH   Chmiel zwyczajny

UKRAINIAN   Хміль звичайний (Xmil' zvyčajnyj)

BELARUSIAN   Хмель звычайны (Xmel' zvyčajny)

LITHUANIAN   Paprastasis apynys

RUSSIAN   Хмель обыкновенный (Xmel' obyknovennyj), хмель вьющийся (xmel' v'juščijsja)

GERMAN   Echte Hopfen

HEBREW   כשותנית (chshutanit)

TATAR   Гади колмак (Gadi kolmak)

As we've noted previously, Ashkenazi Jews often had alcohol concessions in the Pale of Settlement. Bohemia is one of the world's great beer producers, and before the Second World War, Ashkenazim (farmers, vendors, and brewers) played an enormous role in the hops trade (cultivation, commerce, and beer production). Over the centuries, many Eastern European brewers have augmented their beers with medicinal herbs such as mugwort and juniper. Contemporary Lithuanian Jewish folk healers rely on hops as a sedative for nervous tension, insomnia, dyspepsia, and loss of appetite, as well as to treat coughs, fevers, diarrhea, and rheumatism. According to Müller-Dietz, hops are a mild sedative in Russian folk medicine; externally, they are used to treat abscesses and wounds. In Russian homeopathy, hops are employed in cases of diarrhea and inflammation of the bladder and urinary tract.

HYPERICUM PERFORATUM | ST. JOHN'S WORT

FAMILY Hypericeae

YIDDISH שדים–שיץ (sheydim shits)

POLISH Dziurawiec zwyczajny, ziele świętojańskie, ziele Świętego Jana, dziurawiec pospolity, ruta polna, krzyżowe ziele, arlika, przestrzelon, dzwonki Panny Marii

UKRAINIAN Звіробій звичайний (Zvirobij zvyčajnyj), стокровиця (stokrovycja), калмицький чай (kalmyc'kyj čaj), зілля свєтоянське (zillja svetojans'ke), заяча крівця (zajača krivcja)

BELARUSIAN Святаяннік прадзіраўлены (Svjatajannik pradziraŭleny), святаяннік звычайны (svjatajannik zvyčajny), зелле Святога Івана (zelle Svjatoha Ivana), святаянскае зелле (svjatajanskae zelle), зверабой (zveraboj), расанкі (rasanki), свентаянскае зелле (sventajanskae zelle), святаянкі (svjatajanki), кроўка (kroŭka), дзюравец (dzjuravec), крываўнік (kryvaŭnik), бярозка (bjarozka), заяччa кроў (zajačča kroŭ), красная травіца (krasnaja travica)

LITHUANIAN Paprastoji jonažolė

RUSSIAN Зверобой продырявленный (Zveroboj prodyrjavlennyj), заячья кровь (zajač'ja krov'), зверобой дырявый (zveroboj dyrjavyj), зверобой жёлтый (zveroboj žëltyj), зверобойник (zverobojnik), красная травица (krasnaja travica), кровавец (krovavec), кровца (krovca), хворобой (xvoroboj), зелье светоянское (zel'e svetojanskoe)

GERMAN Echtes Johanniskraut, Hartheu, Johanneskraut

We provided a detailed monograph on this universally beloved herb in *Ashkenazi Herbalism*. St. John's wort is a true panacea: an important ingredient in the trianke, it has been sought for digestive support by both physicians such as ha-Kohen and the anonymous bobes surveyed by Talko-Hryncewicz, Osadcha-Janata, and others. For opsphrekherins and other healers who relied on charms and divination to get rid of the evil eye, St. John's wort was particularly effective for driving away both fright and the evil eye itself during pregnancy and childbirth.

HYSSOPUS OFFICINALIS | HYSSOP

FAMILY   Lamiaceae

YIDDISH   אזוב (azuv)

POLISH   Hyzop lekarski, izap lekarski, józefek, józefka

UKRAINIAN   Гісоп лікарський (Hisop likars'kyj)

BELARUSIAN   Ісоп лекавы (Isop lekavy), красвень (krasven'), красвяк (krasvjak), крузбень (kruzben'), ізоп (izop)

LITHUANIAN   Vaistinis isopas, juozažolė

RUSSIAN   Иссоп лекарственный (Issop lekarstvennyj)

GERMAN   Ysop

HEBREW   אזוב (azuv)

In biblical times, hyssop was known as a spice. Early twentieth-century herbalist Maude Grieve wrote that hyssop grew in the gardens of Britain for use in the kitchen. When people from the shtetl of Dusiat (present-day Dusetos, Lithuania) went to pick berries after Shavuot, they identified the fruits by the plants they grew near: "bruknes" (Yiddish for lingonberries) were the berries that grew on top of the hyssop plant. In Russian folk medicine, according to Müller-Dietz, hyssop tinctures have served as a tonic, expectorant (in chronic bronchitis), and treatment for abdominal and intestinal ailments; externally, hyssop is a vulnerary. Teller mentions hyssop as part of a headache bathing formula, as a respiratory support formula, and as a fumigant to clear plague-laden air. Ha-Kohen recommends hyssop as part of his complex protocol for the removal of a kaltine.

JUGLANS REGIA | ENGLISH WALNUT

FAMILY   Juglandaceae

YIDDISH   נוסנבוים (nusboym)

POLISH   Orzech włoski

UKRAINIAN   Горіх волоський (Horix volos'kyj), горіх грецький (Horix hrec'kij)

BELARUSIAN   Грэцкі арэх (Hrecki arex), валоскі арэх (valoski arex)

LITHUANIAN   Graikinis riešutmedis

RUSSIAN   Орех грецкий (Orex greckij), волошский орех (vološskij orex), царский орех (carskij orex), греческий орех (grečeskij orex)

GERMAN   Echte Walnuss, Nussbaum, Welschnuss, Baumnuss

HEBREW   אגוז מלך (oguz melech)

TATAR   Әстерхан чикләвеге (Ästerhan čiklävege)

In the Pale of Settlement, a walnut shell was often the container for an amulet; Teller writes of such an apparatus for an herbal ointment against worms, which was placed inside the walnut shell and then bound to the navel. Ha-Kohen, in the section of *Ma'aseh Tuviyah* devoted to men's sexual health, reports that a groom, in order to protect himself from harm, should hang around his neck an amulet made of a walnut or almond shell that contains a silver coin. In his treatise on medicinal trees, he praises the walnut for its many virtues, including an alchemical water made from the inside of the shell, and an oil extracted from the nuts, which had the ability to treat leprosy.

In Russian folk medicine, according to Müller-Dietz, extracts of the leaves and the green pericarp are used both internally and externally to treat tuberculosis, scrofula, and rickets. In homeopathy, walnut oil is relied upon as a purgative and vermifuge.

Contemporary Lithuanian Jewish folk healers rely on walnut leaves and nuts as good for metabolism and treating diarrhea. Garber, in mid-twentieth-century Argentina, also recommended walnut leaves, taken as a tea, for good health. My Tarnogród-born grandfather maintained a steady diet of walnuts for his health. The green hulls of the shell are effective against "athlete's foot."

JUNIPERUS COMMUNIS | JUNIPER

FAMILY   Cupressaceae

YIDDISH   קאַדיק (kadik), יאַלאָװיץ (yalovits)

POLISH   Jałowiec pospolity

UKRAINIAN   Яловець звичайний (Jalovec' zvyčajnyj), ялівець звичайний (jalivec' zvyčajnyj)

BELARUSIAN   Ядловец звычайны (Jadlovec zvyčajny)

LITHUANIAN   Paprastasis kadagys, ėglius

RUSSIAN   Можжевельник обыкновенный (Možževel'nik obyknovennyj), верес (veres)

GERMAN   Wacholder, Heide-Wacholder, Machandelbaum, Kranewittbaum, Reckholder, Weihrauchbaum, Feuerbaum

TATAR   Артыш (Artyš), гади артыш (gadi artyš)

Seventeenth-century Jewish physicians recommended versatile juniper for many ailments. Issachar bar Teller advises that the resin ("sandracha") of the juniper tree should be burned as incense and inhaled through a funnel to treat runny noses or head colds (he maintained that powdered juniper sprinkled on the head had the same effect). In times of plague, he called for juniper to be burnt in the hearth, "otherwise one should fumigate the house with juniper berry, hyssop, oregano, rosemary, marjoram, basil, lavender, apple peel, etc." The middle layer of juniper wood served as a poultice for eczema. Ha-Kohen also praises the multifaceted juniper: as a topical oil it would relieve abdominal pain brought on by digestive problems. Dauliūtė reports that contemporary

Lithuanians recall that smoking homes and buildings with consecrated juniper branches was formerly the most common traditional apotropaic ritual to drive away evil spirits.

This traditional and still current rite is an echo of a very ancient Jewish apotropaic refue to smoke away all manner of evil spirits and witchcraft. One remedy, documented by Max Grunwald, the pioneering Jewish ethnographer, is preserved in the manuscript of an eighteenth-century Hebrew-language remedy book (note that some plants are given their "Judendeutsch" names):

> *Fumigate the patient with the following: aristolochia ("Grün Ostrilizia Kraut"), hyssop, horehound, "Gülden Wiederschan" [maidenhair fern?], parsley, juniper, carob, "Auslesen" ["selections"?], "Mare" [bitter night-shade or mistletoe], dwarf everlast, artemisia, rue, vervain, castor, ase-foetida, white frankincense, mastic, oregano ("tost"), nigella seeds, cedar wood, barley spike, stag's horn, sulfur. Cut everything up and mix it together. Then fumigate with it for nine days straight, evening, morning, and midday, including just before the beginning of the Sabbath and at the end of the Sab-bath. Place it in a container and fumigate the patient's entire body with it, which will drive out all bewitchment and evil spirits.*

According to Aleksandrowicz, junipers are associated with a sacred site in Sieniawa, Poland (close to my grandfather's birthplace of Tarnogród), a Lipka Tatar cemetery that was the site of pilgrimage for Tatars, Christians, and Jews for miles around, for a visit to this cemetery would heal afflictions, particularly the kołtun/kaltine. Christian women would tie towels or red ribbons to the juniper bushes that grew in the cemetery to get pregnant.

Juniper berries are a spice and, in today's Poland, an increasingly popular flavoring for beer.

LAVANDULA OFFICINALIS | LAVENDER

FAMILY Lamiaceae

YIDDISH לאַוונדל (lavendl), לאַוונדע (lavende)

POLISH Lawenda

UKRAINIAN   Лаванда (Lavanda)

BELARUSIAN   Лаванда (Lavanda)

LITHUANIAN   Levanda

RUSSIAN   Лаванда (Lavanda)

GERMAN   Lavendel

HEBREW   אזוביון (azubiun), לבנדר (lavender)

TATAR   Ләвән (Läven), лаванда (lavanda), милә үшә (milä ùšä)

In Russian folk medicine, according to Müller-Dietz, lavender oil liniment has been used to treat rheumatism. Lavender dries quickly and well, making it a good candidate for export since large quantities of the flowers are light and easy to package and transport. Teller recommends it as part of an herbal tablet recipe to help against dizziness, to be made by crushing several plants in lavender or rose water and then having the mixture further prepared at the apothecary. He also recommends a distilled lavender tonic to strengthen the heart and as a fumigant against the plague. In a formula to combat scrofula, ha-Kohen relied upon French lavender (*Lavandula stoechas*), one of the ingredients in the renowned medieval Four Thieves Vinegar (the other standard ingredients include peppermint, rosemary, juniper, cinnamon, lemon, and cloves).

In 1940s Buenos Aires, the Polish Jewish herbalist Khone Garber wrote that the plant was widespread in Europe and well known as a nerve stimulant, headache soother, and, as in Russian folk medicine, it served as a rheumatic pain reliever when extracted in alcohol and rubbed on the affected areas of the body.

Of the lavender species, my favorite to work with is *Lavandula angustifolia*, formerly *Lavandula officinalis*. This plant aroma is extremely relaxing and refreshing. In the summer I like to add a pinch of lavender flowers to chamomile and linden tea and steep this blend cold for a few hours. In winter months, adding the flowers to a warm footbath with calendula, chamomile, and hops is a perfect way to get ready for sleep. Small sachets of lavender placed in drawers will ward off insects.

LEVISTICUM OFFICINALE | Lovage

FAMILY   Apiaceae

YIDDISH   ליוביסטיק (liubistik), ליבשטיקל (libshtikl)

POLISH   Lubczyk ogrodowy

UKRAINIAN   Любисток лікарський (Ljubystok likars'kyj)

BELARUSIAN   Любіста лекавая (Ljubista lekavaja), любіста аптэчная (ljubista aptečnaja), любісцік (ljubiscik), любісцік аптэчны (ljubiscik aptečny), любчык (ljubčyk), ладук (laduk), сардэчнік (sardečnik), любім (ljubim)

LITHUANIAN   Vaistinė gelsvė

RUSSIAN   Любисток аптечный (ljubistok aptečnyj), любисток лекарственный (ljubistok lekarstvennyj)

GERMAN   Liebstöckel, Garten-Liebstöckel

Lovage is an aromatic herb in the Apiaceae (or Umbelliferae) family native to the Mediterranean region. The plant has been eaten as a sweet herb, and as an integral ingredient in the Romanian soup known as ciorbă, but as a medicinal herb it enjoyed more popularity in earlier times for its root's healing attributes.

For example, Teller calls on lovage in his formula to bathe an aching head along with the flowers of chamomile, rue, sage, dill, wormwood, linden, and hyssop. He also understood it to help with colic (grimn), applied as an infusion with brandy to painful areas, especially around the navel.

In the Polish lands at the turn of the twentieth century, in the town of Łysianka, lovage treated stopped menstruation; in Nowa-Uszyca the plant was sought out in cases of fevers. Among contemporary Lithuanian Jewish folk healers it is taken to improve digestion.

LINUM USITATISSIMUM | FLAX

FAMILY Linaceae

YIDDISH לײַן (layn)

POLISH Len zwyczajny

UKRAINIAN Льон звичайний (L'on zvyčajnyj), льон-довгунець (l'on-dovhunec')

LITHUANIAN Sėjamasis linas

RUSSIAN Лён обыкновенный (Lën obyknovennyj), лён посевной (lën posevnoj)

GERMAN Gemeiner Lein, Saat-Lein, Haarlinse, Flachs

HEBREW פשתן (pishtan)

Flax is the plant from which linen fabric is woven. In the Pale of Settlement, over the centuries, flax was a highly valued commodity. In fact, its species name, usitatissimum, means "most useful." In addition to the herb's role in textiles, its seeds also yield the beneficial linseed oil. Both of these products were often found in the kitchens and medicine cabinets of the Pale. Teller and ha-Kohen each call on the plant's virtues in their many formulations: linen cloth as a poultice, as a container in which to boil herbs in wine or other liquids, or, as a fumigant, when burnt (e.g., against erysipelas); and linseed, crushed or pressed, as part of medicinal formulations. In the New World, the emigré herbalist Khone Garber writes that the herb calmed pain and soothed sore throats. Garber also notes that linseed flour was made from the seeds of the plant and employed in winter to make cataplasms or compresses for recurrent chest catarrhs and other cold conditions. He offers the following recipe: "A quarter of a kilo of flax seed flour is mixed with a tablespoon of water (mixing constantly) and then left on the fire until it begins to boil. Then the bran is tied in a cloth and placed upon the sick person."

In addition, Garber informs readers that the substance was applied as a compress to accelerate the healing of ulcers.

Contemporary Lithuanian Jewish folk healers find flax seeds to improve the healing of stomach ulcers, relaxing the organ and reducing pain.

My mother once told me that my grandmother used to make a kind of simple cheese from milk that was placed in a cloth bag—I'm not sure how this worked without the milk dripping completely out of the bag, but maybe dairy products in the Old Country were much thicker with cream on the top? This she hung over a warm oven, which allowed the liquid to evaporate over a few days, leaving behind a kind of rudimentary cheese. I'm guessing that the bag my grandmother used for this process was made from linen.

A caveat about flax seeds: some people are more sensitive to them than others, so consider eliminating them from your diet if you feel queasy after consuming anything that contains these seeds.

MENTHA PIPERITA | PEPPERMINT

FAMILY Lamiaceae

YIDDISH פעפערמינץ (fefermints), ענגלישע מענטע (englishe mente)

POLISH Mięta pieprzowa

UKRAINIAN М'ята перцева (M'jata perceva)

LITHUANIAN Pipirmėtė

RUSSIAN Мята перечная (Mjata perečnaja), мята холодная (mjata xolod-naja), мята английская (mjata anglijskaja)

GERMAN Pfefferminze

HEBREW נענע (nene), נענע מנתה (nene mintah), נענע הריפה (nene harifah)

TATAR Борыч бәтнек (Boryč bätnek)

In the Mishnah, this plant, employed as a spice, was known as minta, whereas in the Jerusalem Talmud, it is called na'ana, a term identical to its Arabic name. Scholar Marek Tuszewicki informs us that a sixteenth-century pamphlet attributed to Eliasz z Grodziska, or Eliyahu Guttmacher, the tsadik of Gratz, called for mint as one of the herbal ingredients in an incense burned in the house to protect its inhabitants from an epidemic.

Teller wrote of the herb's affinity for digestion, whereas ha-Kohen saw peppermint as more versatile and included it in his formulations for melancholia, scurvy, intestinal worms, cholera, and to comfort pregnant women during their first trimester of pregnancy. By the nineteenth century, in the Polish lands, the herb continued to be offered by folk healers for stomach catarrhs, in a compress to relieve headaches, and, echoing ha-Kohen, an infusion of the herb was given to prevent the spread of cholera.

Contemporary Lithuanian Jewish herbalists find this plant valuable for curbing bacterial growth and reducing headaches. Peppermint tea is offered to those with gastrointestinal discomforts. These folk healers find the herb to have a calming effect on the stomach in the presence of nervous disorders, and they also give it as a rinse for infections of the upper respiratory tract. In contrast, Lithuanian Muslim folk healers find the herb most helpful for treating urinary maladies, nervous system disorders, and also diseases of the digestive system.

In more contemporary folk medicine in the former Pale, Lithuanian traditional healers, according to Vasiliauskas, find peppermint to be a helpful diaphoretic and diuretic; they also offer a preparation to treat stomach acidity.

Russian folk medicine, per Müller-Dietz, employs the herb's leaves as a stomach soother, for colic of the small intestine, as a carminative, a cholagogue, and to treat inflammation of the upper respiratory tract, toothache, neuralgia, and migraines.

NICOTIANA TABACUM | TOBACCO

FAMILY   Solanaceae

YIDDISH   טיטין (titin), טאביק (tabik), מאכארקע (makhorke) (*Tabacum rusticana*)

POLISH   Tytoń szlachetny

UKRAINIAN   Тютюн справжній (Tjutjun spravžnij)

LITHUANIAN   Paprastasis tabakas

RUSSIAN   Табак обыкновенный (Tabak obyknovennyj)

GERMAN   Virginischer Tabak

HEBREW   טבק (tabak)

ROMANI   Drab

Strictly speaking, tobacco is not a kitchen herb. And I would argue it is not an herb associated as much with women in the Pale of Settlement as it is with men. But as some might say, "Who doesn't enjoy a good smoke after a fine meal?" You might call tobacco a kitchen-adjacent herb.

Tobacco arrived in the Pale from the New World after the voyages of Christopher Columbus. Once established, it found a very enthusiastic fanbase in its various forms. Many yizkors detail how the plant was grown, dried, processed, and consumed. In addition to smoking varieties, snuff was also extremely popular, and manufacturers throughout Eastern Europe, both large and small, offered their own proprietary preparations and special flavorings.

Roma throughout Europe found this new plant to be so significant and powerful that "drab," the Romani word for any grass or herb, became a common term for tobacco.

Ha-Kohen's early account of tobacco is fascinating because his historic knowledge of the plant appears flawed, probably due to its relatively recent addition to the materia medica of the era. For example, he mistakenly believed tobacco originated in India, specifically the "Island of Dabaco," and offered its names, now mostly obsolete, in several languages. The terms he consistently invokes in his formulations are "nicotziana," "tutun," and "dabaku," but it's difficult to tell if he is applying them interchangeably. These inconsistencies are frustrating, but fortunately in later centuries, folk medicine practitioners do distinguish among different varieties, each one known for its own unique application and strengths.

Ha-Kohen found tobacco helpful for digestive concerns, as an emetic to purify the chest, head, and stomach, as a fever reducer, for respiratory relief, and as part of his multistep formula to counteract a kaltine. Externally, the plant's leaves were applied as bandages for wounds, including those associated with gout or leprosy. Perhaps ha-Kohen's most remarkable passage regarding tobacco concerns a recipe for treating smallpox. He cryptically mentions that "the women of this country" add into their remedies a certain type of worm egg (see *Sambucus nigra*, p. 173), but he was unable to find this ingredient in any of the official medical literature of the era. Could this be a reference to the elusive and often maligned women folk healers, the opshprekherins?

Centuries later, in the shtetls, a poem by Walter L. Field from Golub-Dobrzyn (present-day Poland) recalled snuff as invoking the sneeze reflex, a well-known folk midwife's method for hastening childbirth:

Teeth were pulled with howl and squeeze.
Snuff—an aid to bring on a sneeze.
Beinkes [bankes] *and herbs, health to restore;*
Hot poultice and Shmaltz to heal a sore;
The midwife was first the baby to adore.

In the Polish lands of the turn of the twentieth century, "bakun" leaves soaked in alcohol were given for colic in the shtetl of Sanok. For fevers, "machorka," a tobacco of lesser quality and therefore cheaper, was the emetic ingredient in fever-reducing formulas. Another method for reducing fevers required a pinch of tobacco, wrapped in paper, to be worn around the patient's neck for nine days before the packet was burned. Lest the patient be cursed with this fever forever, let alone be cured of it, they were not to be told what they were wearing around their neck, and in fact, had they been told, they might never have rid themselves of their fever. Smoking tobacco was also given for infectious diseases. In Talne (present-day Ukraine), "bakun" was part of an ointment made with a fat to be rubbed on the skin for unspecified conditions. For both eye pain and toothache, it was common in the region to take snuff.

Among the Karaim of Trakai and Panavėžys (Yiddish Ponevezh), Zajączkowski tells us that one nineteenth-century healer claimed the best remedy for occasional coughing was cigarette ash to be drunk in cold water.

NIGELLA SATIVA | Black Caraway

FAMILY   Ranunculaceae

YIDDISH   טשערניטשקע (tshernitshke)

POLISH   Czarnuszka siewna

UKRAINIAN   Чорнушка посівна (Čornuška posivna), чорнушка сійна (čornuška sijna), кмин чорний (kmyn čornyj)

LITHUANIAN   Sėjamoji juodgrūdė

RUSSIAN   Чернушка посевная (Černuška posevnaja), калинджи (kalindži), сейдана (sejdana), седана (sedana), черный тмин (černyj tmin), римский кориандр (rimskij koriandr)

GERMAN   Echter Schwarzkümmel, römischer Koriander, Schwarzkümmel

HEBREW   קצח תרבותי (ketzot tarbuti)

Black caraway was part of ha-Kohen's complex formulation to treat kaltines (unusually, he referred to it by its Slavic names "čarnuška" and "gerniška"). In the nineteenth-century Pale of Settlement, according to Talko-Hryncewicz, folk healers in Zwinogródka put a little sac of nigella seeds on a woman's labia to counteract sterility; they also made a compress of nigella seeds soaked in vinegar to apply to the temples in case of headaches. In Jurkow, the smoke from burning nigella seeds was inhaled to treat a runny nose.

In Russian folk medicine, according to Müller-Dietz, nigella has been employed as a diuretic, emmenagogue, and vermifuge. It has also been a remedy against head- and toothaches, facial paralysis, catarrhs of the eyes, and gall bladder ailments.

OCIMUM BASILICUM | Basil

FAMILY   Lamiaceae

YIDDISH   באַזיליק (bazilik)

POLISH Bazylia pospolita, bazylia wonna, bazylik ogrodowy, bazylijka zwyczajna, balsam, bazyliszka polska

UKRAINIAN Васильки справжні (Vasyl'ky spravžni), васильок духмяний (vasyl'ok duxmjanyj), базилік (bazylik)

BELARUSIAN Базілік камфорны (Bazilik kamforny), базілік (bazilik)

LITHUANIAN Kvapusis bazilikas

RUSSIAN Базилик душистый (Bazilik dušistyj), базилик обыкновенный (bazilik obyknovennyj), базилик огородный (bazilik ogorodnyj), базилик камфорный (bazilik kamfornyj)

GERMAN Basilikum, Basilie, Basilienkraut, Königskraut

HEBREW ריחן מצוי (reichan matzui)

TATAR Затлы рәйхан (Zatly räjxan)

Basil's aerial parts are relied upon in traditional Russian folk medicine against debilities and fevers. Herb infusions are taken to improve digestion. According to ha-Kohen, basil is a sudorific. In the late nineteenth-century Pale of Settlement, in the shtetl of Taraszcza, a basil brew was employed to stop abundant menstrual discharge. Among the Gagauz, according to Kvilnkova, basil wreaths serve as magical medicine to treat (unspecified) illnesses.

OLEA EUROPAEA | OLIVE

FAMILY Oleaceae

YIDDISH אײלבירט (aylbirt), מאסלינע (masline), אליבֿן בוים (olivn boim)

POLISH Oliwka europejska, oliwnik europejski, oliwka uprawna, drzewo oliwne

UKRAINIAN Маслина європейська (Maslyna evropejs'ka), оливкове дерево європейське (olyvkove derevo evropejs'ke)

BELARUSIAN Масліна еўрапейская (Maslina eŭrapejskaja), масліна культурная (maslina kul'turnaja)

LITHUANIAN Europinis alyvmedis

RUSSIAN Олива европейская (Oliva evropejskaja), маслина культурная (maslina kul'turnaja), маслина европейская (maslina evropejskaja), оливковое дерево (olivkovoe derevo)

GERMAN Olivenbaum, Echter Ölbaum

HEBREW זית אירופי (zayt ayrupi)

TATAR Зәйтүн (Zäjtùn), европа зәйтүне (evropa zäjtùn)

It's impossible, in this limited space, to convey how very important olive was to the peoples of the Pale of Settlement, both in the kitchen and medicinally. Teller and ha-Kohen each write of its oil as moisturizing or softening the body when dryness causes distress, such as in a clyster for a "stitch in the side," or applied heated and topically to relieve wracking pains in the limbs. Ha-Kohen also called upon the tree's bark to heal lesions in the mouth, to treat bruises and eye problems, and to support women's health.

The Polish ethnobotanical surveys of the late nineteenth century bear witness to how indispensable this herb was in the Pale. For example, in Zwinogródka, it was part of a formula (otherwise unspecified) applied by a midwife to the navel of a woman in labor whose unborn baby was dangerously positioned. The remedy was supposed to have miraculously lent the woman extra strength and realigned the child so as to speed its safe delivery.

Olive's powerful role in the folk medicine of the Pale can be gleaned from the varied remedies reported in the surveys: to reduce lactation, it was mixed with crushed garlic and consumed; to quell coughs, Jews of the region often drank melted butter in milk, but sugar in olive oil was also a common treatment. For rheumatic ache in the hands, in the town of Skwira, a few heads of garlic were crushed to a pulp in a mortar and pestle, and then mixed with a little olive oil into a thick ointment, which was applied to the painful area; for toothache, in the vicinity of Zwinogródka, ground frog fried in olive oil was smeared on the affected tooth. Similarly, according to Zajączkowski, Karaim remedy books call for plasters of worms, snails, or frogs cooked in olive oil to treat wounds. Around Płoskirow, olive oil on a piece of cotton wool was placed in the ear to treat tinnitus. These are just a few of the myriad treatments that included this versatile herb.

In 1940s Argentina, olive oil was remembered by the immigrant herbalist Garber as a pharmacy preparation with camphor for rubbing on the skin (for unspecified reasons). He also wrote that leaves from the olive tree were known as a tonic for the heart, for kidney health, and for treating rheumatic pain.

ORIGANUM VULGARE | OREGANO

FAMILY Lamiaceae

YIDDISH אָריגאַן (origan), מייראַן (mayran), מאַיאָראַן (mayoran)

POLISH Lebiodka pospolita

UKRAINIAN Материнка звичайна (Materynka zvyčajna)

BELARUSIAN Мацярдушка звычайная (Macjarduška zvyčajnaja), мацердушка (macerduška), мацержанка (maceržanka), душанка (dušanka), мята глухая (mjata hluxaja), мята палявая (mjata paljavaja), лябёдка (ljabëdka), мацеранка (maceranka), зянощца (zjanoščka), мята лясная (mjata ljasnaja), пчалалюб (pčalaljub), бабіна душыца (babina dušyca), мацярынка (macjarynka), дзікі маяран (dziki majaran)

LITHUANIAN Paprastasis raudonėlis

RUSSIAN Душица обыкновенная (Dušica obyknovennaja), материнка (materinka), ладанка (ladanka), мацердушка (macerduška), душница (dušica), зеновка (zenovka), матрешка (matreška)

GERMAN Oregano, Echter Dost, Gemeiner Dost, Gewöhnlicher Dost, Dostenkraut, Wohlgemut, Müllerkraut, Wilder Majoran

HEBREW אורגנו (origanu)

TATAR Гади мәтрүшкә (Gady mätrùškä)

We should state that marjoram, another extremely important medicinal and culinary plant in Jewish culture throughout history, is also an Origanum species. While the two are synonymous in different cultures and languages, both Teller and ha-Kohen take pains to distinguish them: Teller includes oregano in five recipes, and marjoram in seven; Ha-Kohen recommends marjoram as part of his complex formulation to treat the kaltine.

Contemporary Lithuanian Jewish folk healers rely on oregano to help with expectoration. According to Vasiliauskas, in Lithuanian folk medicine, oregano treats epilepsy, paralysis, stomach aches, colds, and mild coughs.

In Russian folk medicine, according to Müller-Dietz, oregano promotes sweating and gallbladder and urinary tract function. It is also relied upon in cases of ileus (intestinal atony) and as an expectorant.

PAPAVER SOMNIFERUM | POPPY

FAMILY Papaveraceae

YIDDISH מאָן (mon)

POLISH Mak lekarski

UKRAINIAN Мак городній (Mak horodnij, мак снодійний (mak snodijᴦyj)

BELARUSIAN Мак снатворны (Mak snatvorny), відук (viduk), ᴍак праўдзівы (mak praŭdzivy), мак-самасей (mak-samasej), мак (mak), хароɯы мак (xarošy mak), мак-цякун (mak-cjakun)

LITHUANIAN Daržinė aguona

RUSSIAN Мак снотворный (Mak snotvornyj), мак опийный (mak opijᴨyj)

GERMAN Schlafmohn

HEBREW פרג האופיום (parag ha-upium), פרג תרבותי (parag tarbuti), פרג מרדים (parag mardim)

Poppies are a wild and cultivated plant in the Pale of Settlement. We have come across many remedies documented among Ashkenazim and their neighbors that exploit the narcotic effects of *Papaver somniferum*, but other species, such as *Papaver Rhoeas*, were and still are highly valued for their tiny black seeds, an essential topping for so many delicious baked treats, such as cakes, breads, and bagels.

PETROSELINUM SATIVUM | PARSLEY

FAMILY   Apiaceae

YIDDISH   פעטרישקע (petrishke), פיעטרעשקע (pietreshke)

POLISH   Pietruszka zwyczajna

UKRAINIAN   Петрушка кучерява (Petruška kučerjava), петрушка городня (petruška horodnja)

BELARUSIAN   Пятрушка кучаравая (Pjatruška kučaravaja), пятрушка (pjatruška)

LITHUANIAN   Petražolė

RUSSIAN   Петрушка кудрявая (Petruška kudrjavaja), петрушка курчавая (petruška kurčavaja)

GERMAN   Petersilie, Peterle, Peterli, Peterling, Petergrün, Silk, Felsensilge, Steineppich

HEBREW   פטרוזיליה (petrozilyah)

Parsley appears no less than forty-seven times in the *Vilna Vegetarian Cookbook*, testimony from Fania Lewando's legendary pre-war eatery. Both Teller and ha-Kohen were enthusiastic proponents of this herb, especially with regard to the urinary tract.

Teller employs the plant for women's health, to treat urinary tract stones, and for eczema. Ha-Kohen advises incorporating parsley into treatments for urinary system health in pregnant women.

Parsley was a staple of the Ashkenazi table. Berl Rabakh's inventory of women's occupations in Sonik (now Sanok, Poland) included a פיעטרעשקע־ווייבל

(pietreshke-vaybl), a parsley-lady, who at market every Thursday sold parsley and other herbs, along with bunches of greens for making soup. Some
of Rabakh's other women's trades include the רופֿאטע (rufate) who applied
bankes (cupping) and healed with "babske refues"; the טוקערין (tukerin) who
worked in the mikvah and the women's bath, where she trimmed toenails; the
opshprekherin, who could remove an evil eye; the קװעטשערין (kvetsherin), the
presser, who in the summertime pressed fruit to make syrups; the הײװן־װײבל
(hayvn-vaybl), the yeast-lady, who didn't actually sell yeast but some other
fermented material (probably sourdough) to use as a substitute for yeast. There
were also the אוגערקע־װײבל (ugerke-vaybl), to whom everyone went to buy good
sour pickles, and the אויפֿצִיערין (oyftsierin), the stringer, who made strings and
bands of pearls, a "gilgul of the shterntikhl (headcovering worn by Orthodox
women) at the time."

In Russian folk medicine, according to Müller-Dietz, parsley has been
an important herb for treating the urinary tract, jaundice, and quickening the
course of an illness; it is also effective against intermittent fevers, malaria,
scarlet fever, and measles.

And, like dill, who doesn't like to sprinkle a little parsley in their chicken soup?

RAPHANUS RAPHANISTRUM SATIVUS | Wild Radish

FAMILY Brassicaceae

YIDDISH רעטעך (retekh)

POLISH Rzodkiew świrzepa

UKRAINIAN Редька дика (Red'ka dyka)

BELARUSIAN Рэдзька палявая (Redz'ka paljavaja), рэдзька дзікая
(redz'ka dzikaja), рапуха (rapuxa), свірэпа (svirepa), свірэпка (svirepka)

LITHUANIAN Dirvinis ridikas

RUSSIAN Редька полевая (Red'ka polevaja), редька дикая (red'ka dikaja)

SORBIAN Hóŕčičnik

GERMAN Acker-Rettich, Hederich, Wilder Rettich

HEBREW צנון מצוי (tsenun matzui)

Many yizkor memory books contain accounts of canning, and radish preserves appear again and again as a particular delicacy on the Ashkenazi Jewish table. In the kitchen, the mortar and pestle did double duty, grinding plants for preserves and for medicines. The wild radish has been gathered in Poland for centuries, along with wild mustard and burdock. There are many folk remedies around the Pale of Settlement that rely upon radish, but we'll limit ourselves to mentioning that Wlislocki reports that Roma in Eastern Europe in the nineteenth century would treat nightmares and asthma with radish juice and mustard flour, kneaded into small balls of dough.

RHODIOLA ROSEA | GOLDEN ROOT

FAMILY Crassulaceae

YIDDISH רויזן–וואָרצל (royzn-vortsl)

POLISH Różeniec górski

UKRAINIAN Оливник рожевий (Olyvnyk roževyj), родіола рожева (rodiola roževa), золотий корінь (zolotyj korin'), рожанка властива (rožanka vlastyva), олівник (olivnyk), омега (omega)

BELARUSIAN Ружавая радыёла (Ružavaja radyёla), залаты корань (zalaty koran')

LITHUANIAN Rausvoji rodiolė

RUSSIAN Родиола розовая (Rodiola rozovaja), родянка

SORBIAN Róžotka

GERMAN Rosenwurz

Rhodiola, which was identified as one of several important adaptogens by the Soviet pharmacologist Izrail' Brexman in the 1960s, has a lengthy history in Eastern Europe, including as an edible green and a flavoring for alcoholic beverages. Remarkably, ha-Kohen includes it in his plant glossary.

Most common in Siberia and the Russian Far East, rhodiola also grows wild in southeastern Europe (ha-Kohen probably encountered it here), and was to be found in the Tatra mountains of Polish Galicia in the nineteenth century. According to Shikov et al., rhodiola rhizomes and roots, cooked with butter, are a side dish for meals in some parts of Russia; the plant is also an additive for teas. Today this adaptogenic plant is overharvested and considered endangered.

RIBES NIGRUM | BLACK CURRANT

FAMILY   Grossulariaceae

YIDDISH   פּאָרעטזקע (poretzke)

POLISH   Porzeczka czarna

UKRAINIAN   Смородина чорна (Smorodyna čorna)

BELARUSIAN   Парэчкі чорныя (Parečki čornyja), смарода (smaroda), смародыня (smarodynja), смуродзіна (smurodzina), парэчка чорная (parečka čornaja), смарода чорная (smaroda čornaja)

LITHUANIAN   Juodasis serbentas

RUSSIAN   Смородина черная (Smorodina černaja)

GERMAN   Johannisbeere, Schwarze Ribisel

HEBREW   ענבי שועל (envi shuel)

Berry picking was a shared activity throughout the Pale of Settlement. My grandparents would go raspberry picking in the woods around Józefów. The yizkor books are replete with stories of picking currants (poretzkes), blackberries (shvartse yagdes), raspberries (malines), strawberries (pozhimkes), lingonberries (bruknes), bilberries (blo-yagdes or shikur-nislekh, "drunk nuts"), cranberries (spalgines), gooseberries (agres), and more. Entire families would go into the forests every weekend, picking berries from dawn to dusk.

In the nineteenth century, Deriker reports, folk healers in Russia recommended a tea of Ribes leaves against scrofula.

RUMEX ACETOSA | SORREL

FAMILY Polygonaceae

YIDDISH שטשאװ (shtshav), כטשוף (khetshūf); Schaechter's transliterated names include shtshavey, shtshav, kvasets, shtshuf, khtshuf, shtshavye, shtshavel, shtshavl, tsvey, tshakhets, amper, shtshov

POLISH Szczaw zwyczajny

UKRAINIAN Щавель кислий (Ščavel' kyslyj), щавель звичайний (ščavel' zvyčajnyj)

BELARUSIAN Шчаўе кіслае (Ščaŭe kislae), шчаўе звычайнае (ščaŭe zvyčajnae), шчаўе звычайнае (ščaŭe zvyčajnae), кісляніца (kisljanica), шчавей (ščavej), шчаўнік (ščaŭnik), шчавель (ščavel'), шчаўе (ščaŭe), шчавель праўдзівы (ščavel' praŭdzivy), кісліца (kislica)

LITHUANIAN Valgomoji rūgštynė

RUSSIAN Щавель кислый (Ščavel' kislyj), щавель обыкновенный (ščavel' obyknovennyj)

GERMAN Wiesen-Sauerampfer, Sauerampfer, Sauerlump

HEBREW חומעה מצויה (khumeh matzuih), חומעת שדה (khumet shodah), חומעת גינה (khumet ginah)

My grandmother's wild-foraged sorrel soup (shchav, or green borscht) was a family favorite. I'll never forget the time I took a walk with her in Sacramento and watched in amazement as she suddenly bent down and plucked something green from a crack in the sidewalk. When I asked in surprise what she was doing, she told me this was shchav. We took the leaves home and my grandmother washed them and prepared the most delicious green borscht I have ever tasted. As medicine, sorrel was a popular remedy in the Pale of Set-tlement, and throughout Russia: in the nineteenth century, around Novgorod, ground sorrel root and soot from the hearth were applied to treat conditions such as acne and other skin diseases.

According to Pastušenkov, modern Russian folk medicine has relied on sorrel to treat diarrhea, wounds that are slow to heal, fevers, scalp diseases, and furuncles.

Equally important in the folk medicine of the Pale is a related species, *Rumex crispus* (curly dock or mare sorrel). According to Zajączkowski, this sorrel was a very important healing plant among the Karaim; they relied on boiled mare sorrel leaves to help digestion and the seeds to deal with constipation. The leaves were also incorporated into a steam. One recipe went as follows: "For internal pains (stomach diseases) the following remedy is to take an oak acorn, crush the grain, and drink with vodka and pepper, then boil the seed of mare sorrel (*Rumex acutus*, "atnyn ščavniginiń urłuğun") and drink it—it does good."

Crushed mare sorrel root they applied to ulcers, including syphilitic ulcers, in a plaster of rose oil and saffron. Simply drinking a wine or water decoction was even better. Mare sorrel seed decoctions were a common Karaim remedy for ameliorating toxic snake or insect bites, or as a prophylactic anesthetic in anticipation of being bitten.

In cases of leprosy or scabies, and other skin conditions (including chipped fingernails), Karaim healers would boil mare sorrel root in vinegar, or crush the root to be mixed with saltpeter powder and vinegar, and apply as an ointment. Crushed sorrel also helped with excessive menstrual discharges. Boiled mare sorrel taken in wine was an effective tooth rinse and ameliorated jaundice

Similar to sage, Karaim also applied mare sorrel root vinegar decoctions to treat lumps behind the ear or beneath the throat.

In Lithuania and Poland, Zajączkowski tells us that Karaim healers were renowned for their famous "Karaim root," which they called učur koreni, "accident root" (which suggests magical power), relied upon as a remedy for fear paralysis, epilepsy, St. Vitus's dance, and other neurological ailments. It is likely that the Karaim root is a Rumex species, either the hybrid *Rumex pratensis* or *Rumex hydrolapatham*, which neighboring Lithuanians know as Švoja Šaknis, "Švoja River root."

RUTA GRAVEOLENS | RUE

FAMILY   Rutaceae

YIDDISH   רוטע (rute), רויטן (roytn)

POLISH   Ruta zwyczajna

UKRAINIAN   Рута запашна (Ruta zapašna), рута садова (ruta sadova), рута городня (ruta horodnja), рута пахуча (ruta paxuča)

BELARUSIAN   Рута духмяная (Ruta duxmjanaja), рута пахучая (ruta paxučaja), бута пахучая (buta paxučaja), рута (ruta), зіма-зелень (zima-zelen')

LITHUANIAN   Žalioji rūta

RUSSIAN   Рута душистая (Ruta dušistaja), рута пахучая (ruta paxučaja)

GERMAN   Weinraute

HEBREW   פיגם (peygam), רוטה (rutah)

I have understood rue to be particularly important for magical protection and for women's health. Both Teller and ha-Kohen include rue in formulas for uterine concerns.

In Russian folk medicine, according to Müller-Dietz, rue has been a treatment for rheumatism of the joints, and for sciatica. Among both Jews and their neighbors in the Pale of Settlement, it was an important apotropaic plant, often warding off malevolent forces, including the evil eye and the walking dead.

Syrian rue (*Peganum harmala*, Yiddish פּעגאַן, pegan), a psychoactive plant not native to the Pale, was also important to Eastern European folk healers and may have been introduced by either Jews or Tatars. In the Ukrainian ethnobotanical surveys conducted between the wars, Osadcha-Janata tells us, *Peganum harmala* was singled out as a

> weed which has come from the Crimea to southern Ukraine (it occurs as far north as Kirovsk). It grows on the steppes, along river banks and in the Sivash region (coastal salt marshes), and it is often found at the site of former Tatar settlements. European medicine early used the seeds of this plant for the treatment of eye diseases, as a vermifuge, as a soporific, etc. The peoples of the

*East have also held this plant in the highest esteem since time immemorial . . .
we noticed that in twelve villages in the districts of Melitopol and Kherson
the inhabitants, the natives as well as newcomers were using the roots of
P. harmala for the treatment of rheumatism and nervous affections* [sic].

In 1940s Argentina, the emigré herbalist Khone Garber wrote of rue: "Very
widespread in European countries, one of the best known plants. Since ancient
times, rue leaf has been used to relieve abdominal cramps and to normalize
menstruation in women."

Among contemporary Lithuanian Jewish herbalists, *Ruta graveolens*
has broad applications for women's health and soothing the pain of gout and
rheumatism.

After our first book was published, I became aware of a folk healer or
opshprekherin, currently available for telephone consultations. When I called
to ask about her method for removing the evil eye, she told me that rue was
one of the ingredients she worked with to heal her clients—presumably for the
nervous afflictions brought on by the ayn hore—although she didn't specify
which plant she meant.

Rue has for centuries been a popular kitchen herb, particularly along the
Mediterranean. Today it is most commonly ingested in European liqueurs
(mostly grappas and amaros, but also in commercially produced spirits of
Poland and Ukraine).

SESAMUM INDICUM | SESAME

FAMILY Pedaliaceae

YIDDISH קונזשוט (kunzhut), סומסום (sumsum)

POLISH Sezam indyjski

UKRAINIAN Кунжут індійський (Kunžut indijs'kyj), кунджуд
(kundžud), сезам (sezam)

BELARUSIAN Кунжут (Kunžut), сезам (sezam)

LITHUANIAN Indinis sezamas

RUSSIAN   Кунжут индийский (Kunžut indijskij)

GERMAN   Sesam

HEBREW   שֻׁמְשֻׁם (shumshum), סוּמְסוּם (sumsum)

Sesame is a well-known and ancient ingredient in diasporic Jewish cuisines. My Poland-born grandmother always had little rectangular individually wrapped sesame and honey candies for us to snack on. I recently found packets of these same candies at a grocery store and was at first surprised to notice they're made in Poland. I never wondered why my grandmother was so fond of these sweets, but it's now obvious they must have been a reminder for her of her youth in that country.

Sesame, a plant native to sub-Saharan Africa, is an important source of oil for both cooking and medicine. Each plant yields countless tiny strongly flavored seeds that enhance the taste of foods worldwide, including halva and many varieties of bagel toppings. It is lightweight and easily transported, and it's not hard to imagine sesame's journeys along the spice routes.

SINAPIS ALBA | WHITE MUSTARD

FAMILY   Brassicaceae

YIDDISH   ווײַסער זענעפֿט (vayser zeneft)

POLISH   Gorczyca biała

UKRAINIAN   Гірчиця біла (Hirčycja bila)

LITHUANIAN   Baltoji garstyčia

RUSSIAN   Горчица белая (Gorčica belaja), английская белая горчица (anglijskaja belaja gorčica)

GERMAN   Weißer Senf, Gelbsenf

Aside from providing a piquant seasoning to meats and vegetables, "mustard plasters" are attested quite often in the yizkors of the Pale of Settlement for treating a variety of health concerns.

SOLANUM TUBEROSUM | POTATO

FAMILY Solanaceae

YIDDISH (יע)קאַרטאָפֿל (kartofl(ie)); Schaechter also lists the following trans-literated names: bilves, bulbe, bulve, kartople, erdepl, ekhpl, riblekh, bar-bulyes, zhemikes, mandeberkes, banderkes, krumpirn

POLISH Ziemniak

UKRAINIAN Картопля (Kartoplja), бульба (bul'ba), бараболя (barabolja)

BELARUSIAN Бульба (Bul'ba)

LITHUANIAN Valgomoji bulvė

RUSSIAN Паслен клубненосный (Paslen klubnenosnyj), картофель (kar-tofel'), бульба (bul'ba), картопля (kartoplja)

GERMAN Kartoffel, Erdapfel

Like the tomato in Italian cuisine, it's hard to believe that the potato hasn't been eaten in Eastern Europe since time immemorial. A New World plant, it arrived in the region just a little more than three centuries ago but did not become a staple of the field and table until the early nineteenth century; Ash-kenazim seem to have been the "early adopters." This starchy favorite (baked, fried, roasted, distilled) is celebrated in a classic Yiddish folk song:

> *Zuntik bulbes (Sunday potatoes)*
> *Montik bulbes (Monday potatoes)*
> *Dinstik un mitvokh bulbes (Tuesday and Wednesday potatoes)*
> *Donershtik un fraytik bulbes (Thursday and Friday potatoes)*
> *Shabes in a novene a bulbe-kugele (for a change a potato kugel on the*
>   *Sabbath)*
> *Zuntik vayter bulbes! (Sunday potatoes again!)*

In the Pale of Settlement, placing slices of the humble potato on the fore-head of the sick would lower fevers. As each slice heated, a fresh one replaced it, eventually bringing a temperature down. Dry compresses of grated potatoes, beets, or carrots were applied to burns around Kyiv.

In modern Russian folk medicine, according to the twentieth-century Soviet phytopharmacologist Pastušenkov, potatoes are good for treating gastritis and gastric or duodenal ulcers, as well as constipation, inflammations of the mouth and pharynx, and externally to treat burns and wounds. In traditional Polish folk medicine, according to Fischer, remedies include applying potato slices to the temple to cure headaches and relying on boiled or baked potato compresses to treat sore throats (the steam of boiling potatoes can also be inhaled); grated raw potatoes soothe burns.

Throughout, we've mentioned vodka as an ingredient in many decoctions and infusions. Zajączkowski reports that among the Karaim, for women's health, vodka (neat), poured across the edge of a knife into a glass and drunk three times a day, combined magic ritual with a well-loved stomach-warming agent.

SYZYGIUM AROMATICUM | CLOVE

FAMILY Myrtaceae

YIDDISH נעגעלע (negele)

POLISH Czapetka pachnąca

UKRAINIAN Гвоздика (Hvozdyka)

BELARUSIAN Гваздзiковае дрэва (Hvazdzikovae dreva)

LITHUANIAN Kvapnusis gvazdikmedis

RUSSIAN Гвоздичное дерево (Gvozdičnoe derevo), гвоздики (gvozdiki)

GERMAN Gewürznelkenbaum

HEBREW ציפורן (tsiporen)

Clove is a standard ingredient in the trianke. Another plant introduced to Eastern Europe via the spice trade, clove is known in Yiddish as negele (nail), owing to its appearance. Ashkenazi Jews recognize the scent of cloves is similar to the roots of the European *Geum urbanum* (wood avens), which in Yiddish is called kamu-negelekh ("like little nails").

Because "nail" nomenclature is so frequently applied to morphologically similar but taxonomically dissimilar plants (Syzygium in the Myrtaceae, Geum in the Rosaceae, and Dianthus in the Caryophyllaceae families), folk remedies for clove may sometimes be obscure. However, Talko-Hryncewicz reports that in Włodzimierz, an eye leucoma could be treated with a teaspoon of ground coffee and sugar sifted through muslin and mixed with two finely ground cloves; the scent of clove was thought to "blow away" the leucoma. Could this have been a remedy borrowed from a Tatar siufkacz?

THEOBROMA CACAO | CHOCOLATE

FAMILY   Malvaceae

YIDDISH   שאָקאָלאַד–בוים (shokolad-boym)

POLISH   Czekolada, kakao

UKRAINIAN   Шоколад (Šokolad)

BELARUSIAN   Шакалад (Šakalad)

LITHUANIAN   Šokoladas

RUSSIAN   Какао (Kakao), шоколадное дерево (šokoladnoe derevo)

GERMAN   Kakao, Schokolade

Since 1500, chocolate has been a worldwide treat. Jewish traders and merchants of the Pale imported and sold cacao and chocolate in the nineteenth century. Jewish pharmacists in Poland sold cocoa oil suppositories. Popular medical guides, such as Dr. Meir Gottlieb's Yiddish-language *Populere algemeyne hygiene* (Popular General Hygiene; Warsaw, 1908), recommended drinking hot cocoa for its nutritional value and high fat content. Chocolate, like red wine, contains anti-oxidants, which are associated with maintaining heart health.

THYMUS VULGARIS | THYME

FAMILY   Lamiaceae

YIDDISH   טימיאַן (timian)

POLISH   Macierzanka tymianek

UKRAINIAN   Чебрець садовий (Čebrec' sadovyj)

BELARUSIAN   Чабор звычайны (Čabor zvyčajny)

LITHUANIAN   Vaistinis čiobrelis

RUSSIAN   Тимьян обыкновенный (Tim'jan obyknovenyj)

GERMAN   Echter Thymian, Römischer Quendel, Kuttelkraut

HEBREW   קורנית (koranit), טימין (timin)

In my own practice, I like to protect and support the lungs with a thyme steam if someone in my household comes down with a cold or flu. It's one of our favorite kitchen spices, making soups, salads, and fish more flavorful. In the folk medicine of the Pale of Settlement, its importance is summed up by a traditional healer from early twentieth-century Suwałki, Poland, who claimed, "Jest na wszystko pomocna" (It's helpful for everything).

VACCINIUM MYRTILLUS | BILBERRY
VACCINIUM OXYCOCCOS | CRANBERRY
VACCINIUM VITIS-IDAEA | LINGONBERRY

FAMILY   Ericaceae

YIDDISH   באָרעפֿקע (borefke)

POLISH Borówka czarna

UKRAINIAN Чорниця звичайна (Čornycja zvyčajna), черниця (cernycja), борівка (borivka), бурівка (burivka), чорні ягоди (čorni jahody), чорничник (čornyčnyk), афина (afyna), яфина (jafyna), яфин (jafyn)

BELARUSIAN Чарніцы (Čarnicy), чарніца (čarnica), чорніцы (čornicy), чорныя ягады (čornyja jahady), чарнушкі (čarnuški)

LITHUANIAN Mėlynė

RUSSIAN Черника (Černika), черника обыкновенная (černika obyknovennaja), черника миртолистная (černika mirtolistnaja)

GERMAN Heidelbeere, Blaubeere, Besinge, Esing, Schwarzbeere, Mollbeere, Waldbeere, Bickbeere, Staulbeere, Heubeere

HEBREW אוכמנית שחורה (okhmanit shechurah)

Communal berry-picking outings are not only part of my family stories, but are a cultural universal across the history of the Pale of Settlement. The European berries of the Vaccinium genus (bilberry, cranberry, and lingonberry) are among the most important healing plants of the region, particularly in children's health, as they satisfy the three main requirements of treating illness in children: they are effective, gentle, and delicious.

Across the Pale, fresh *Vaccinium myrtillus* (European blueberry) berries were given to children to relieve diarrhea; for this ailment, the dried berries, grown in Polesia, were also a popular offering at markets across Ukraine.

Contemporary Lithuanian Jewish folk healers also recommend both the berries and leaves of *Vaccinium myrtillus* (Yiddish טשערניצקעס, tshernitskes) as a treatment for diarrhea as well as irritation or inflammation of the mucous membranes of the mouth and throat. They rely on it in general to improve eyesight and lower blood sugar. They also employ the berries and leaves of *Vaccinium vitis-idaea* (Yiddish באָרעפקעס, borefkes) to reduce bladder inflammation. A great majority of the healers surveyed in Kvedaravičiūtė's research include *Vaccinium oxycoccus* (also known as *Oxycoccus palustris*: Yiddish

זשערעכל־נעס (zherekhlines), גאָגעלעך (gogelekh)); they take the fruit to help reduce stomach acidity and strengthen immunity.

Contemporary Lithuanian healers from the formerly majority-Jewish region of Kaišiadorys rely on the berries, which can be eaten to treat diarrhea, address loss of appetite, improve vision, and regulate blood sugar in diabetes.

VITIS VINIFERA | COMMON GRAPE VINE

FAMILY   Vitaceae

YIDDISH   וויין (vayn), טרויבן (troybn)

PCLISH   Winorośl właściwa

UKRAINIAN   Виноград справжній (Vinohrad spravžnij), виноград звичайний (vinohrad zvyčajnyj)

BELARUSIAN   Вінаград культурны (Vinahrad kul'turny), вінаград (vinahrad), вінаград еўрапейскі (vinahrad eŭrapejski)

LITHUANIAN   Tikrasis vynmedis

RUSSIAN   Виноград культурный (Vinograd kul'turnyj)

GERMAN   Weinrebe

HEBREW   גפן היין (gefen ha-yayn)

Wine is as rooted in much of the Pale of Settlement as it is elsewhere in the world. Large-scale wine grape cultivation has taken place around the Black Sea, including Moldova, Ukraine, and Crimea, for thousands of years. Along with wine's ritual significance among the region's many peoples, from wine at Pesach to communion, its most common role in regional folk medicine has been as a vulnerary, especially the application of grape leaves to heal wounds. Grape leaves also keep dill pickles crisp. Wine's healing powers are acknowledged by the frequency with which it is utilized as an extracting liquid for herbal tinctures.

ZINGIBER OFFICINALE | GINGER

FAMILY Zingiberaceae

YIDDISH אינגבער (ingber), אימבער (imber)

POLISH Imbir lekarski

UKRAINIAN Імбир лікарський (Imbyr likars'kyj), імбир садовий (imɔyr sadovyj), имберець (ymberec'), инбирець (ynbyrec')

LITHUANIAN Tikrasis imbieras

RUSSIAN Имбирь аптечный (Imbir' aptečnyj), имбирь лекарственный (imbir' lekarstvennyj), имбирь настоящий (imbir' nastojaščij), имбирь обыкновенный (imbir' obyknovennyj)

GERMAN Ingwer, Ingber, Imber, Immerwurzel, Ingwerwurzel

Jewish spice merchants in the Pale of Settlement sold ginger, one of the most often employed components in the trianke. In my tea blends, especially in the winter, I like to mince fresh (Peruvian) ginger into most formulas for its warming qualities. If I have a scratchy throat, a strong ginger-based tea usually helps resolve any possible infections.

AFTERWORD

ONCE AGAIN, WE COME TO THE END of a book overwhelmed by the rich legacy of communal healing that we have all inherited. *Woven Roots* grew ineluctably out of the world we uncovered in *Ashkenazi Herbalism*. We finished our first book knowing we were omitting far more than we could include, and we've arrived at the same point once again.

We might have included far more of the "woo" that we uncovered. In addition to the many magical folk beliefs of the Pale, we struggled to fit in some of the fascinating, and apposite, observations of ha-Kohen, who covers a great number of topics that require further and greater investigation, such as the many physical forms a human may take when we're born into this world. For example, some concepts he discusses include "hermaphrodite," "androgyny" and the "tumtum," a term that appears in rabbinic literature, referring to a person of indeterminate sex because their genitalia are difficult to identify. Ha-Kohen also describes what he refers to "in the language of Sepharad" as "sir na di la mar" (siren of the sea), and "in the language of Ashkenaz" as "vashir man oder vashir vayb" (water man or water woman), rusalki like those against whom children of the Pale of Settlement could be protected with calamus; and still more fabulous entities, such as the "barumits," the Vegetable Lamb of Tartary, a mythological plant of central Asia believed to grow sheep (and sheep's wool) as its fruit. Ha-Kohen also demonstrates what strikes us as a more than nodding familiarity with Unani healing traditions of Iran, which should be examined more closely.

If *Ashkenazi Herbalism* emerged through a single keyhole, *Woven Roots* coalesced a palace's worth of such tantalizing glimpses, making this book challenging, yet fun and exciting, to research and write, and we look forward to spending more time exploring and mapping this world.

Many people helped us immeasurably throughout this journey. We are grateful to the Librarians Association of the University of California (LAUC), which funded some of our research travels. The amazing Jennifer Harbster made sure we could spend highly productive hours at the Library of Congress.

The wonderful staff at UC Davis's Shields Library (Jason Newborn, Susan Sullivan, and their colleagues) were able to locate and deliver even the most obscure publications. Axel Borg provided a rich table and richer conversation to make our way through Eastern European history and food cultures. Many libraries around the world have thoughtfully digitized their collections in recent years, making much of this research even easier. Much gratitude to Rokhl Kafrissen not only for her support but for her valuable advice in navigating digital Yiddish-language newspaper archives. And to Marek Tuszewcki, for his kind words and support, bardzo dziękujemy un a sheynem dank.

We would like to send out our thanks and appreciation to everyone who, since 2021, has asked us to take part in the conversation around ancestral healing, in person, on the air, on film, and on podcast recordings.

We are grateful to Yunnie Snyder, who named our herbal collective (and thence our title) Woven Roots.

We also owe a debt of gratitude to a number of cafés, without which this work could not have progressed: In Davis, we are sorry to say farewell to Common Grounds; Coffee Works in Sacramento has been a workshop in its own right. In Victoria, we spent many productive hours in Moka Coffeehouse, Grindstone, and Pancho's.

Debra Felman has been an angel of inspiration and generosity to us.

Our families have been with us throughout, and Murray Cohen, Andrea Houtman, Alex Levy, and Mark Torpey in particular have delivered the family lore, so unexpected and yet so necessary, to advance this book.

We owe a huge debt of gratitude to everyone at North Atlantic Books who believed in this project and made our work so much better than it would otherwise have been: Shayna Keyles, Janelle Ludowise, Emily Shapiro, Bevin Donahue, Julia Sadowski, Sarah Serafimidis, Drew Cavanaugh, Alla Spector, Susan Bumps, Emma Cofod, Matthew Hoover, Kelly Bolding, and Joe Finlaw.

And, of course, all our love to our son Nathanael, who put up with so much.

Our role in recovering this world is to be conduits, nothing more. We are very aware and grateful that we live within this world among plants that protect and support us. We remain humble students, in constant awe of the majesty of the plants that nurture our health, our hearts, and our common humanity.

A NOTE ON OUR SOURCES

One spring day, 15 years ago, I (AP) visited the Warburg Library in London in search of some old medico-folkloric papers focusing on the Mediterranean area. While I was searching for this, I noticed a hidden, old, dusty, monograph, which captured my attention since it was located at the edge between the Mediterranean and the Eastern European sections. It was Leopold Glück's work on folkloric medicine and ethnobotany in Bosnia, probably the first modern ethnobotanical work ever written in Southeastern Europe (Glück 1894); I had never heard of it before, neither had I ever found this reference, and I still remember the trepidation with which I copied the monograph and ran home to read it.

ANDREA PIERONI AND CASSANDRA L. QUAVE, eds.,
Ethnobotany and Biocultural Diversities in the Balkans

THE WORK TO WHICH CONTEMPORARY ETHNOBOTANISTS Andrea Pieroni and Cassandra Quave refer in this epigraph is Leopold Glück's "Skizzen aus der Volksmedecin und dem medicinischen Aberglauben in Bosnien und der Hercegovina," a study that also informed our own work. The latter half of the nineteenth century (and the early decades of the twentieth) was a time when the mandate to document traditional cultures around the world was likely at its apogee (many of the ideological positions that motivated this research are questionable at best, but we are grateful for their role in preserving in many cases soon-to-be-vanished cultures). The importance of libraries in preserving and making accessible this body of knowledge is inestimable. We also walked a path to the Warburg Library (and to the Wellcome Library not too far away) that contributed to our journey through the world of plant healing.

This book, unlike our previous one, appears without endnotes. However, a perusal of our bibliography should make clear the many sources we relied upon when assembling our research. We have opted to provide general textual references to our sources: for instance, a reference to Talko-Hryncewicz will take the reader to his *Zarysy lecznictwa ludowego na Rusi południowej* (1893).

In a number of instances, we followed Talko-Hryncewicz's footnotes back to even earlier sources, some extending back to the early nineteenth century. Our main sources for documenting plant-based folk medicine among Ashkenazi Jews and their neighbors throughout the Pale of Settlement and throughout Eastern Europe are listed here.

For information gleaned from the yizkor memory books, we have provided both the "standard" (Polish, Belarusian, Lithuanian, Ukrainian) place name and the town's Yiddish name (e.g., Mława/Mlave).

The library of yizkor books, particularly those that have been translated by the generous labor of the Jewishgen community, has also been invaluable: references to a particular yizkor (e.g., Zawiercie) should be understood to refer back to the Jewishgen collections at www.jewishgen.org/yizkor, unless otherwise specified.

We've also tried to make this multilingual material less forbidding, in part by transliterating names and terms from the Hebrew, Yiddish, Ukrainian, Russian, and Belarusian. Sometimes our transliteration schemas (scientific for Cyrillic, YIVO for Yiddish) come into conflict: e.g., Berdyčiv versus Bardtichev. In most instances, we use Yiddish rather than Hebrew terms (e.g., Yiddish refue over Hebrew refuah). Any errors in transliterations, as well as translations, are our own.

We hope this approach to acknowledging the many works of scholarship, literature, remembrance, and poetry in which we immersed ourselves makes for an informative and enriching—but not cumbersome—reading experience.

Alksnis, J. "Materialien zur lettischen Volksmedizin, gesammelt, in Deutsche übersetzt und geordnet." *Historische Studien aus dem Pharmakologischen Institut der Kaiserlichen Universität Dorpat*, 1894: 166.

Aronson, Emil. "Ueber die Volksheilmittel der Letten von pract. Arzt zu Libau." *Magazin herausgegeben von der Lettisch-Litterärischen Gesellschaft* (1891): 185.

Dauliūtė, Roberta. *Telšių rajono etnofarmacinis tyrimas*. [Unpublished master's thesis] Kaunas: 2018.

Demitsch, Wassily, Anton Alfred von Henrici, I. Alksnis, and R. Kobert. *Historische Studien zur Russischen Volksmedizin*. Leipzig: Unveränderter Nachdrück, 1968.

Deriker, Vasilij Vasil'evič. *Sbornik narodnovračebnyx sredstv, znaxarjami v Rossii upotrebljaemyx*, Sanktpeterburg: 1866.

Dykewomon, Elana. *Beyond the Pale*. 2nd edition. Vancouver, BC: Raincoast Books, 2003.

Fischer, Adam. *Rośliny w wierzeniach i zwyczajach ludowych: Słownik Adama Fischera*. Edited by Monika Kujawska. Wrocław: Polskie Towarzystwo Ludoznawcze, 2016.

Garber, Chane. *Mentshn, flantsn un refues*. Buenos Ayres, 1945.

Glacun, Jaroslav. *Likars'ki roslyny Prykarpattja*. Kyïv: N. Terletsky, 2015.

Grieve, Maude. *A Modern Herbal: The Medicinal, Culinary, Cosmetic and Economic Properties, Cultivation and Folk-Lore of Herbs, Grasses, Fungi, Shrubs, and Trees with All Their Modern Scientific Uses*. New York: Dover Publications, 1971.

Grunwald, Max. "Kleine Beiträge zur jüdischen Volkskunde." *Mitteilungen zur Jüdischen Volkskunde* 3, 4, no. 24 (1907): 118.

Gudelytė, Ugnė. *Tradiciškai Lietuvoje augintų dekoratyvinių augalų etnofarmacinis tyrimas*. [Unpublished master's thesis] Kaunas: 2010.

Henneberg, Maria, and Maria Stasiulewicz. "Herbal Ethnopharmacology of Lithuania, Vilnius region. 3: Medicament and Food." In *Médicaments et climents: approche ethnopharmacologique, International Conference on Ethnomedicine* 2, no. 11 (1993): 243.

Henrici, Ant. Alf. v. "Weitere Studien über Volksheilmittel verschiedener in Russland lebender Völkerschaften." *Historische Studien aus dem Pharmakologischen Institut der Kaiserlichen Universität Dorpat* (1894): 1.

Kašinskij, Ivan Grigor'evič. *Russkij lečebnyj travnik, ili Opisanie otečestvennyx vračebnyx rastenij, celebnymi kačestvami zamenjajuščix čužezemnye i upotrebljaemyx dlja lečenija vnutrennix i naružnyx boleznej, osnovannoe na nabljudenijax prežnix i novejšix opytnyx vračej, s prisovokupleniem csostavnyx dejstvitel'nejšix lekarstv i ekonomičeskix zamečanij, dlja vsex sostojanij, raspoloženyj azbučnym porjadkom*. Moskva: Tip. S. Orlova, 1862.

Kats Ṭoviyah, and Stamparia Bragadina. *Ma'aseh Toviyah: Kolel Ha-Arba'a 'Olamot: Ve-Nelek Le-Hameshah Hekekim: He-Helek Ha-Rishon Medaber Be-'Ule Ha-'Eliyon She-Hu 'Olam Ha-Ruhani: Ha-Sheni Be-'Olam*

Ha-Emtsa'i She-Hu 'Olam Ha-Galgalim. Bevenetsi'a [Venice]: Nella Stamparia Bragadina, 1708.

Knab, Sophie Hodorowicz. *Polish Herbs, Flowers & Folk Medicine.* Revised edition. New York: Hippocrene Books, 2020.

Krebel, Rudolph. *Volksmedicin und Volksmittel verschiedener Völkerstämme Russlands.* Leipzig and Heidelberg: C. Winter'sche Verlagshandlung, 1858.

Kryczyński, Stanisław. *Tatarzy litewscy: Próba monografii historyczno-etnograficznej.* Warszawa: Drukprasa, 1938.

Kurinsky, Samuel. *The Glassmakers: An Odyssey of the Jews: The First Three Thousand Years.* New York: Hippocrene Books, 1991.

Kvederavičiūtė, Austina. *Lietuvos Žydų Bendruomenės Naudotų Natūralių Vaistingųjų Medžiagų Etnofarmacinis Tyrimas.* Kaunas: Technologijos ir Socialinės Farmacijos Katedra, 2019.

Kvilinkova, Elizaveta Nikolaevna. *Zagovory, magija i oberegi v narodnoj medicine gagauzov.* Kišinev: Elan Incorporated, 2010.

Lewando, Fania. *The Vilna Vegetarian Cookbook.* Translated by Eve Jochnowitz. New York: Schocken Books, 2015.

Löw, Immanuel. *Flora der Juden.* Hildesheim: Georg Olms Verlagsbuchhandlung, 1967.

Manafova, Ruhangiz. *Musulmonų (Totorių ir Azerbaidžaniečių), Gyvenančių Lietuvos Teritorijoje, Naudojamų Vaistingųjų Medžiagų, Etnofarmacinis Tyrimas.* Kaunas: Lietuvos Sveikatos Mokslų Universitetas Medicinos Akademija, 2014.

Moldenke, Harold N., and Alma L. Moldenke. *Plants of the Bible.* Waltham, MA: Chronica Botanica Co., 1952.

Müller-Dietz, Heinz, and Kurt Rintelen. *Arzneipflanzen in der Sowjetunion,* Berlin: Osteuropa-Institut, 1960.

Oczykowski, Romuald. "Poszukiwania. Lecznictwo ludowe," *Wisła* 10, no. 1 (1896): 121.

Osadča-Janata, Natalija. *Ukraïns'ki narodni nazvy roslyn.* Nju-Jork: Ukraïns'ka vil'na akademija nauk u SŠA, 1973.

Ossadcha-Janata, Natalia. *Herbs Used in Ukrainian Folk Medicine*. New York: Research Program on the USSR and the New York Botanical Garden, 1952.

Petkevičius, Rolandas, Joanna Typek, and Maciej Bilek. "Jan Kazimierz Muszyński (1884–1957) prekursorem badań etnobotanicznych na Litwie." *Etnobiologia Polska*, 4 (2014): 55.

Ratkevičiūtė, Kristina. *Kaišiadorų Rajonu Etnofarmacinis Tyrimas*. Kaunas: Lietuvos Sveikatos Mokslų Universitetas, 2018.

Rulikowski, Edward. "Zapiski etnograficzne z Ukrainy." *Zbiór Wiadomości do Antropologii Krajowej*, 3 (1879): 62.

Schaechter, Mordkhe. *di geviksn-velt in yidish [Plant Names in Yiddish]*. New York: YIVO, Institute for Jewish Research, 2005.

Talko-Hryncewicz, Julian. *Zarysy Lecznictwa Ludowego na Rusi Południowej*. Kraków: Nakladem Akademii Umiejętności, 1893.

Teljat'ev, Viktor Vasil'evič. *Poleznye rastenija Central'noj Sibiri*. Irkutsk: Vostočno-Sibirskoe knižnoe izdatel'stvo, 1987.

Teller, Issachar bar. *The Wellspring of Living Waters: A Medical Self-Help Book*. Translated and annotated from the Yiddish by Arthur Teller. New York: Tal Or Oth, 1988.

Tuszewicki, Marek. *A Frog Under the Tongue: Jewish Folk Medicine in Eastern Europe*. Translated by Jessica Taylor-Kucia. London: Littman Library of Jewish Civilization, in association with Liverpool University Press, 2021.

Veckenstedt, Edmund. *Wendische Sagen, Märchen Und Abergläubische Gebräuche, Gesammelt Und Nacherzählt Von Edm. Veckenstedt*. Graz: Leuschner und Lubensky, 1880.

Weiss, Nelly. *The Origin of Jewish Family Names: Morphology and History*. English edition. Bern: P. Lang, 2002.

Wlislocki, Heinrich von. *Aus dem Inneren Leben der Zigeuner, Ethnologische Mitteilungen*. Berlin: E. Felber, 1892.

Wlislocki, Heinrich von. *Volksglaube und Religiöser Brauch der Zigeuner*. Münster: Aschendorff, 1891.

Wulle, Stefan. *Bilsenkraut und Bibergeil: zur Entwicklung des Arzneischatzes: Begleitheft und Auswahlbibliographie zur Ausstellung vom 30.4. bis 19.6.*

1999; 50 Jahre DFG-Sondersammelgebiet Pharmazie. Univ.-Bibliothek, 1999.

Zajączkowski, Ananiasz. "Teksty i studia folklorystyczne." *Myśl Karaimska*, 12 (1938): 41.

Zevin, Igor Vilevich, Nathaniel Altman, and Lilia Vasilevna Zevin. *A Russian Herbal: Traditional Remedies for Health and Healing.* Rochester, Vermont: Healing Arts Press, 1997.

APPENDIX

PALE OF SETTLEMENT TOWNS WITH SIGNIFICANT ASHKENAZI JEWISH POPULATIONS CIRCA 1900

CURRENT NAME, COUNTRY	YIDDISH NAME	TALKO-HRYNCEWICZ NAME	OSADCHA-JANATA NAME	JEWISH POPULATION (%) (1897)
Balta, Ukraine	Balte	n/a	Balta	57
Bełchatów, Poland	Belkhatov	n/a	n/a	75
Berdychiv, Ukraine	Berdichev/ Barditchev	Berdyczow	Berdichiv	80
Bila Cerkva, Poland	Shvarts-Timeh	Biała Cerkiew	Bila Tserkva, Belaya Tserkov'	53
Borščiv, Ukraine	Borshtshiv	Borszczów	n/a	42
Čerkasy, Ukraine	Cherkoss	Czerkasy	Cherkasy	37
Chełm, Poland	Khelm	Chełm	n/a	56
Čyhyryn, Ukraine	Cherin	Czehryń	n/a	30
Dmytre, Ukraine	n/a	Dmytrze	n/a	n/a
Hrodna, Belarus	Grodne	n/a	n/a	69
Husakiv, Ukraine	Husakov	Hussakowa	n/a	30
Jarun', Ukraine	n/a	Jurkow	n/a	n/a
Jędrzejów, Poland	Yendzhev	n/a	n/a	40
Józefów, Poland	Yozefov	n/a	n/a	72
Kam'janec'-Podil's'kyj, Ukraine	Komenets/ Kamenits	Kamieniec	Kamenets-Po-dolski	40
Kaniv, Ukraine	Kanev	Kaniow	Kaniv	30
Korosten', Ukraine	Korosten	n/a	Korosten	48
Krasyliv, Ukraine	Kresilev	n/a	Krasiliv	37
Kyiv, Ukraine	Kiev	Kijow	Kiiv	13
Ladyžyn, Ukraine	Ladizhin	n/a	Ladizhin	49
Lepel' Belarus	Lieplie	n/a	n/a	50

CURRENT NAME, COUNTRY	YIDDISH NAME	TALKO-HRYNCEWICZ NAME	OSADCHA-JANATA NAME	JEWISH POPULATION (%) (1897)
Lityn, Ukraine	Litin	Lityń	Lityn	41
Lypovec', Ukraine	Lipovetz	Lipowiec	n/a	48
Lysyanka, Ukraine	Lisinka	Łysianka	n/a	40
Maxnivka, Ukraine	Makhnovka	Machnówka	Komsomolsk	46
Nova-Ušycja, Ukraine	Nay-Ushitsah, Oyshits	Nowa-Uszyca	n/a	56
Perejaslav, Ukraione	Prejaslov	Perejesław	n/a	39
Radomyšl', Ukraine	Rademishl	Radomyśl	n/a	69
Ryžanivka, Poland	Rizinivka	Ryżanówka	n/a	33
Sanok, Poland	Sonik	Sanok	n/a	42
Savran, Ukraine	Savran	n/a	Savran	54
Sieradz, Poland	Sheradz	n/a	n/a	31
Smarhon, Belarus	Smorgon	n/a	n/a	76
Smykivci, Ukraine	n/a	Smykowce	n/a	n/a
Starokostjantyniv, Ukraine	Olt-Kosntin	n/a	Starokonstantiv	61
Stebliv, Ukraine	Steblev	Steblów	n/a	25
Stryj, Ukraine	Stri	Stryj	n/a	42
Talne, Ukraine	Talna	Talne	n/a	57
Tarnów, Poland	Tarne	Tarnów	n/a	43
Ternopil, Ukraine	Tarnapol	Tarnopol	Tarnopol	51
Trojaniv, Ukraine	Troyanov	n/a	Troyaniv	19
Troškūnai, Lithuania	Trashkon	n/a	n/a	78
Turobin, Poland	Turbin	n/a	n/a	63
Uman', Ukraine	Uman	Humań	Uman	58
Utena, Lithuania	Utian	n/a	n/a	75
Vasyl'kiv, Ukraine	Vaslkev	Wasylków	n/a	40

CURRENT NAME, COUNTRY	YIDDISH NAME	TALKO-HRYNCEWICZ NAME	OSADCHA-JANATA NAME	JEWISH POPULATION (%) (1897)
Verxnij Doroživ, Ukraine	Dorozuv	Dorożów	n/a	13
Vicebsk, Belarus	Vitebsk	Witebsk	n/a	52
Vil'šany, Ukraine	Olshan, Vilshana	Olszana	n/a	20
Vinnytsja, Ukraine	Vinitza	Winnica	Vinnitsya	38
Volodymyr, Ukraine	Ludmir	Włodzimierz	n/a	73
Xarkiv, Ukraine	Kharkov	Charków	Kharkiv	20
Xerson, Ukraine	Khersun	Chersoń	Kherson	30
Xmel'nyc'kyj, Ukraine	Proskurov	Płoskirow	n/a	60
Zakopane, Poland	Zakopona	Zakopane	n/a	n/a
Zalužžja, Ukraine	n/a	Załuże	n/a	n/a
Zbaraž, Ukraine	Zbarazh	Zbaraż	n/a	47
Zlatopil', Ukraine	Zlatopol	Zołotopol	n/a	79
Zvenyhorodka, Ukraine	Zvenigorodka	Zwinogródka	Zvinohorodka	38
Zviahel', Ukraine	Zvil	Zwiahel	n/a	55
Žytomyr, Ukraine	Zhitomir	n/a	Zhitomir	47

BIBLIOGRAPHY

Alksnis, J. "Materialien zur lettischen Volksmedizin, gesammelt, in Deutsche übersetzt und geordnet." *Historische Studien aus dem Pharmakologischen Institut der Kaiserlichen Universität Dorpat*, 1894: 166.

Allan, Nigel. "Illustrations from the Wellcome Library: A Jewish Physician in the Seventeenth Century." *Medical History* 28, no. 3 (1984): 324.

Arends, Johannes. *Volkstümliche Namen der Drogen, Heilkräuter, Arzneimittel und Chemikalien.* Heidelberg: Springer, 2005.

Bächtold-Stäubli, Hanns, and Eduard Hoffmann-Krayer. *Handwörterbuch des deutschen Aberglaubens.* Berlin: De Gruyter, 1987.

Balkienė, Monika. "Bloga akis šiuoiaikinėje Lietuvoje." *Liaudiès kultura* 5, no. 146 (2012): 54.

Balsevičiūtė, Rita. "XX a. pirmosios pusès aukštadvario apylinkės lietuvių ir kitataučių etniškumo sampprata renkantis gydymosi praktikas." *Res Humanitariae*, 26 (2019): 110.

Baumgarten, Elisheva. "Appropriation and Differentiation: Jewish Identity in Medieval Ashkenaz." *AJS Review* 42, no. 1, April (2018): 39.

Baumgarten, Elisheva. "Ask the Midwives: A Hebrew Manual on Midwifery from Medieval Germany." *Social History of Medicine* 32, no. 3 (2019): 712.

Baumgarten, Elisheva. *Mothers and Children: Jewish Family Life in Medieval Europe.* Princeton: Princeton University Press, 2004.

Baumgarten, Jean. "L'impression de livres yiddish à Frankfort aux XVIIe et XVIIIe siècles." *Bulletin du centre du recherche français à Jérusalem*, 20 (2009): 1.

Baumgarten, Jean. "Un livre de médecine en yiddish: le *Beer Mayim Hayyim* c'Issachar ber Teller (Prague, seconde moitié du XVIIe siècle)." *Revue des études juives* 168, no. 1 (2009): 103.

Bergel, Josef. *Die Medizin der Talmudisten nebst einem Anhänge: Die Anthropologie der alten Hebräer.* Leipzig/Berlin: Verlag von Wilhelm Friedrich, 1885.

Berkoff, Anita Engle. "A Jewish Glass-Blower from Spain." *Miscelánea de estudios árabes y hebraicos. Sección Hebreo* (1966): 43.

Bersohn, Mathias. *Słownik biograficzny uczonych Żydów Polskich XVI, XVII i XVIII wieku*. Warszawa: Piotr Laskaver, 1905.

Bersohn, Mathias. *Tobiasz Kohn, lekarz polski w XVII wieku*. Kraków: Czas, 1872.

de Blécourt, Willem. "Between the Devil and the Host: Imagining Witchcraft in Early Modern Poland." *Folklore* 125, no. 3 (2014): 374.

Blumgarten, Aaron S. *Materia Medica for Nurses*. New York: The Macmillan Company, 1922.

Bohdanowicz, L. "The Polish Tatars." *Man,* September–October (1944): 116–121.

Bos, Gerrit, and Guido Mensching. "A 15th Century Medico-Botanical Synonym List (Ibero-Romance-Arabic) in Hebrew Characters." *Panace@* 7, no. 24, Diciembre (2006): 261.

Bos, Gerrit. "'Balādhur' (Marking-Nut): A Popular Medieval Drug for Strengthening Memory." *Bulletin of the School of Oriental and African Studies* 59, no, 2 (1996): 229.

Brill, Robert H. "Some Chemical Observations on the Cuneiform Glassmaking Texts," *Annales du 5e Congrès de l'Associatión Internationale pour l'Histoire du Verre*. Liège: Edition du Secretariat Général, 1972: 329.

Brown, Jeremey. "The Medicine of Tuviya Cohen in Comparison and Contrast." *Ma'ase Tuviya (Venice 1708): Tuviya on Medicine and Science*. Edited by Kenneth Collins, Samuel Kottek, and Helena Paavilainen. Jerusalem: Muriel and Philp Berman Medical Library, 2021: 129.

Caballero-Navas, Carmen. "The Care of Women's Health and Beauty: An Experience Shared by Medieval Jewish and Christian Women." *Journal of Medieval History* 34, no. 2 (2008): 146.

Caballero-Navas, Carmen. "El saber y la práctica de la magia en el judaísmo hispano medieval." *Clio & Crimen: Revista del centro de historia del crimen de Durango*, 8 (2011): 73.

Caballero-Navas, Carmen. "Medicine Among Medieval Jews: The Science, the Art, and the Practice." In *Science in Medieval Jewish Cultures,* edited by G. Freudenthal. Cambridge: Cambridge University Press, 2017: 320.

Caro, Georg. *Sozial- und wirtschaftsgeschichtliche der Juden im Mittelalter und der Neuzeit.* Leipzig: G. Fock, 1908.

Černiauskaitė, Dalia. "Metaforos funkcijos lietuvių užkalbėjimuose." *Tautosakos darbai* 20, no. 27 (2004): 151.

Cohen-Hanegbi, Naama. "Learning Practice from Texts: Jews and Medicine in the Later Middle Ages." *Social History of Medicine* 32, no. 4 (2019): 659.

Dafni, Amots, and Barbara Böck. "Medicinal Plants of the Bible—Revisited." *Journal of Ethnobiology and Ethnomedicine,* 15 (2019): 57.

Dafni, Amots et al. "Myrtle, Basil, Rosemary and Three-Lobed Sage as Ritual Plants in the Monotheistic Religions: An Historical-Ethnobotanical Comparison." *Economic Botan* 74, no. 3 (2020): 330.

Dalby, Andrew. *Dangerous Tastes: The Story of Spices.* Berkeley: UC Press, 2000.

Dan Demeter. "Volksglauben und Gebräuche der Juden in der Bukowina." *Zeitschrift für österreichische Volkskunde,* 2 (1896): 81.

Danzer, Diviš. *Židovstvo v obchodě s chmelem.* Praha: Tiskem Jos. R. Vilímka v Praze - Nákladem Diviše Danzera, 1890.

Dannaway, Frederick R. "Strange Fires, Weird Smokes and Psychoactive Combustibles: Entheogens and Incense in Ancient Traditions." *Journal of Psychoactive Drugs* 42, no. 2 (2010): 485.

Dembińska, Maria. *Food and Drink in Medieval Poland: Rediscovering a Cuisine of the Past.* Translated by Magdalena Thomas, revised and adapted by William Noys Weaver. Philadelphia: University of Pennsylvania Press, 1999.

Domańska, Aneta. "Metody leczenia chorób wśród ludu polskiego w XIX wieku. Próba bilansu." *Zeszyty wiejskie,* 32 (2016): 309.

Duschak, Moritz. *Zur Botanik des Talmud.* Pest: Selbstverlag des Verfassers, 1871.

Dynner, Glenn. *Yankel's Tavern: Jews, Liquor, and Life in the Kingdom of Poland.* Oxford: Oxford University Press, 2014.

Dziekan, Marek M. "History and Culture of Polish Tatars." In *Muslims in Poland and Eastern Europe: Widening the European Discourse on Islam,* edited by Katarzyna Górak-Sosnowska. Warszawa: University of Warsaw, 2011: 27.

Easley, Thomas, and Steven H. Horne. *The Modern Herbal Dispensatory: A Medicine-Making Guide*. Berkeley, CA: North Atlantic Books, 2016.

Eliach, Yaffa. *There Once Was a World: A Nine-Hundred-Year Chronicle of the Shtetl of Eishyshok*. Boston: Little, Brown, 1998.

Feldman, W. M. *The Jewish Child: Its History, Folklore, Biology, and Sociology*. London: Bailliére, Tindal & Cox, 1917.

Fiore, Cristina, et al. "A History of the Therapeutic Use of Licorice in Europe." *Journal of Ethnopharmacology* 99, no. 3 (2005): 317.

Fischel, Walter J. "Azarbaijan in Jewish History." *Proceedings of the American Society for Jewish Research*, 22 (1953): 1.

Fischel, Walter J. "The Jewish Merchants Called Radanites." *Jewish Quarterly Review* 42, no, 3 (January 1952): 321.

Fischel, Walter J. "The Spice Trade in Mamluk Egypt: A Contribution to the Economic History of Medieval Islam." *Journal of the Economic and Social History of the Orient* 1, no. 2 (April 1958): 157.

Fischer, Adam. *Rośliny w wierzeniach i zwyczajach ludowych: Słownik Adama Fischera*. Edited by Monika Kujawska. Wrocław: Polskie Towarzystwo Ludoznawcze, 2016.

Fischer, Josef Ludwig. *Handbuch der Glasmalerei: für Forscher, Sammler und Kunstfreunde wie für Künstler, Architekten und Glasmaler*. Leipzig: Verlag von Karl W. Wiersemann, 1914.

Fliginskikh, Ekaterina E., Svetlana L. Yakovleva, and Ksenia Y. Babyina. "Superstitions as Part of the Frame 'Pregnancy and Birth' in the English, Russian, and Mari Languages: Postliminary Level." In *Issues and Trends in Interdisciplinary Behavior and Social Science*. London: CRC Press, 2018: 185.

Fried, Moses. "Volksmedizinisches und Diätetisches aus Ostgalizien." *Mitteilungen zur jüdischen Volkskunde* 13, no. 4 (1910): 167.

Geller, Ewa. "A New Portrait of Early Seventeenth-Century Polish Jewry in an Unknown Eastern Yiddish Remedy Book." *European Judaism: A Journal for the New Europe* 42, no. 2 (Autumn 2009): 62.

Gellman, Uriel. "Popular Religion and Modernity: Jewish Magic Books in Eastern Europe in the Nineteenth Century." *Polin: Studies in Polish Jewry*, 33 (2021): 185.

Gladstar, Rosemary. *Rosemary Gladstar's Herbal Recipes for Vibrant Health: 175 Teas, Tonics, Oils, Salves, Tinctures, and Other Natural Remedies for the Entire Family*. North Adams, MA: Storey, 2008.

Glauber-Zimra, Samuel. "Summoning Spirits in Egypt: Jewish Women and Spiritualism in Early Twentieth-Century Cairo." *Nashim: A Journal of Jewish Women's Studies & Gender Issues*, 38 (Spring 2021): 25.

Glück, Leopold. "Skizzen aus der Volksmedecin und dem medicinischen Aberglauben in Bosnien und der Hercegovina." *Wissenschaftliche Mittheilungen aus Bosnien und der Hercegovina*, 2 (1894): 394.

Green, Monica H. "Conversing with the Minority: Relations among Christian, Jewish, and Muslim Women in the High Middle Ages." *Journal of Medieval History*, 34 (2008): 105.

Green, Monica H. *The Trotula: A Medieval Compendium of Women's Medicine*. Philadelphia: University of Pennsylvania Press, 2001.

Grieve, Maude. *A Modern Herbal: the Medicinal, Culinary, Cosmetic and Economic Properties, Cultivation and Folk-Lore of Herbs, Grasses, Fungi, Shrubs, and Trees with All Their Modern Scientific Uses*. New York: Dover, 1971.

Griffin, Clare. "Disentangling Commodity Histories: *Pauame* and Sassafras in the Early Modern Global World." *Journal of Global History*, 15, 1 (2020): 1.

Griffin, Clare. *Mixing Medicines: The Global Drug Trade and Early Modern Russia*. Montreal: McGill QUP, 2022.

Griffin, Clare. "Plants and Medicine." In *A Cultural History of Plants in the Seventeenth and Eighteenth Centuries, Vol 4*, edited by Jennifer Milam. London, New York: Bloomsbury Academic, 2022: 111.

Griffin, Clare Louise. *The Production and Consumption of Medical Knowledge in Seventeenth-Century Russia: The Apothecary Chancery*. London: University College, London, 2012. (Unpublished dissertation)

Griffin, Clare. "Russia and Early Modern Medicine." *Kritika: Explorations in Russian and Eurasian History* 12, no. 4 (Fall 2011): 967.

Griffin, Clare. "Russia and the Medical Drug Trade in the Seventeenth Century." *Social History of Medicine* 31, no. 1 (2016): 2.

Grunwald, Max. "Altjüdisches Gemeindeleben." *Mitteilungen zur jüdischen Volkskunde*, 29 (1926): 599.

Grunwald, Max. "Aus dem jüdischen Kochbuch." *Mitteilungen zur jüdischen Volkskunde*, 31/32 (1929): 40.

Grunwald, Max. "Aus Philo." *Mitteilungen zur jüdischen Volkskunde*, 14, 4, 40 (1911): 137.

Grunwald, Max, ed. *Die Hygiene der Juden. Im Anschluss an die internationale Hygiene-Ausstellung Dresden 1911*. Dresden: Verlag der historischen Abteilung der internationalen Hygiene-Ausstellung Dresden 1901, 1911.

Grunwald, Max. "Jüdische Mystik," *Mitteilungen zur jüdischen Volkskunde*, 25 (1923): 371.

Grunwald, Max. "Schnorrer." *Mitteilungen zur jüdischen Volkskunde*, 29 (1926): 574.

Gudanavičius, St. *Vaistiniai augalai*. Vilnius: Valstybinė Politines ir Mokslinės Literatūros Leidykla, 1960.

Guesnet, François. "Body, Place, and Knowledge: The Plica Polonica in Travelogues and Experts' Reflection around 1800." *Central Europe* 17, no. 1 (2019): 54.

Gunda, Béla. "Gypsy Medical Folklore in Hungary." *Journal of American Folklore* 75, no. 296 (April–June 1962): 131.

Hajnáczky, Tamás. "The Forced Assimilation Gypsy Policy in Socialist Hungary." *Romani Studies* 30, no. 1 (2020): 49-87.

Halikowski Smith, Stefan. "'Profits Sprout Like Tropical Plants': A Fresh Look at What Went Wrong with the Eurasian Spice Trade c. 1550–1800." *Journal of Global History*, 3 (2008): 387.

Hanchuk, Rena Jeanne. *The Word and Wax: A Medical Folk Ritual among Ukrainians in Alberta*. Edmonton: Huculak Chair of Ukrainian Culture and Ethnography; Canadian Institute of Ukrainian Studies Press, 1999.

Henrici, Ant. Alf. v. "Weitere Studien über Volksheilmittel verschiedener in Russland lebender Völkerschaften." *Historische Studien aus dem Pharmakologischen Institut der Kaiserlichen Universität Dorpat* (1894): 1.

Heyde, Jürgen. "The Jewish Economic Elite in Red Ruthenia in the Fourteenth and Fifteenth Centuries." *Polin*, 22 (2010): 156.

Heyde, Jürggen. "Komunikacja elit na Rusi Czerwonej w połowie XV wieku." *Żydzi i judaizm we współczesnych badaniach polskich Tom IV.* Kraków: Polska Akademia Umiejętności, 2008: 109.

Horowitz, Elliott. "Coffee, Coffeehouses, and the Nocturnal Rituals of Early Modern Jewry." *AJS Review* 14, no. 1 (Spring 1989): 17.

Hryniewiecki, Bolesław. *Tentamen Florae Lithuaniae. Zarys Flory Litwy.* Warszawa: Nakładem Towarzystwa Naukowego Warszawskiego, 1933.

Jacob, Irene, and Walter Jacob, eds. *The Healing Past: Pharmaceuticals in the Biblical and Rabinic World.* Leiden, New York, Köln: E. J. Brill, 1993.

Jánošíková, Magdaléna. "United in Scholarship, Divided in Practice: (Re-) Translating Smallpox and Measles for Seventeenth-Century Jews." *Isis* 113, no. 2 (June 2022): 289.

Jessel, Andrea. "Die 'heylsame Dreck-Apotheke' des Doktor Paullini." *Pflege-zeitschrift,* 74 (2021): 66.

Jones, Louis C. "The Evil Eye among European-Americans." *Western Folklore* 10, no. 1 (January 1951): 11.

Jones, Louis C. "Practitioners of Folk Medicine." *Bulletin of the History of Medicine* 23, no. 5 (1949): 480.

Jütte, Daniel. "'They Shall Not Keep Their Doors or Windows Open': Urban Spaces and the Dynamics of Conflict and Contact in Premodern Jewish-Christian Relations." *European History Quarterly* 42, no. 2 (2016): 209.

Kahl, Thede. "Der böse Blick: Ein gemeinsames Element im Volksglauben von Christen und Muslimen." In *Religion und Magie in Ostmitteleuropa,* edited by Thomas Wünsch. Münster: Lit Verlag, 2008: 321.

Kahn, Fritz. *Das Versehen der Schwangeren in Volksglaube und Dichtung.* Frankfurt am Main: J. F. Sauerländer's Verlag, 1912.

Kaminski, Patricia, and Richard Katz. *Flower Essence Repertory: A Comprehensive Guide to North American and English Flower Essences for Emotional and Spiritual Well-Being.* Nevada City, CA: Flower Essence Society, Earth-Spirit, Inc., 2019.

Kapaló, James Alexander. *Text, Context and Performance: Gagauz Folk Religion in Discourse and Practice.* Leiden, Boston: Brill, 2011.

Kaps, Klemens. "Grain, Flour, Beer, and Liquor: Commodity Chains, Labor Relations and Economic Developments in Habsburg Galicia, 1772–1913." In *Global Commodity Chains and Labor Relations*, edited by Andrea Komlosy and Goran Musić. Leiden: Brill, 2021: 107.

Katz, Jordan R. "Jewish Midwives, Wise Women, and the Construction of Medical-Halakhic Expertise in the Eighteenth Century." *Jewish Social Studies* 26, no. 2 (2021): 1.

Kisa, Anton. *Das Glas im Altertume in 3 Teilen*. Leipzig: Hiersmann, 1908.

Klaniczay, Gábor. "Healers in Hungarian Witch Trials." In *Witchcraft and Demonology in Hungary and Transylvania*, edited by G. Klaniczay and É. Pócs. London: Palgrave, 2017: 111.

Klymasz, Andrea Karen. *Folk Medicine: A Ukrainian-Canadian Experience*. Winnipeg: University of Manitoba, 1991. (Unpublished dissertation)

Knab, Sophie Hodorowicz. *Polish Herbs, Flowers & Folk Medicine*. Revised edition. New York: Hippocrene, 2020.

Kobert, R. "Ueber Sarsaparille." *Deutsche Medizinische Wochenschrift*, 8, 26, 30 June (1892): 601.

Koroloff, Rachel D. *The Beginnings of Russian Natural History: The Life and Work of Stepan Petrovich Krasheninnikov (1711–1755)*. Corvallis: Oregon State University, 2007. (Unpublished thesis)

Koroloff, Rachel D. "Juniper: From Medicine to Poison and Back Again in 17th-Century Muscovy." *Kritika: Explorations in Russian and Eurasian History* 19, no. 4 (2018): 697.

Koroloff, Rachel. *Seeds of Exchange: Collecting for Russia's Apothecary and Botanical Gardens in the Seventeenth and Eighteenth Centuries*. Urbana-Champaign: University of Illinois, 2014. (Unpublished dissertation)

Koroloff, Rachel. "*Travniki, Travniki,* and *Travniki*: Herbals, Herbalists, and Herbaria in Seventeenth-Century and Eighteenth-Century Russia." *Bibliothika: E-Journal of Eighteenth-Cetnury Russian Studies*, 6 (2018): 58.

Krauss, S. "Aus der jüdischen Volksküche." *Mitteilungen zur jüdischen Volkskunde* 18, no. 1 (1915): 1.

Krawll, M. D. "Jewish Folk Medicine: Science or Superstition?" *Jewish Exponent*, 30 (December 1983): 22.

Kujawska, Monika, Łukasz Łuczaj, and Joanna Typek. "Fischer's *Lexicon of Slavic Beliefs and Customs*: A Previously Unknown Contribution to the Ethnobotany of Ukraine and Poland." *Journal of Ethnobiology and Ethnomedicine* 11, no. 85 (2015).

Kujawska, Monika, Piotr Klepacki, and Łukasz Łuczaj. "Fischer's *Plants in Folk Beliefs and Customs*: A Previously Unknown Contribution to the Ethnobotany of the Polish-Lithuanian-Belarusian Borderland." *Journal of Ethnobiology and Ethnomedicine* 13, no. 20 (2017).

Kujawska, Monika, and Ingvar Svanberg. "From Medicinal Plant to Noxious Weed: *Bryonia Alba* (Cucurbitaceae) in Northern and Eastern Europe." *Journal of Ethnobiology and Ethnomedicine* 15, no. 22 (2019).

Kulakauskienė, Dorilė. "Užkalbėjimai." *Darbai ir dienos*, 31 (2002): 277.

Kvederavičiūtė, Austina. *Lietuvos Žydų Bendruomenės Naudotų Natūralių Vaistingųjų Medžiagų Etnofarmacinis Tyrimas*. Kaunas: Technologijos ir Socialinės Farmacijos Katedra, 2019. (Unpublished master's thesis)

Laurikienė, Nijolė. "Sambariai Arba Trejos Devynerios." *Liaudies Kultūra*, 2 (2009): 9.

Lechler, George. "The Tree of Life in Indo-European and Islamic Cultures." *Ars Islamica*, 4 (1937): 369.

Lehmhaus, Lennart, and Matteo Marielli. *Collecting Recipes: Byzantine and Jewish Pharmacology in Dialogue*. Boston, Berlin: De Gruyter, 2017.

Lepicard, Etienne. "An Alternative to the Cosmic and Mechanic Metaphors for the Human Body? The House Illustration in *Ma'aseh Tuviyah* (1708)." *Medical History*, 52 (2008): 93.

Lev, Efraim, and Zohar Amar. "Ethnopharmacological Survey of Traditional Drugs Sold in the Kingdom of Jordan." *Journal of Ethnopharmacology* 82, no. 2/3 (2002): 131.

Lev, Ephraim. "Drugs Held and Sold by Pharmacists of the Jewish Community of Medieval (11-14th Centuries) Cairo According to Lists of *Materia Medica* found at the Taylor-Schechter Genizah Collection, Cambridge." *Journal of Ethnopharmacology* 110, no. 2 (2007): 275.

Lev, Efraim, and Zohar 'Ammār. *Practical Materia Medica of the Medieval Eastern Mediterranean According to the Cairo Genizah*. Leiden: Brill, 2008.

Lev, Ephraim. "Reconstructed *Materia Medica* of the Medieval and Ottoman Al-Sham." *Journal of Ethnopharmacology* 80, no. 2/3 (2002): 167.

Levi, Moric. *Sefardi u Bosni*. Beograd: Savez jevrejskih opština Jugoslavije, 1969. Levinson, A. "A Medical Cyclopedist of the Seventeenth Century." *Bulletin of the Society of Medical History of Chicago*, 2 (January 1917): 27.

Lévy, Isaac Jack, and Rosemary Lévy Zumwalt. *Ritual Medical Lore of Sephardic Women: Sweetening the Spirits, Healing the Sick*. Urbana, Chicago: University of Chicago Press, 2002.

Levy, Juliette de Baïracli. "The Gypsies of Turkey." *Journal of the Gypsy-Lore Society* 3, no. 31 (1952): 5.

Levy, Juliette de Baïracli. "Gypsy Herbalists in France and England," *Journal of the Gypsy-Lore Society* 3, no. 30 (1950): 23.

Lewicka, Magdalena, "The Literature of the Tatars of the Grand Duchy of Lithuania: Characteristics of the Tatar Writings and Areas of Research." *Journal of Language and Cultural Education* 4, no. 1 (2016).

Libera, Zbigniew. "Etnobotanika, etnomedycyna i etnografia w Polsce." *Medycyna Nowożytna* 29, no. 1 (2023): 205.

Libera, Zbigniew. "Oczy i widzenie (fragment semiotyki antropologii popularnej Europy środkowej i wschodniej w XIX i XX wieku)." In *Polacy i świat kultury i zmiana. Studia historyczne i antropologiczne oficrowane Profesor Halinie Firkowskiej-Francii*, edited by J. Lencznarowicz, J. Pezda, and A. Zięba. Kraków: Księgarnia Akademicka, 2016: 550.

Lichocka, Halina. "Historia pierwiastka narkotycznego." *Analecta* 13, no, 1/2 (2004): 113.

Lilienthal, Regina. "Das Kind bei den Juden." *Mitteilungen zur jüdischer Volkskunde* 11, no. 1 (1908): 1.

Lobo, Ricardo Alexandre de Araujo Monteiro, Ana Cristina Bastos Nigro Monteiro Lobo, Antônio Fernando Morais de Oliveira, and Laise de Holanda Cavalcanti Andrade. "Ethnomedicinal Plants for Veterinary Use in Gypsy Communities of the Northeast of Brazil." *Boletin Latinoamericano y del Caribe de Plantas Medicinales y Aromáticas* 19, no. 2 (2020): 179

Los, Karina. *Natūraliųjų Vaistingųjų Medžiagų, Naudotų Vilniaus Krašte 2016–2017 Metais, Etnofarmacinis Tyrimas*. Kaunas: Lietuvos Sveikatos

Mokslų Universitatis, Farmacijos Fakultetas, 2018. (Unpublished master's thesis)

Löw, Immanuel. *Flora der Juden*. Hildesheim: Georg Olms Verlagsbuchhandlung, 1967.

Löw, Immánuel. *Zsidó Folklór Tanulmányok*. Szeged: Néprajai és Kulturális Antropologiai Tanszók, 2014.

Löwinger, Adolf. "Der böse Blick," *Mitteilungen zur jüdischen Volkskunde*, 29, no. 1011 (1926): 551, 567.

Łuczaj, Łukasz, Jarosław Dumanowski, Cecylia Marszałek, and Fabio Parasecoli. "Turmeric and Cumin Instead of Stock Cubes: An Internet Survey of Spices and Culinary Herbs Used in Poland Compared with Historical Cookbooks and Herbals." *Plants* 12, no. 3 (2023): 591.

Łuczaj, Łukasz et al. "Wild Edible Plants of Belarus: From Rostafiński's Questionnaire of 1883 to the Present." *Journal of Ethnobiology and Ethnomedicine* 9, no. 21 (2013).

Macht, Davis I. "Calendula or Marigold in Medical History and in Shakespeare." *Bulletin of the History of Medicine* 29, no. 6 (November–December 1955): 491.

Mačus, Adomas. "Pirmieji lietuvos botanikai ir augalų tyrinėtojai." *Farmacijos zinios*, 1 (1938): 6.

Madej, Tomasz et al. "Juniper Beer in Poland: The Story of the Revival of a Traditional Beverage." *Journal of Ethnobiology* 34, no. 1 (2014): 84.

Manafova, Ruhangiz. *Musulmonų (Totorių ir Azerbaidžaniečių), Gyvenančių Lietuvos Teritorijoje, Naudojamų Vaistingųjų Medžiagų, Etnofarmacinis Tyrimas*. Kaunas: Lietuvos Sveikatos Mokslų Universitetas Medicinos Akademija, 2014. (Unpublished thesis)

Mansikka, Viljo J. *Litauische Zaubersprüche*. Helsinki: Suomalainen Tiedeskatemia / Academia Scientiarum Fennica, 1929.

Marcus, Ivan G. *Rituals of Childhood: Jewish Acculturation in Medieval Europe*. New Haven: Yale University Press, 1996.

Marzell, Heinrich. "Heilkräuter in der deutschen und der südslawischen Volksmedizin." *Sudhoffs Archive für Geschichte der Medizin und der Naturwissenschaften* 34, no. 1/4 (1941): 133.

Maslauskaitė, Rimantė. *1921–1928 m. Lietuvoje Gamintų Patenruotų Preparatų Receptūros Tyrimos*. Kaunas: Lietuvos Sveikatos Mokslų Universitetas, 2018.

Meir, Nathan M. *Stepchildren of the Shtetl: The Destitute, Disabled, and Mad of Jewish Eastern Europe, 1800–1939*. Stanford, CA: Stanford University Press, 2020.

Miškinienė, Galina. "The Distinctive Features of the Traditional Rites of the Lithuanian Tatars in the Second Half of the Twentieth Century." *Tatarica (History and Society)*, 5 (2015): 127.

Miškinienė, Galina. "Features of the Lithuanian Tatars' Traditional Rites, in the Early 20th Century: A Wedding Ceremony (Based on the Lithuanian Tatars' Manuscripts Written in Arabic Script)." *Tatarica*, 14 (2020): 23.

Morawski, Stanisław, Adam Czartkowski, and Henryk Mościcki. *Kilka Lat Młodości Mojej W Wilnie <1818–1825>*. Warszawa: Biblioteka polska, 1924.

Motiekaitytė, Vida, and Zenonas Venckus. "Treatment of Heart and Circulation Disorders Using Autochthonous Medicinal Plants of Lithuania." *Professional Studies: Theory and Practice* 5, no. 20 (2019): 34.

Motley, Timothy J. "The Ethnobotany of Sweet Flag, Acorus Calamus (Araceae)." *Economic Botany* 48, no. 4 (October–December 1994): 397.

Müller-Dietz, Heinz, and Kurt Rintelen. *Arzneipflanzen in der Sowjetunion*. Berlin: Osteuropa-Institut, 1960.

Müler-Ebeling, Claudia, Christian Rötsch, and Wolf-Dieter Storl. *Hexermedizin: Die Wiederentdeckung einer verbotenen Heilkunst: Schamarische Traditionen in Europa*. Aarau, CH: AT Verlag, 1998.

Nadel-Golobič, Eleonora. "Armenians and Jews in Medieval Lvov. Their Role in Oriental Trade 1400–1600." *Cahiers du monde russe et soviétique* 20, no. 3/4 (July–December 1979): 345.

Nosallovsky, Michael. "Folk Beliefs, Mystics, and Superstitions in Ashkenazi and Karaite Tombstone Inscriptions from Ukraine." *Markers*, 26 (2009): 120.

Oczykowski, Romuald. "Poszukiwania. 1. Lecznictwo ludowe." *Wisła* 10, no. 1 (1896): 121.

Ort, Jan. "Belonging, Mobility, and the Socialist Policies in Kapišová, Slovakia." *Romani Studies* 32, no. 1 (2022): 23.

Ossadcha-Janata, Natalia. *Herbs Used in Ukrainian Folk Medicine*. New York: Research Program on the USSR and the New York Botanical Garden, 1952.

Ostling, Michael. "Witches' Herbs on Trial." *Folklore* 125, no. 2 (August 2014): 179.

Penkala-Gawęcka, Danuta. "Maladies populaires et médecine complémentaire en Cachoubie." *Ethnologie Française* 40, no. 2 (March 2010): 295.

Petran, Madalina, Dorin Dragos, and Marilena Gilca. "Historical Ethnobotanical Review of Medicinal Plants Used to Treat Children's Diseases in Romania (1860s–1970s)." *Journal of Ethnobiology and Ethnomedicine* 16, no. 15 (2020).

Pieroni, Andrea, and Cassandra L. Quave, eds. *Ethnobotany and Biocultural Diversities in the Balkans: Perspectives on Sustainable Rural Development and Reconciliation*. New York: Springer, 2014.

Phillips, Sarah D. "Waxing Like the Moon: Women Folk Healers in Rural Western Ukraine." *Folklorica* 9, no. 1 (2004): 13.

Pócs, Éva. *Between the Living and the Dead: A Perspective on Witches and Seers in the Early Modern Age*. Budapest: Central European Press, 1999.

Podolinská, Tatiana Zachar, and Tomáš Hrustič. "Religiosity and Spirituality among the Gypsy/Roma in Twentieth-Century Europe: Theoretical Framing and Ethnographic Perspectives." *Romani Studies* 31, no. 2 (2021): 143.

Prakofjewa, Julia, et al. "Diverse in Local, Overlapping in Official Medical Botany: Critical Analaysis of Medicinal Plant Records from the Historical Regions of Livonia and Courland in Northeast Europe, 1829–1895." *Plants* 11, no. 8 (2022): 1064.

Pranskuniené, Zivile. "Ethnobotanical Study of Cultivated Plants in Kaišiadorys District, Lithuania: Possible Trends for New Herbal Based Medicines." *Evidence-Based Complementary and Alternative Medicine*, 14 (2019): 70.

Pranskuniené, Zivile, et al. "Home Gardens as a Source of Medicinal, Herbal, and Food Preparations: Modern and Historical Approaches in Lithuania." *Applied Sciences* 11, no. 21 (2021): 9988.

Preuss, Julius. *Biblisch-Talmudische Medizin: Beiträge zur Geschichte der Heilkunde und der Kultur überhaupt*. Berlin: Verlag von S. Karger, 1921.

Preuss, Julius. *Biblical and Talmudic Medicine*. Translated and edited by Fred Rosner, MD. Lanham, MD: Rowman & Littlefield, 2004 (1978).

Rabakh, Berl. vaybershe parnoses in sonik. *Yidishe shprakh* 24, no. 1 (June 1964): 26.

Rabinowitz, Louis I. "The Routes of the Radanites." *Jewish Quarterly Rev ew* 35, no. 3 (January 1945): 251.

Rechtman, Abraham. *The Lost World of Russia's Jews: Ethnography and Folklore in the Pale of Settlement*. Translated by Nathaniel Deutsch and Noah Barrera. Bloomington: Indiana University Press, 2021.

Romaniello, Matthew P. "'Tobacco! Tobacco!' Exporting New Habits to Siberia and Russian America." *Sibirica* 16, no. 2 (Summer 2017): 1.

Romaniello, Matthew P. "True Rhubarb? Trading Eurasian Botanical and Medical Knowledge in the Eighteenth Century." *Journal of Global History* 11, no. 1 (2016): 3.

Rosner, Fred. *The Medical Legacy of Moses Maimonides*. Hoboken: KTAV, 1998.

Rotaru, Julieta. "Considerations about the 'Turkish Gypsies' as Crypto-Muslims in Wallachia." In *Romani History and Culture: Festschrift in Honor of Prof. Dr. Vesselin Popov*, edited by Khristo Kiuchukov, Sofiia Zakhova, and Ion Duminica. München: Lincom GmbH, 2021: 75.

Ruderman, David B. "Medicine and Scientific Thought: The World of Tobias Cohen." In *The Jews of Early Modern Venice*, edited by Robert C. Davis and Benjamin David. Baltimore: Johns Hopkins University Press, 2001: 191.

Ruhräu, John. "Pediatric Biographies: Tobias Katz, 1652–1727." *American Journal of Diseases of Children* 47, no. 2 (1934): 399.

Ryan, William F. "Maimonides in Muscovy: Medical Texts and Terminology." *Journal of the Warburg and Courtauld Institutes*, 51 (1988): 43.

Shikov, Alexander N., et al. "Medicinal Plants of the Russian Pharmacopoeia: Their History and Applications." *Journal of Ethnopharmacology* 154, no. 3 (April 2014): 481.

Simonsen, David. "Les marchands juifs appelés 'Radanites.'" *Revue des études juives* 54, no. 107 (July–September 1907): 141.

Spector, Naomi. *The Jewish Book of Flowers.* Pennsauken Township, NJ: BookBaby, 2023.

Steele, Robert. "A Mediaeval Panacea." *Proceedings of the Royal Society of Medicine*, 10 (1917): 93.

Stein, Sarah Abrevaya. "Botánica Sephardica." *Comparative Studies in Society and History* 64, no. 3 (2022): 611.

Stein, Sarah Abrevaya. "The Queen of Herbs: A Plant's Eye View of the Sephardic Diaspora." *Jewish Quarterly Review* 113, no. 1 (Winter 2022): 119.

Steni, Diana L., Sarah Kielt Costello, and Karen Polinger Foster, eds. *The Routledge Companion to Ecstatic Experience in the Ancient World.* Abingdon, New York: Routledge, 2022.

Stichler-Alegria, Tischa. "Hatte die Zootherapie ägyptischer und babylonischer Pharmakopoen Einfluss auf die Dreck-Apotheke des 17. Jahrhunderts." *Isimu*, 10 (2007): 183.

Supady, Jerzy. "Działalność lekarska Juliana Talko-Hryncewicza." *Analecta Studia i Materiały z Dziejów* 10, no. 19 (2001): 153.

Supady, Jerzy. "Zasługi polskiego lekarza i antropologa Juliana Talko-Hryncewicza dla nauki rosyjskiej." *Archivum Historii i Filozofii Medycyny*, 75 (2012): 131.

Sutherland, Anne. "Health and Illness among the Rom of California," *Journal of the Gypsy Lore Society*, series 5, 2, no. 1 (February 1992): 19.

Temeseváry, Rudolf. *Volksbräuche und Aberglauben in der Geburtshilfe und der Pflege des Neugeborenen in Ungarn: Etnografische Studien.* Leipzig: Th. Grishen's Verlag, 1900.

Theissen, Ulrich. "'Ein bezauberndes Hustenkraut': Zu den Bezeichnungen des Alant (Inula helenium L.) in den slawischen Sprachen, vor allem in Bulgarischen." *Zeitschrift für Balkanologie* 42, no. 1/2 (2006): 226.

Tilhagen, Carl-Herman. "Food and Drink among the Swedish Kalderaša Gypsies." *Journal of the Gypsy Lore Society*, series 3, 36 (1957): 25.

Trachtenberg, Joshua. *Jewish Magic and Superstition.* Philadelphia: University of Pennsylvania Press, 2004 (1939).

Tuszewicki, Marek. "Non-Jewish Languages of Jewish Magic: On Homeliness, Otherness, and Translation." In *Jewish Translation, Translating Jewishness*, edited by Magdalena Waligórska and Tara Kohn. Berlin, Boston: de Gruyter, 2018: 135.

Udziela, Marjan. *Medycyna i przesądy lecznicze ludu polskiego*. Warszawa: Skład głowny w księgarni M. Arota, 1891.

Valodzina, Tatiana. "Plica Polonica in Belarusian Beliefs and Incantations." *Incantatio: An International Journal on Charms, Charmers, and Charming*, 4 (2014): 59.

Vasiliauskas, Juozas. *Vaistažolių Galia*. Vilnius, Lithuania: Politika, 1991.

Vesey-Fitzgerald, Brian. "Gypsy Medicine." *Journal of the Gypsy Lore Society*, series 3, 23 (1944): 21.

Weinbaum, Batya. "What the Gypsy Women Probably Tell the Female Anthropologist: A Critical Response to Judith Okeley's Own or Other Culture." *Femspec* 11, no. 1, (2010): 44.

Weinreich, Max. "Holekrash: A Jewish Rite of Passage." In *Folklore International: Essays in Traditional Literature, Belief, and Custom in Honor of Wayland Debs Hand*, edited by C. Sommer and W. D. Hand. Hatboro: Folklore Associates, 1967: 243.

Wengeroff, Pauline. *Memoirs of a Grandmother: Scenes from the Cultural History of the Jews of Russia in the Nineteenth Century*. Translated and edited by Shulamit S. Magnus. Stanford, CA: Stanford University Press, 2010–2014.

Yoffie, Leah Rachel. "Popular Beliefs and Customs among the Yiddish-Speaking Jews of St. Louis, Mo." *Journal of American Folklore* 38, no. 149 (July–September 1925): 375.

Zaidman-Mauer, Daniella. "'May God Shield Us from the Plague.' Vernacular Remedies for the Plague from Moyshe Kalish's Yiddish Self-Help Medical Book *Seyfer Yeruin Moyshe* (Amsterdam 1679)." *Zatot*, 19 (2002): 144.

Zedler, Johann Heinrich, Jacob August Franckenstein, Paul Daniel Longolius, Johann Peter von Ludewig, and Carl Günther Ludovici. *Grosses Vollständiges Universal Lexicon Aller Wissenschafften Und Künste, Welche*

Bisshero Durch Menschlichen Verstand Und Witz Erfunden Und Verbessert Worden. Halle und Leipzig: Verlegts Johann Heinrich Zedler, 1754.

Zevin, Igor Vilevich, Nathaniel Altman, and Lilia Vasilevna Zevin. *A Russian Herbal: Traditional Remedies for Health and Healing.* Rochester, VT: Healing Arts Press, 1997.

Zimmels, Hirsch J. *Magicians, Theologians, and Doctors: Studies in Folk-Medicine and Folk-Lore as Reflected in the Rabbinical Responsa (12th–19th Centuries).* London: Edward Golston & Son, 1952.

Zinger, Nimrod. "'Who Knows What the Cause Is?': 'Natural' and 'Unnatural' Causes for Illness in the Writings of the Ba'alei Shem, Doctors, and Patients among German Jews in the Eighteenth Century." In *The Jewish Body: Corporeality, Society, and Identity in the Renaissance and Early Modern Period,* edited by Maria Diemling and Giuseppe Veltri. Leiden: Brill, 2009.

INDEX

ABOUT THE AUTHORS

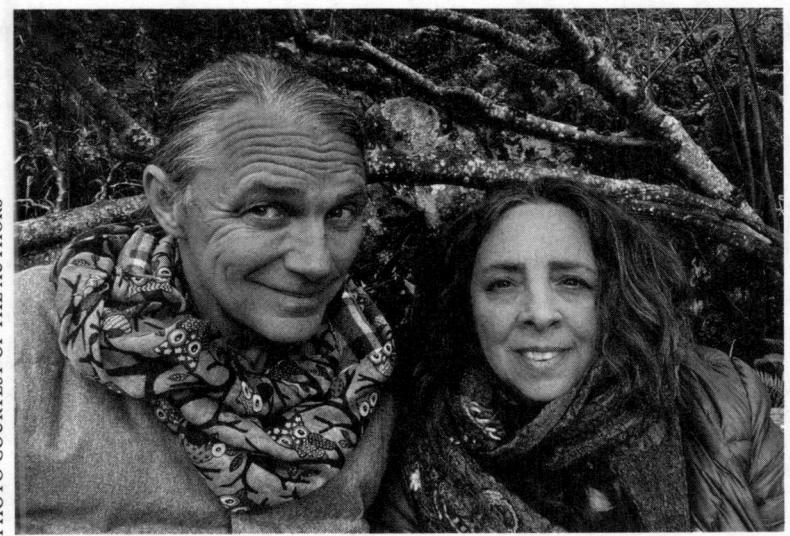

DEATRA COHEN and ADAM SIEGEL are the co-authors of *Ashkenazi Herbalism: Rediscovering the Herbal Traditions of Eastern European Jews*. Deatra trained as a clinical herbalist at the Berkeley Herbal Center, co-founded a Western Clinical Herbal collective, and is currently part of a community herbal project. Adam is a linguist, translator, and bibliographer. In their research, Deatra and Adam are dedicated to recovering the lost or forgotten shared plant healing cultures of Jews and their neighbors in the historic Pale of Settlement. They continue to explore the rich diasporic symbiosis of plants and peoples in both the Old World and the New.

ABOUT NORTH ATLANTIC BOOKS

North Atlantic Books (NAB) is an independent, nonprofit publisher committed to a bold exploration of the relationships between mind, body, spirit, and nature. Founded in 1974, NAB aims to nurture a holistic view of the arts, sciences, humanities, and healing. To make a donation or to learn more about our books, authors, events, and newsletter, please visit www.northatlanticbooks.com.